Medical Textiles

Textile Institute Professional Publications

Series Editor: Helen D. Rowe for The Textile Institute

Care and Maintenance of Textile Products Including Apparel and Protective Clothing
Rajkishore Nayak, Saminathan Ratnapandian

Radio Frequency Identification (RFID) Technology and Application in Fashion and Textile Supply Chain
Rajkishore Nayak

The Grammar of Pattern
Michael Hann

Standard Methods for Thermal Comfort Assessment of Clothing
Ivana Špelić, Alka Mihelić Bogdanić, Anica Hursa Sajatovic

Fibres to Smart Textiles: Advances in Manufacturing, Technologies, and Applications
Asis Patnaik and Sweta Patnaik

Flame Retardants for Textile Materials
Asim Kumar Roy Choudhury

Textile Design: Products and Processes
Michael Hann

Science in Design: Solidifying Design with Science and Technology
Tarun Grover and Mugdha Thareja

Textiles and Their Use in Microbial Protection: Focus on COVID-19 and Other Viruses
Jiri Militky, Aravin Prince Periyasamy, Mohanapriya Venkataraman

Dressings for Advanced Wound Care
Sharon Lam Po Tang

Medical Textiles
Holly Morris and Richard Murray

For more information about this series, please visit:
www.routledge.com/Textile-Institute-Professional-Publications/book-series/TIPP

Series Page
Textile Institute Professional Publications

The aim of the ***Textile Institute Professional Publications*** is to provide support to textile professionals in their work and to help emerging professionals, such as final year or master's students, by providing the information needed to gain a sound understanding of key and emerging topics relating to textile, clothing and footwear technology, textile chemistry, materials science, and engineering. The books are written by experienced authors with expertise in the topic and all texts are independently reviewed by textile professionals or textile academics.

The textile industry has a history of being both an innovator and an early adopter of a wide variety of technologies. There are textile businesses of some kind operating in all countries across the world. At any one time, there is an enormous breadth of sophistication in how such companies might function. In some places where the industry serves only its own local market, design, development, and production may continue to be based on traditional techniques, but companies that aspire to operate globally find themselves in an intensely competitive environment, some driven by the need to appeal to followers of fast-moving fashion, others by demands for high performance and unprecedented levels of reliability. Textile professionals working within such organisations are subjected to a continued pressing need to introduce new materials and technologies, not only to improve production efficiency and reduce costs, but also to enhance the attractiveness and performance of their existing products and to bring new products into being. As a consequence, textile academics and professionals find themselves having to continuously improve their understanding of a wide range of new materials and emerging technologies to keep pace with competitors.

The Textile Institute was formed in 1910 to provide professional support to textile practitioners and academics undertaking research and teaching in the field of textiles. The Institute quickly established itself as the professional body for textiles worldwide and now has individual and corporate members in over 80 countries. The Institute works to provide sources of reliable and up-to-date information to support textile professionals through its research journals, the ***Journal of the Textile Institute***[1] and ***Textile Progress***,[2] definitive descriptions of textiles and their components through its online publication ***Textile Terms and Definitions***,[3] and contextual treatments of important topics within the field of textiles in the form of self-contained books such as the ***Textile Institute Professional Publications***.

References

1. http://www.tandfonline.com/action/journalInformation?show=aimsScope&journalCode=tjti20
2. http://www.tandfonline.com/action/journalInformation?show=aimsScope&journalCode=ttpr20
3. http://www.ttandd.org

Medical Textiles

Holly Morris and Richard Murray

CRC Press
Taylor & Francis Group
Boca Raton London New York

CRC Press is an imprint of the
Taylor & Francis Group, an **informa** business

First edition published 2022
by CRC Press
6000 Broken Sound Parkway NW, Suite 300, Boca Raton, FL 33487-2742

and by CRC Press
2 Park Square, Milton Park, Abingdon, Oxon, OX14 4RN

Library of Congress Cataloging-in-Publication Data

Names: Morris, Holly, author. | Murray, Richard, author.
Title: Medical textiles / Holly Morris, Richard Murray.
Description: Boca Raton : CRC Press, 2021. | Series: Textile Institute professional publications | Includes bibliographical references and index. | Summary: "This book addresses advances in medical textiles to stimulate collaborative research and development in the field of medical textiles and to equip researchers with an understanding of the steps they need to take to ensure that their efforts are carried out in such a way as to improve their effectiveness and enhance the prospects for their implementation. The book provides essential reading for textile professionals, biomedical engineers, and others involved in the research, design and engineering of medical and healthcare appliances, and for those employed in the medical profession wishing to gain new insights into the wealth of materials at their disposal"-- Provided by publisher.
Identifiers: LCCN 2021035281 (print) | LCCN 2021035282 (ebook) | ISBN 9780367772734 (hardback) | ISBN 9780367772734 (paperback) | ISBN 9781003170570 (ebook)
Subjects: LCSH: Biomedical materials. | Biomedical materials--Research.
Classification: LCC R857.M3 M67 2021 (print) | LCC R857.M3 (ebook) | DDC 610.28--dc23
LC record available at https://lccn.loc.gov/2021035281
LC ebook record available at https://lccn.loc.gov/2021035282

ISBN: 978-0-367-77274-1 (hbk)
ISBN: 978-0-367-77273-4 (pbk)
ISBN: 978-1-003-17057-0 (ebk)

DOI: 10.1201/9781003170570

Typeset in Times
by Deanta Global Publishing Services, Chennai, India

Holly is dedicating this, her first textbook, to her late grandfather, Geoffrey Rex Iliffe. Not only did he relish listening to her antics, he offered some of the wisest guidance based on years of experience. Some of his last advice, typical of style and given on the driveway of his home when Holly had returned from NZ to spend a final afternoon with him, were this "Life is a rollercoaster at times and it's better to ride it and hold on tight than it is to watch it." So it has been with this venture into the growing field of medical textiles.

Working on the topic has required a considerable amount of tenacity and innovation, so Holly also dedicates the book to all of those personal friends and professional colleagues who have supported her through a few very creative years.

Richard would wish to dedicate this text to the healthcare professionals in his family both past:

Mary Murray (District Nurse), Nancy Holmes (Health Visitor), Capt. W.A. Holmes (RAMC), Elizabeth Johnson (Health Visitor), Liz Murray (Health Visitor), Leslie Murray (Dental Nurse),

and present:

Margaret Murray (Day Centre Manager), Inowattie Lacey (Staff Nurse), Steven Forman (Principal Medical Advisor, HSE), Catherine Forman (Regional Lead Infection Prevention & Control Nurse for Community Services) and Elaine Murray (Senior Care Assistant),

and to Dr Toby Williams, Consultant Neuroradiologist, and the Neuroradiology Department team at Salford Royal NHS Foundation Trust in thanks for their excellent treatment.

Contents

Preface

Often, books about medical textiles address recent advances in research and the development of particular products that use textile materials to make those products work. This textbook is somewhat different in that it aims not only to ensure that recent advances are addressed but also to make certain that the context for their development can be appreciated and understood not only by medical practitioners and healthcare personnel but also by textile scientists and technologists. The idea is to stimulate collaborative research and development in the field of medical textiles and to equip researchers with an understanding of the steps they need to take to ensure that their efforts, be they to develop new devices for implantation or items for external application, are carried out in such a way as to improve their effectiveness and enhance the prospects for their implementation. There is good reason to believe that it would be most helpful for healthcare managers, administrators, government officials, and politicians to read this book and use it to guide both policy and practice because their role in healthcare is so crucial in bringing about changes in healthcare practice. Their contribution to healthcare is often overlooked, but just like the healthcare professionals they guide and support, they deserve to be praised when they act upon research findings such as those set down here and be open to criticism when they do not, because research findings are worth little if they fail to be taken into account or are not implemented. One of the case studies is intended to illustrate what healthcare managers, administrators, government officials, and politicians, as well as healthcare professionals should have to hand to help them to deal with emergencies; it takes the reader through exemplary research, guidance, and advice, which should be addressed at all management levels in both the healthcare sector and in government to minimise the negative impact of a crisis.

To understand what has already been achieved in the field of medical textiles can be a great help in understanding what still needs to be done, how that might be achieved, and what obstacles may need to be overcome to achieve the implementation of new developments. To that end the book provides the reader with a short history of medical textiles and sets this within the context of the history of medicine. Particular attention is given to the key concepts of the latter part of the 19th century, namely antisepsis and asepsis, and associated developments since then.

The authors believe that it is a good idea for medical practitioners and other healthcare professionals to have a sound knowledge of those key aspects of textile science and technology that confer the properties special to textiles such as their tensile strength and flexibility and how such properties might be able to be finely adjusted during fibre formation or by fabric finishing. Consequently, the book sets out important aspects of textile science from polymers through fibres and filaments to fabrics and their finishing to match the needs of particular medical applications. Because of relatively recent advances in electrospinning and associated techniques concerned with the miniaturisation of weaving and braiding processes and tissue engineering, particular attention has been paid to the production and applications of nanofibres as well as to the uses made of materials in nano-particulate form, particularly those intended to provide antimicrobial effects in the treated textiles.

The authors also believe that it is helpful for textile scientists, technologists, and designers to acquire an understanding of medicine sufficient for them to transfer some of their specialist knowledge and expertise into the healthcare setting. The book takes the stance that there is a continuing need for products to be designed and developed to support ongoing changes in approach to each of the key aspects of healthcare, namely caring for the patient, protecting patients and healthcare staff, maintaining patient function, comfort, and mobility, and where necessary, providing external artificial support. To help to establish a working level of understanding of medicine, the book addresses medical textiles and the conditions they are intended to help, alleviate, or correct under chapter headings about implants, non-implanted applications, and extracorporeal devices. The functions of the associated organs are explained first so that the reader can understand the context and the performance that will be required of the medical textile device. The chapter about medical textiles in health and hygiene products deals with medical textiles for the protection of patients and healthcare personnel with a strong focus on how pathogens may be transferred by aerosols or cross-contamination, how such transfer may be prevented, and whether, or how well, attempts to date have succeeded in preventing the transfer of pathogens. Attention is paid to the importance of detailed planning of experimental work to ensure that the test methods employed match the conditions which apply in practice and improve the outcomes in the practical setting. Guidance is given not only about appropriate approaches to ensure that this is the case, but also to standard tests that can help researchers to monitor the effectiveness of treatments and to instances where the standard tests fall seriously short and the testing regimes require further development. Attention is drawn to both the financial and environmental costs of the throwaway culture which has been encouraged within healthcare settings since the 1960s and provides detail about the value of adopting re-useable items instead of disposables for items used in high volumes and/or in arranging for the decontamination and reuse or remanufacture of all other medical devices.

Just as is the case with treatments intended to improve hygiene control, so it is with medical devices; detailed planning of experimental work and immaculate record-keeping are essential in enabling a new product to become approved and accepted. How to address the requirements is given detailed attention. Case studies are used to illustrate how medical textiles are applied in practice.

Acknowledgements

This textbook would not have been possible without the help and thoughts of colleagues and friends. We would like to acknowledge the following who were directly involved in writing and reviewing sections of the textbook pertinent to their field.

Professor Peter Ogrodnik for writing a chapter on the current regulations process for medical devices.

Dr Khaleel Hamdulay, who improved the section on vascular grafts and provided an excellent clinical example of an unusual presentation of the limitations of modern medicine currently.

Mr Francisco Barbosa, who kindly wrote the section on soft tissue ligament and tendon reconstruction based on his interest in soft tissue knee surgery.

Mr Steve Lindley, who spends his time finishing general surgical training and pursuing his interests in hernial repair in less economically developed countries with Operation Hernia and Hernia International.

Professor Douglas Tincello, who has dedicated his professional lifetime to the management and improvement of urogynaecology and prolapse repair.

Dr Afrah Riaz and Miss Aneesa Rahim, who wrote the section on eye pathology and ocular implants.

Associate Professor Mohammad Tajul Islam for reviewing and expanding the section on resorbable scaffolds.

Mr Miran Pankhania for his otorhinolaryngology expertise and knowledge on how to stop someone bleeding from difficult to reach areas!

Ms Nora Nugent for her expertise on the management of burns and the role compression garments hold.

Mr Ayaaz Ebramjee, who kindly reviewed, edited, and expanded the section on orthotics.

Dr Andrew Suchowersky and Dr Anand Segar, who wrote the section on the management of scoliosis with bracing.

Ms Alexandra Thompson for contributing a section on dental floss.

Dr Matthew Charlton and Dr Daniel Fleet, both of whom were exceptionally busy in one of the United Kingdom's busiest ECMO centres, yet still found time to pen the relevant section despite the ongoing COVID pandemic.

Dr Hussain Allawati for reviewing the section on the kidney and pancreas and replacement options.

Thanks are also extended to Helen Rowe, who helped piece together the initial proposal and to the editorial team at CRC Press for their expertise.

Holly remains indebted to her mentors over the years for their expertise, supervision, and encouragement.

The authors do not personally endorse any of the products mentioned within this textbook.

Authors

Ms Holly Morris holds dual professional registration across the medical and textile industries. Internationally trained, Holly is a registered medical professional currently completing higher surgical training in Trauma and Orthopaedics with a subspeciality interest in Hand Surgery. She is a Member of the Royal College of Surgeons of Edinburgh.

Holly's childhood love of textiles led her to gain a formal textile qualification through a Master of Applied Science at the University of Otago, Dunedin, New Zealand. Her thesis centred on the role of textile technology in implantable bioscaffolds used within regenerative medicine and was co-supervised by Professor Raechel Laing and Professor David Gwynne-Jones. Since her return to the United Kingdom to complete higher surgical training in Trauma and Orthopaedics, near her family in the textile-infused East Midlands, she has continued to develop an interest in the field of medical textiles.

As a Fellow of the Textile Institute, Holly already has several publications in professional literature including, most recently, a review of the "Medical Textiles" sector which appears in the Textile Progress series. Her interests centre around the importance of upholding patient safety to the highest standards while welcoming innovation and technological progress, sustainability, and the development of new devices.

Holly is involved with a Master's and PhD programme in medical device design and supervises postgraduate students. In addition, she is currently part of ENG4, a Not-For-Profit collaboration of professionals and volunteers designing and developing garments for the COVID-19 pandemic. The group was awarded the 2021 Institute of Engineering Designers' Gerald Frewer Memorial Trophy. Holly enjoys mentoring juniors within the medical profession and has a healthy regard for fellow nonconformists.

Professor Richard Murray was Pro-Vice Chancellor International and Dean of the Hollings Faculty at the Manchester Metropolitan University (MMU) in the United Kingdom for 15 years before becoming Emeritus Professor in 2011.

Richard graduated in textile chemistry from the University of Leeds and, combining protein chemistry with electron microscopy, carried out research into wool fibre fine structure for his PhD before continuing his research in textile physics, publishing papers on wool, cotton, polyester, Kevlar 49, and carbon fibre fine structures before moving to Edinburgh to pursue a lecturing career and to develop research into fabric care and high-performance garment design. During that time, Queen Margaret College where he worked had the widest range of healthcare courses in the United Kingdom, and one of Richard's duties was to guide them in the development of their diploma courses into bachelor's degree programmes, hence his continuing interest in textiles and health, and his research into aspects of clothing comfort and function.

During his time in Edinburgh, Richard was the member for Scotland on the Consumer Standards Advisory Committee of the British Standards Institution, represented the Scottish University sector on the General Teaching Council for Scotland, was Chairman of the Scottish Section of the Textile Institute, and worked as Technical Director for two small companies in England. At MMU, one of Professor Murray's priorities was to establish new partnerships with leading universities in China, particularly with those undertaking teaching and research on textiles and garment design and technology. He became a Visiting Professor at several Chinese universities including Donghua, Huizhou, and GDUT, delivering lectures and presentations to university staff, students, and to business representatives on a regular basis. Richard is the Chairman of the Textile Institute Publications Committee and the editor of its research review journal, *Textile Progress*. He maintains his research interests as a member of Professor Kuo-bing Cheng's textile research team, 'GLORIA,' at Feng Chia University in Taiwan.

1 Introduction

As defined by The Textile Institute, a medical textile is "a textile structure which has been designed and produced for use in any of a variety of medical applications, including implantable applications" (The Textile Institute, 2021). The field of medical textiles is one of the fastest growing parts of the technical textiles sector of the textile industry, with products ranging from personal protective equipment (PPE) through to bandage materials, and replacement parts for the human body to bioscaffolds for tissue engineering. This book provides details about the roles for which textiles can be employed in the healthcare sector as well as reviewing current developments within the field. Due to advances in technology, and mainly, but not only, in nanotechnology, the technical medical textile sector is undergoing rapid progression and expansion particularly in fields such as wound healing, pressure and bandaging garments, and implantable textiles. In addition, there is growth in medical devices aided by the incorporation of a growing range of durable and effective antimicrobial agents and in the development of smart garments intended to provide remote monitoring of patient's vital functions. Population growth, an ageing population, and rising standards of living will all continue to fuel the growth of this sector.

A total of 3,238 papers about medical textiles were published between 2000 and 2021 according to a search of the record provided by PubMed®/Medline® (PubMed.gov 2021), of which over half of the total (2,075) emerged in the last 5 years. The largest category in the past 20 years, antimicrobial textiles, accounted for 2,077 papers in total. The papers reported research on both the development and incorporation of the antimicrobial agents to bring about the desired antimicrobial effects and on the efficacy of the resultant textiles/garments. The intended applications of the antimicrobial textiles ranged from barrier fabrics in uniforms for healthcare personnel and in their personal protective equipment, through sutures and implantable items, to wipes, dressings for wound care, and hospital textiles in general. The surge in published research on antimicrobial topics over the past 5 years can be attributed, at least in part, to advances in nanotechnology (Mishra et al. 2014, 133–226), enabling the incorporation of the active antimicrobial agent in nanoparticle form into the textile either during spinning of the fibre-forming polymer or through finishing treatments. Helpfully, the nanoparticles can be applied to fabrics intended for medical use without detrimental effects on their textile properties. Regarding effectiveness, such treatments with antimicrobial agents in the form of nanoparticles can demonstrate high levels of antimicrobial activity coupled with excellent durability (both in use and through repeated cycles of laundering), much better

DOI: 10.1201/9781003170570-1

than metal salts or adsorbed quaternary ammonium compounds for example, which work by leaching from the treated fabric and therefore become diminished by laundering. The fully developed versions of antimicrobial nano-finishes can therefore find widespread application. In this regard, nanosilver (nano-Ag) treatments can be thought of as leading the way. Despite concerns (even in this case) over possible leaching of the nanosilver from the garment onto the skin of the wearer (which it would be wise to keep under review), skin contact has been shown to be not so great a problem (Liao, Li, and Tjong 2019, 449; Mahltig and Haase 2012, 1262–1266). As for loss into the environment at the end of the textile's useful life, given consideration of the complete lifetime assessment, concerns are reduced, and overall, nanosilver treatments can be judged to have made a positive contribution to health and to establish a secure and substantial niche in the market for antimicrobial textiles (Pourzahedi, Vance, and Eckelman 2017, 7148–7158). That may be so, but there are now several other nano-particulate agents and combinations of agents demonstrating similarly high levels of effectiveness, and pre-treatments with chitosan or carbon nanotubes, for example, are being shown to enhance not only uptake of the active agents, but also their effectiveness and durability. For protective clothing for healthcare workers, however, rather than any single agent, the antibacterial treatments that are expected to show the most benefit in practice are multifunctional finishes which combine antimicrobial action with surface modification to enable the fabric to repel/shed hazardous liquids such as bodily fluids (Mitchell, Spencer, and Edmiston 2015, 285–292). Unfortunately, however, up to the present time, despite great enthusiasm being expressed in research papers about the high level of antibacterial activity as shown by standard test methods for several treatments for medical textiles, antimicrobial effectiveness is not exhibited by those antimicrobial-treated materials when they are used in the PPE garments worn by healthcare personnel during surgery or patient care.

Finishing treatments including antimicrobial treatments on textiles are addressed in Chapter 5, but will also be discussed elsewhere in the context of each particular application. What is interesting to note is that while there might have been a substantial surge in the development of antibacterial treatments for textiles, the same level of activity does not explicitly apply to viruses. Although there was a single reference to virus removal (in water treatment) by liquid filters (Schabikowski 2019, 4373–4382) and a small number to surgical respirators, there was only one reference to work engaged specifically in the development of an antiviral textile barrier material aimed at forming part of the healthcare workers' PPE. Parthasarathi and Thilagavathi engaged with trying to more fully address improved protection from potential infection by viruses, using a bacteriophage as a surrogate virus, and unlike the test methods for antibacterial activity, this test does appear to more closely represent the range of conditions experienced by PPE during surgery and patient care and the authors were confident that they had developed an effective barrier material for this kind of use (Parthasarathi and Thilagavathi 2015, 1095–1105).

Electro-spun nanofibres are relatively slow to produce compared to outputs from traditional wet, dry, or melt-spinning processes. Nevertheless, they are worth the effort because of the very particular properties they possess on account of their fine diameter which allows for the production of structures that possess extremely high surface areas combined with great flexibility. The electrospinning process is well-established and can be applied to a wide range of polymers given suitable solvents and sufficient polymer-chain entanglement. Although they can readily be collected and used in the form of a web, such webs are very weak and tricky to handle, so most interest lies in collection in the form of continuous bundles or yarns of nanofibres, bundles which can be of very neat construction and may be twisted together to yield twofold nanofibre yarns for example. Also, yarns can be created by coating a conventional filament yarn with nanofibres to bring together in that core-spun yarn characteristics not achievable alone; such core-spun yarns have the strength of the conventional yarn combined with the surface characteristics of the nanofibres. If, however, the core is made from a soluble polymer, dissolving that core can yield hollow yarns (of interest as reservoirs for drug delivery). Electro-spun yarns made from synthetic absorbable polymers (SA polymers) now play a significant role in medical textiles both as scaffolds for tissue engineering and in drug delivery. That achievement is due in great part to the way the massive surface areas and the porosities of electro-spun fibrous assemblies/fabrics provide such excellent scaffolds for cell proliferation and growth during the period that the steadily degrading electro-spun-polymer yarn bundle is needed to continue to offer support (Mokhtari et al. 2016, 191–207). The sought-after performance from these particular materials arises, therefore, not only from the nano-fibrous nature of the textile support but also from the properties conveyed into the structure by the SA polymer. Accordingly, there has been a significant amount of work carried out on candidate SA polymers and the best ways of preparing the fibrous materials to achieve repair without the need to engage in further surgical procedures to remove the support once it has achieved the desired effect.

REFERENCES

Liao, Chengzhu, Yuchao Li, and Sie Chin Tjong. "Bactericidal and cytotoxic properties of silver nanoparticles." *International Journal of Molecular Sciences* 20, no. 2 (2019): 449.

Mahltig, Boris, and Hajo Haase. "Comparison of the effectiveness of different silver-containing textile products on bacteria and human cells." *Journal of The Textile Institute* 103, no. 11 (2012): 1262–1266.

Mishra, Rajesh, J. Militky, Vijaykumar Baheti, Juan Huang, B. Kale, Mohanapriya Venkataraman, V. Bele, V. Arumugam, Guocheng Zhu, and Yan Wang. "The production, characterization and applications of nanoparticles in the textile industry." *Textile Progress* 46, no. 2 (2014): 133–226.

Mitchell, A., M. Spencer, and C. Edmiston Jr. "Role of healthcare apparel and other healthcare textiles in the transmission of pathogens: A review of the literature." *Journal of Hospital Infection* 90, no. 4 (2015): 285–292.

Mokhtari, F., M. Salehi, F. Zamani, F. Hajiani, F. Zeighami, and M. Latifi. "Advances in electrospinning: The production and application of nanofibres and nanofibrous structures." *Textile Progress* 48, no. 3 (2016): 119–219.

Parthasarathi, V., and G. Thilagavathi. "Development of tri-laminate antiviral surgical gown for liquid barrier protection." *Journal of The Textile Institute* 106, no. 10 (2015): 1095–1105.

Pourzahedi, Leila, Marina Vance, and Matthew J. Eckelman. "Life cycle assessment and release studies for 15 nanosilver-enabled consumer products: Investigating hotspots and patterns of contribution." *Environmental Science & Technology* 51, no. 12 (2017): 7148–7158.

PubMed. "PubMed.gov." 2021. Accessed May 22, 2021. https://pubmed.ncbi.nlm.nih.gov

Schabikowski, Mateusz, Alicja Cichoń, Zoltán Németh, Władysław Kubiak, Dariusz Kata, and Thomas Graule. "Electrospun iron and copper oxide fibers for virus retention applications." *Textile Research Journal* 89, no. 21–22 (2019): 4373–4382.

The Textile Institute. "Textile terms and definitions." 2021. Accessed January 7, 2021. https://www.ttandd.org/content/textile-terms-and-definitions.

2 The Development of Textiles in Medicine and the Healthcare Environment over Time

2.1 INTRODUCTION

It is thought that in ancient times, leaves, grasses, and flax may have been used as wound dressings, and it has also been hypothesised that bandages may have been made from wool or linen, but evidence has long since degraded. However, archaeological evidence does show that the Egyptians used linen bandages to splint broken bones and to wrap around bodies in the mummification process (Forrest 1982, 198–205), whilst in China, where historically clothing has been an indicator of societal rank, silk was a material worn only by the privileged, and undyed hemp ramie were the poor person's clothing materials. Later, the poor wore cotton, and although flax was used in sutures, cotton was the fabric for staunching bleeding and for bandages. Lower socio-economic classes in Japan also tended to use coarse fabrics made from hemp or flax.

The first written references to the use of textiles in medicine and healthcare in the West date back to the ancient Greeks; over 130 wounds sustained during the Trojan War, and the management of them, are discussed by Homer in his poem, the *Iliad*. However, it is considered that the attribution of development of medical textiles to the Greeks may be based more on their excellence in record-keeping rather than their own innovation, and that it was in India that much of the initial work was thought to have been carried out, particularly in the case of sutures in India, as indicated by many of the items being listed by the Indian, Susruta (Mackenzie 1973). By the time of Hippocrates (460–375 BCE), a philosophical as well as a practical approach to medicine had developed (Fox 2020).

Whilst these early developments must be regarded as significant, many major innovations are much more recent hence main focus of attention in this chapter is on more-recent key developments, particularly those which have taken place since the mid-1800s.

DOI: 10.1201/9781003170570-2

2.2 PROTECTING THE PATIENTS AND THE HEALTHCARE STAFF

2.2.1 Patient and Practitioner Safety

Whilst the Hippocratic Oath, once sworn as entrance into the medical profession, has now been replaced by the Declaration of Geneva, the fundamental principle in medicine that the health of the patient will be the first consideration remains in place to the present day (World Medical Association 2017). Certainly, patient safety is of paramount importance and due consideration needs to be granted, as there can often be a very fine line between causing serious harm and achieving considerable good. For example, before the introduction of anaesthetics, the emphasis was on the operating surgeon to be swift and accurate, with little emphasis on hygiene due to the poor knowledge of the nature of pathogens. Armed, however, with the new knowledge from 'germ theory' comes the recognition that apart from being properly trained and equipped with the means to help the patient with their surgical techniques, medical practitioners and healthcare workers also need to be provided with adequate personal protection to help themselves to keep working effectively. There was also a recognition that they needed to be trained to systematically apply all necessary steps, not only in terms of immediate surgical-treatment techniques but also in patient aftercare and personal safety. This was not always appreciated or applied; sometimes because the fundamental scientific principles had yet to be established or had been misunderstood, in others, principles were understood but testing and/or training in equipment was insufficient, neglected, or needed to be developed.

Following the French Revolution and the dissolution of traditional hospitals across France, hospitals there were eventually re-established, but in a new form. Here the clinical training of medical students adopted methods such as bedside training as initiated in Padua, but in the more highly systematic manner first established in the late 1600s to early 1700s at Leiden by Herman Boerhaave (his approach influenced training in Austria and Scotland as well as in France). Rather than being solely a place for treating patients, the hospital also became a place of training, learning, and research, so that in time French medical schools were expected to be attached to hospitals. This was how improved practices were propagated. Paris became the centre for medical innovation until the mid-1800s, and surgeons and physicians from the USA and Europe went there to learn and to benefit from its approach to training. It should not, therefore, come as a surprise that it was a French clinician (Pierre-Charles-Alexandre Louis from the La Charité Hospital in Paris) who established a significant step forward in medicine by applying both a scientific and mathematical method to what might now be described as an early form of clinical trial (in this case, assessing the efficacy of the timing of blood-letting) in research published in 1828 (Morabia 2006). Other pioneers emerged, first in France, then Austria, Germany, Switzerland, the UK, and the USA, who, together, were instrumental in establishing systematic training for medical personnel including hygienic treatment methods combined with personal hygiene and the use of personal protective wear. There was also a lot that needed to be done to improve the surroundings within which treatment was taking place, as may be concluded from the image shown in Figure 2.1, taken near the beginning of the 20th century; its appearance is more akin to that of

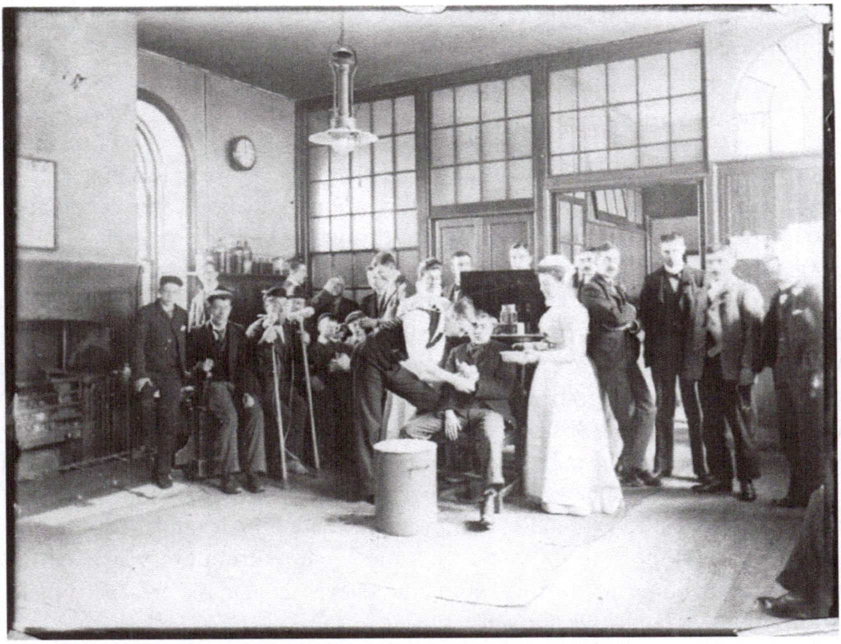

FIGURE 2.1 Guy's Hospital London, Front Surgery, 1897 (COPY 1/428 The National Archives).

a waiting room in a small-town, Victorian railway station than an outpatients department in a major London hospital.

It serves to indicate that the adoption of hygiene recommendations was not immediate, as illustrated by a statistical analysis of 338 un-staged photographs taken mostly in the USA (71%) and Europe (14.5%) from 1863 to 1969 (Adams et al. 2016, 19–24) about the timing of the introduction and adoption of protective wear. They established two key sets of definitions:

(i) They defined the year of 'general acceptance,' 'more probable,' or 'widespread' as the most recent year when the predicted probability of its being worn exceeded 50%.
(ii) They defined the year of 'commonplace,' 'consistently,' or 'routine,' as that when the predicted probability of its being worn exceeded 90%.

Applying those definitions, they showed that the year by which the wearing of the item was *more probable* for surgeons was 1876 for gowns, 1904 for caps, 1911 for gloves, and 1919 for masks. The years by which items were *consistently* being worn by surgeons were 1901 for gowns, 1930 for caps, 1937 for gloves, and 1937 for masks. Anaesthetists were later in their adoption in each case but except for gloves, both surgeons and anaesthetists were wearing all of the other items by the 1950s. Rather than immediate adoption of recommendations then, analysis of the photographs revealed that the probability of wearing caps, gloves, gowns, and masks as operating-theatre wear increased intermittently across the many decades captured in the photographs

2.2.2 The Antiseptic Approach

In the mid-19th century, the English surgeon Joseph Lister, whilst teaching and practising in Glasgow, introduced a new idea that wound infections, which at that time led to high levels of mortality following surgery, were caused by microbes, the minute organisms to which Louis Pasteur had attributed the initiation of changes such as fermentation and putrefaction. As his way of limiting the access of the tiny organisms to patients' wounds during and after surgical operations, Lister not only applied antiseptics directly to the areas being treated but also as sprays during operations, as illustrated in the photograph of an operation being undertaken in Aberdeen by Sir Alexander Ogston, one of his supporters, shown in Figure 2.2. Lister also continually promoted the benefits to be gained from the adoption of the antiseptic approach over many years. As can be seen, there had been no particular attempt otherwise in the operating area at Aberdeen Royal Infirmary, where Sir Alexander Ogston, fourth from the left, was the surgeon in charge, to move away from everyday wear in its usual form at that time, apart from rolling the sleeves up, and the presence of a hand towel over Sir Alexander Ogston's arm.

Sir Alexander was the one who introduced Lister's antiseptic procedure at the Aberdeen Royal Infirmary but it took time for antiseptic application to become widespread, and there were arguments put forward strongly both from supporters and

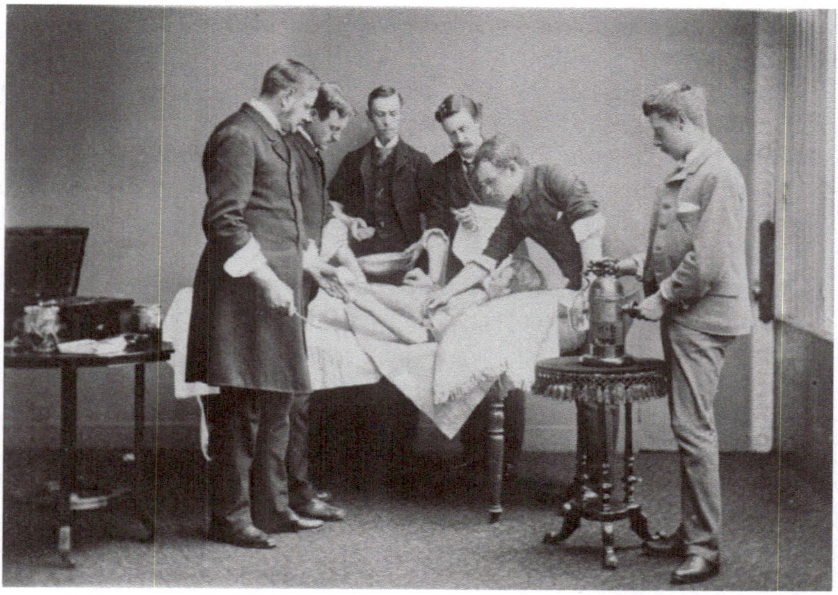

FIGURE 2.2 Surgical procedure at Aberdeen Royal Infirmary (1870s) with Lister's antiseptic spray in action. © Aberdeen City Council (Art Gallery & Museums Collections).

sceptics, an experience not unusual with innovations in other fields. Nevertheless, Lister's persistence through demonstration, promotional lectures, and educational training in antiseptic practices did eventually pave the way towards their approval. Lister did engage in correspondence with Pasteur and they met at the time of the International Medical Congress held in London in 1881, where Pasteur was giving a talk about vaccination. Interestingly, there appeared to be easier acceptance of the application of antiseptics by surgeons elsewhere in Europe, where contemporaries of Lister had already made some use of antiseptics during operations before his sustained push to achieve more widespread adoption.

Also of interest, this time in relation to implantable medical textiles, is the development by Lister of serviceable, antiseptic-treated, absorbable sutures made from catgut (dried sheep's intestine, as used in violin strings) which he intended to be used to replace silk. The silk sutures often gave rise to the formation of pus in a wound. Catgut was not a popular choice amongst surgeons at the time because of its tendency to become too weak to support the wound before sufficient healing had taken place for it to support itself, and Lister was aware of the likelihood of the antiseptic soak causing the catgut to soften and weaken further. Rather than just soaking in antiseptic phenolic solutions, he therefore also treated the antiseptic-soaked catgut sutures with chromic acid or a chromium salt, widely used at the time in histology as a fixative to harden tissue samples prior to thin-sectioning and mounting onto slides for microscope examination. The purpose of the chromium salt treatment was to harden the suture material (in much the same way as in the tanning of leather), thereby slowing down the rate of absorption of the suture once in place, and giving time for the incision to heal before the suture was completely absorbed.

2.2.3 The Aseptic Approach

During the last decade of the 19th century, Gustav Neuber in Germany introduced different means of reducing the risk of infection to that of Lister. Similarly based on an understanding of Louis Pasteur's work and concern regarding high mortality rates caused by post-operative infection (Alexander 1985), Neuber's aseptic approach was intended to prevent pathogens from entering wounds by attempting to ensure that none were present at the time of the operation. His first step in achieving improvement was by creating operating rooms specifically for treating patients with septic wounds; these were kept separate from the rest. Second, he established, in his clinic in Kiel, a system involving the sterilisation of surgical instruments prior to their use together with associated aseptic methods, based on the work of Robert Koch (who was awarded the Nobel Prize in 1905 for his work in this field). However, for the aseptic concept to work in practice, it required attention to be paid to more than just different rooms for different types of surgery and the sterilisation of the surgical instruments, particularly when it began to be recognised that the surgical team and the operating environment might also be sources of pathogens. Carl Flügge in Breslau in Poland, having demonstrated that droplets in respiration carried germs within them, began working with Johann Anton von Mikulicz-Radecki, professor at the University of Breslau. In an attempt to combat transmission, Anton began to wear a cotton gauze face mask covering both mouth and nose in 1897. In the same year, the surgeon Paul Berger in Paris also began wearing a mask in the operating room, but it was Mikulicz-Radecki, a graduate of the University of Vienna who had originally worked and taught at the Billroth School of Surgery in Vienna, who has been credited with establishing the world's first aseptic operating theatre in Breslau (Zajaczkowski 2008).

For those intent on reaping benefits from asepsis, the list of requirements began to grow, such that surgical teams now began to wear sterile gowns, caps, and shoe covers, together with the surgical instruments being sterilised in an autoclave. Attention was also drawn to the need for the surfaces of hospital walls, floors, storage shelves, and cabinets to be easy to clean and to disinfect. With the introduction of surgical gloves at Johns Hopkins Hospital in America, the recognisable elements of the 'close-to-sterile' operating theatre were in place. As with antisepsis, there was no immediate acceptance of the benefits to be derived from creating an aseptic operating environment and although the aseptic approach did begin to influence surgeons' operating wear and hospital design and furnishing in the UK, the response was erratic until the early part of the 20th century. Figure 2.3, of Guy's Hospital, London, taken in 1897 suggests that there, at that time, surgeons might be relying wholly on the antiseptic approach, whereas in the Edinburgh Royal Infirmary in the 1880s, attempts were at least being made to provide some sort of protective barrier

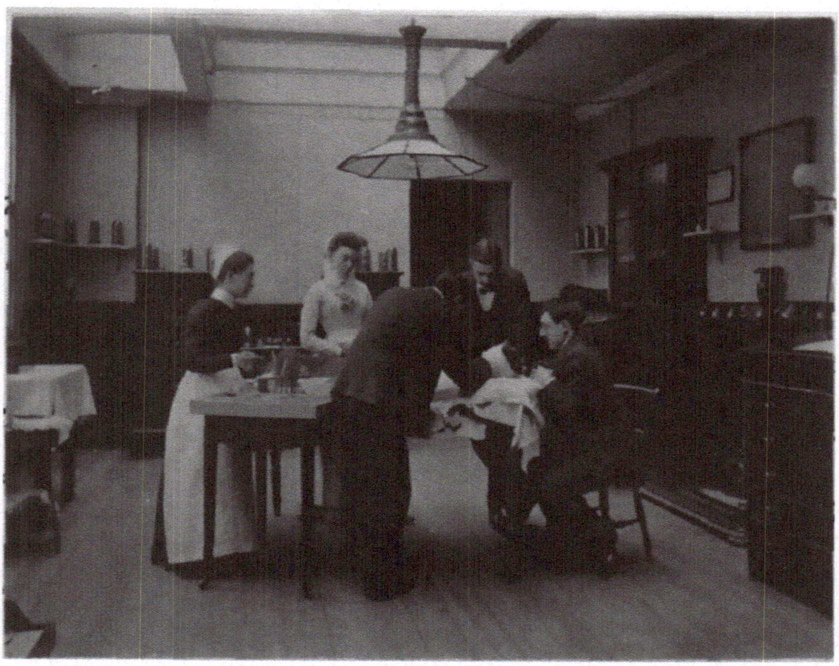

FIGURE 2.3 Guy's Hospital London Operating Theatre 1897 (COPY 1/428; The National Archives).

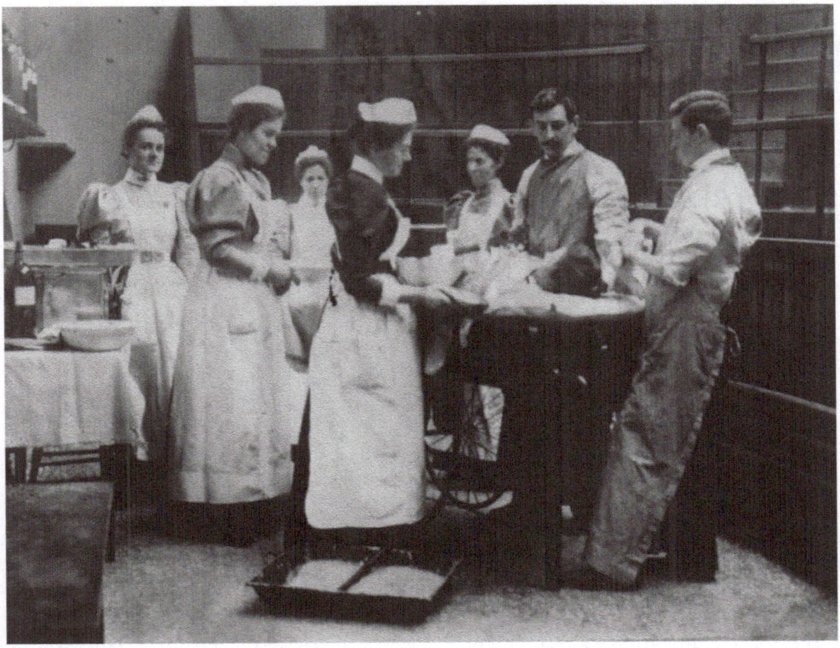

FIGURE 2.4 The Royal Infirmary, Edinburgh (1880s). (Reproduced from The Goldie Scot Collection. by kind permission of the Royal College of Surgeons of Edinburgh, Library and Archive.)

between the patient and the surgeons' street clothes, with what have the appearance of coated or at least densely woven aprons (Figure 2.4).

The 1910 image of the operating theatre at the hospital in Islington, London (Figure 2.5), shows that by that time, white-tiled walls and a smooth floor surface were being employed to create an environment where hygiene could be kept at a good level, the electric lighting positions could be adjusted, and the patient was supported on a simple wheeled trolley and covered by a sheet as was the table in the background. The surgeons were wearing gowns, masks over both mouth and nose, and surgical gloves, but no shoe coverings. Everybody else in the operating room is wearing at least a gown plus functional headwear. There does not appear to have been agreement in the early part of the century about whether the mask should cover both the nose and mouth or just the mouth, because in 1915 at the King George Hospital, the mask, where worn, was only used to cover the mouth (see Figure 2.6).

2.2.4 Surgical Gloves

Although their use was not routinised for patient protection in the hospital setting until the early 20th century at the Johns Hopkins Hospital in Baltimore, USA, surgical gloves have references in the literature dating back to 1758, when a primitive glove was made from the caecum of a sheep in an attempt to reduce tissue laceration

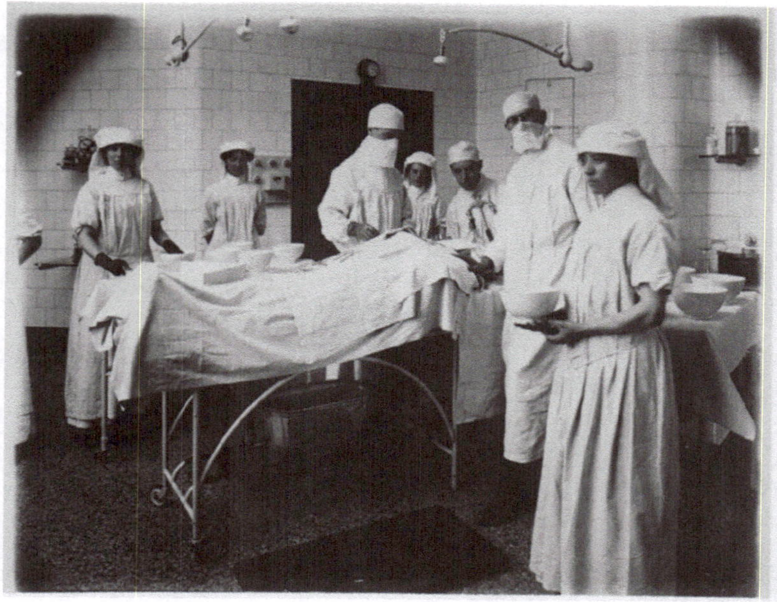

FIGURE 2.5 Operating Theatre, Great Northern Central Hospital, Islington 1910 (COPY 1/547; The National Archives).

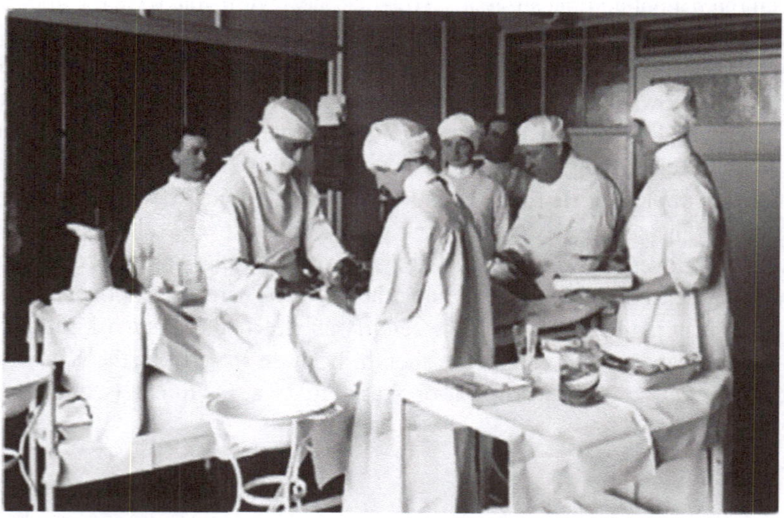

FIGURE 2.6 King George Military Hospital, London, 1915; 4th Floor Theatre Group, Dr Murrison (ENT) operating. (Reproduced by kind permission of the US National Library of Medicine.)

during obstetrics (Spirling and Daniels 2002, 122–124). Following this, the materials used to make gloves evolved through cotton, leather, silk, and rubber (Eisen 2011, 1–20). It is, however, the outstanding American surgeon, William Stewart Halsted, who tends to be credited with the introduction of surgical gloves in 1889 (Spirling and Daniels 2002, 122–124). Given that Halsted was one of the group of four leading lights in medicine recruited to help establish the newly formed Johns Hopkins School of Medicine, it is no surprise that it would be there that the routine use of surgical gloves would be first established, and that he would be the one to take the first step. Rather than to protect the patient, however, he commissioned the gloves to be produced by the Goodyear Rubber Company in New York to protect the hands of his chief surgical nurse, Caroline Hampton, who was developing dermatitis from the sterilisation solutions used on the nurses' and surgeons' hands (a drawback in Lister's successful antiseptic was the aggressive nature of the early phenolic antiseptics; in this case, a solution containing both phenol and mercuric chloride). This was 'true love' and William later married his nurse (Eisen 2011, 1–20). Whilst Caroline inspired other nurses also to begin wearing the rubber gloves in the operating theatre to protect themselves from skin irritation by the antiseptics, Joseph Bloodgood, Halsted's junior, was the first routine wearer of rubber gloves. Having worn them during hernia operations from 1893 and noticed a 100% drop in surgical site infection (Spirling and Daniels 2002, 122–124), Bloodgood was the one who insisted that surgical rubber gloves were worn to protect the patient from becoming infected (Kean 2020) together with the gowns and caps already being worn by some operating theatre staff members in other US hospitals. This was the case, as shown by Figure 2.7, for the New Haven Hospital, but as usual, not by the anaesthetist, nor indeed by the chief surgeon, and no one is wearing gloves.

However, as can be seen below in Figure 2.8, gloves *were* being worn at Johns Hopkins at the time of this contemporary photograph (1904), but not masks. Gloves were quite quickly adopted, and it can be seen that the surgeons carrying out the operations and the nurses directly supporting them at the operating tables in Figures 2.4 and 2.5 in 1910 and 1915 in the UK were also wearing gloves.

With the advent of knowledge of blood-borne diseases, gloves are now also routinely used to protect the healthcare worker outside the operating theatre; in vivo studies have demonstrated that glove material can reduce the transferred blood volume in a needle-stick injury by 46–86% (Mast et al. 1993, 1589–1592).

2.2.5 Surgical Masks

Traditionally, the fabric in surgical masks was made from layers of cotton gauze. Although masks were not evident in the 1904 image at Johns Hopkins shown in Figure 2.8, they were in use in Professor Payr's clinic in Leipzig (see Figure 2.9) at the time of the Clinical Surgical Society Visit to Austrian and German Hospitals and Clinics in 1912 (this prestigious American group included two Honorary Fellows of The Royal College of Surgeons, Edinburgh, which now exhibits a digitised pristine version of the photographic collection from the visit). The members of the Clinical Surgical Society on this visit were effectively following in the footsteps of William

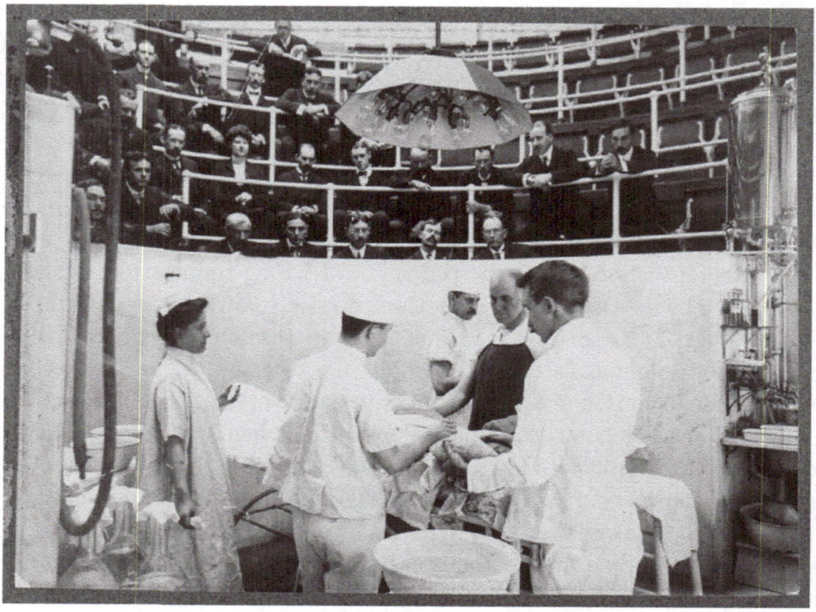

FIGURE 2.7 William Carmalt operating in New Haven Hospital, approximately 1900. (Reproduced by kind permission of the Medical Historical Library, Harvey Cushing/John Hay Whitney Medical Library, Yale University.)

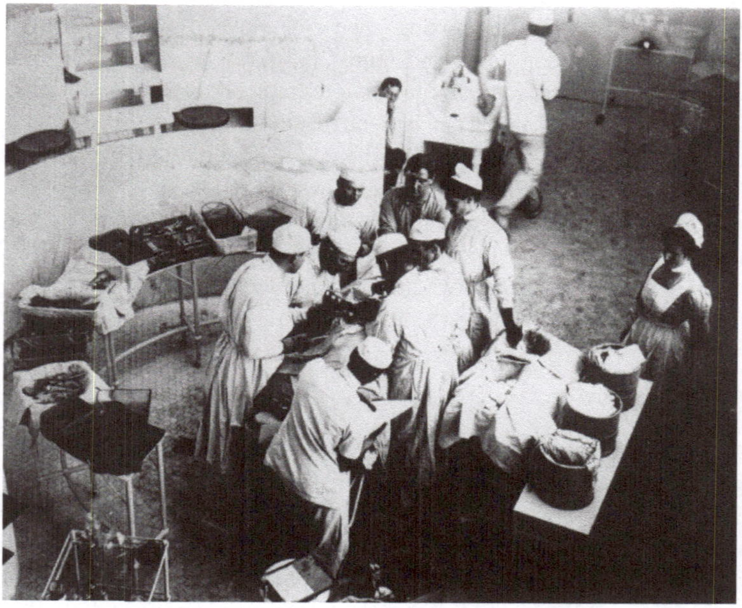

FIGURE 2.8 Johns Hopkins Hospital 'All Star Operation' 1904. (Reproduced by kind permission of the Medical Historical Library, Harvey Cushing/John Hay Whitney Medical Library, Yale University.)

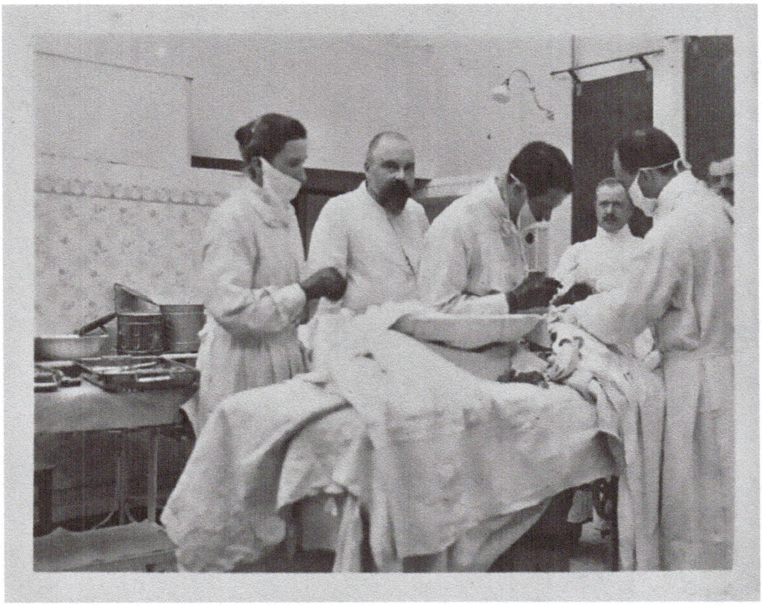

FIGURE 2.9 Professor Payr and Assistants, Leipzig (The Royal College of Surgeons, Edinburgh, Special Collections, Clinical Surgical Society Visit to Austrian and German Hospitals and Clinics, 1912).

Halsted. After graduation from the three-year course at the College of Physicians and Surgeons of New York and 18 months of training at its Belle Vue Hospital, Halsted had gone to Austria and Germany for two years in 1878 to study science and anatomy, and during that time became familiar with and was very impressed by the German system of graduate surgical training (Rankin 2006). Not everyone in the operating theatre in Leipzig was wearing a mask, including Professor Payr himself (he was a pioneer in the treatment of hydrocephalus), and those who were masked were using them to cover the mouth but not the nose; the members of his team involved in carrying out the operation can, however, be seen to be wearing gloves.

During the same series of visits, the audience viewing the operation at Professor Von Eiselsberg's Clinic in Vienna, as seen in Figure 2.10, were mask-free, but the operating group wore both gloves and hats; the hats look as if they would be reasonably effective in controlling the hair. Austrian and German surgeons were amongst those at the forefront of establishing and applying hygienic approaches to surgery and the image indicates that both the antiseptic and aseptic approaches were being implemented there, at least in regard to the operating team, if not to the audience. Professor Von Eiselsberg was one of the leading lights in surgery at this time, the winner of the second Lister Medal in 1927 for his contributions to surgical science, including the establishment of the world's first emergency surgery station in Vienna.

Apart from their use in the surgical setting, there is photographic evidence of masks being worn by the wider public during the 'Spanish influenza' epidemic in 1918, and in the USA it was made compulsory not only for medical personnel to

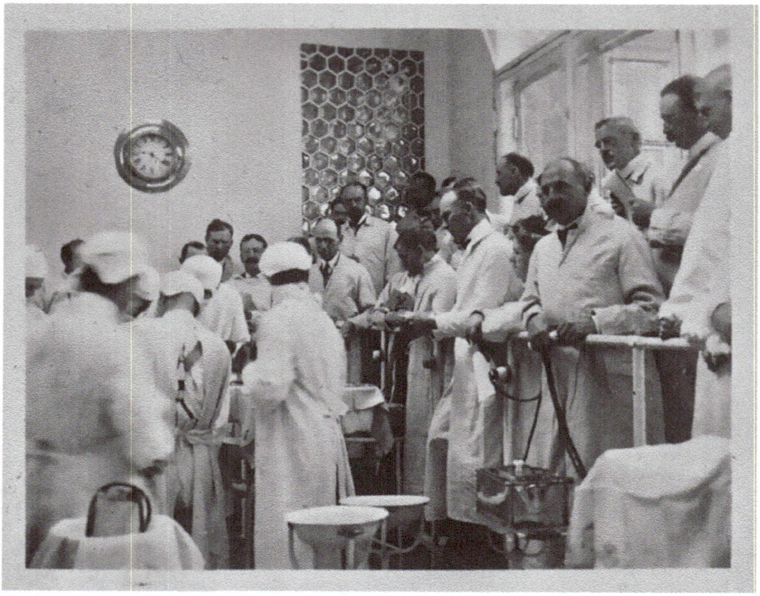

FIGURE 2.10 Professor Von Eiselsberg's Clinic (The Royal College of Surgeons, Edinburgh, Special Collections, Clinical Surgical Society Visit to Austrian and German Hospitals and Clinics, 1912).

wear masks, but also the police (and members of the public in some cities). However, there was some opposition and the response was not sustained afterwards (Strasser and Schlich 2020). Culturally, there has been more inclination amongst the public towards infection-prevention by mask-wearing in China because of its alignment with the Chinese medicine concept of Qi (breath/life force), but it was nothing of great significance until the plague outbreak in Manchuria in 1910. For Japan, the modern habit of mask-wearing followed a different path, starting with the import of wire-framed industrial masks to protect miners and others who worked in dusty surroundings, and it has been the case from the mid-20th century on that mask-wearing by members of the general public is done not only to protect themselves but also so as not to infect others (Vachon 2020). Regarding masks for use in medical settings in the West, testing was first undertaken to try to establish the effectiveness of surgical masks in the 1920s (Meleney and Stevens 1926, 333–342). Such testing was subsequently developed to include aerosols and infected individuals. It was said that there was some evidence of a benefit and this type of cotton-layered arrangement continued to be recommended and used into the 1950s, as shown in the image of *The Pharmaceutical Journal*, November 21, 1953, held in the collection at the UK National Archives (National Archives). Even at this time, there were the beginnings of a move towards disposable masks (paper ones at first) but this gained much more impetus from the mid-1950s in what was labelled at the time by *LIFE* magazine as 'Throwaway Living' (Strasser and Schlich 2020). The advantages in terms of the convenience of disposable items were strongly marketed to the healthcare sector at this point. Particular attention was drawn to similarities in cost and the possibility of moving away completely from the management responsibilities involved with in-house or outsourced institutional laundering and sterilisation. Such claims about the cost effectiveness and competitiveness of disposables have remained the topic of intermittent review and, according to Zins (2006, 73–80) and Sun (2011, 125–135), disputes have been intense even though what appeared to be a sensible, balanced view had already been put forward by Walton that reusables were the better choice for items where there is large-volume use and disposables more suitable for situations where the volumes used were low (Walton 1986, 213–217). The National Institute for Occupational Health published their *Guidelines for Protecting the Safety and Health of Healthcare Workers* in 1988 (NIOSH 1988) which require all healthcare workers in the USA to use protective textiles such as gowns, gloves, drapes, and face masks when in contact with patients to reduce or prevent disease transmission, and all of these items apart from face masks can be either reusable or disposable (face masks are designed to be disposable). Overcash undertook a useful analysis in 2012 combining the findings from six independent lifecycle assessments for gowns and drapes which had been carried out in terms of cost-effectiveness analyses and lifecycle testing. What that particular analysis showed was that there was little cost difference to the hospital/institutional user between using disposable gowns and drapes compared with using reusables, but there were significant differences in terms of negative environmental impact. The environmental problem arises because disposables require proportionately much greater amounts of energy and water per single use (because they are only used once, whereas because reusables are expected to withstand being used and cleaned at least 50 times, only $^{1}/_{50}$th of the energy and water used in their manufacture needs to be accounted for single use of the item). By similar reasoning, disposables can be shown to cause significantly greater emissions of volatile organic compounds (VOCs) in their manufacture than reusables, then at the end of their single-use life, disposables occupy many times the amount of landfill (Overcash 2012). Such considerations override the materials and energy costs associated with laundering and sterilisation steps that have to be taken after each use of a reusable, and their associated effluents (although there are now much more energy-efficient laundering and disinfection methods available such as those which use ozone in the washing machine; JLA 2021). Even so, it would be wrong to assume that reusable medical textiles would always be the best choice; instead it should prove better to match the choice to fit best with the known requirements of the healthcare unit considering that:

(i) reusable medical textiles are the best choice for high-usage situations because with established arrangements for their cleaning and sterilisation, reusable equipment is more cost effective over its lifetime than a disposable type, but that
(ii) at lower volumes of use, disposables are less costly than their reusable counterparts because special small-scale arrangements do not have to be made for their cleaning, sterilisation, or other care and maintenance (Walton 1986, 213–217).

The business case and step-by-step guidance documents to give practical help in developing a sound basis from which to reach a decision about what choice to make for the operating room (Practice Greenhealth 2011) has been developed by Practice Greenhealth™ (Reston, VA, USA).

For surgical masks, despite moves to non-woven synthetic-fibre masks from the late 1960s on, early comparisons of their efficiency were said to show that cotton masks were similarly effective and that mask design, softness, the presence of pleats and more fibre were important features in achieving effectiveness in addition to fibre composition (Quesnel 1975, 936–940). Disposable masks have come under repeated scrutiny and it was concluded from a 2015 Cochrane Review comparing the use of disposable surgical masks with the use of no mask (three randomised trials involving 2,106 patients and monitoring their infection rates following surgery) (Vincent and Edwards 2016) that: *There was no statistically significant difference in infection rates between the masked and unmasked group in any of the trials.*

Debate has continued about the relative effectiveness of face masks across different situations and also their structure and composition. A randomised trial was conducted with adult healthcare workers in high-risk hospital wards in Vietnam in 2015 to check the relative effectiveness of cloth masks vs medical masks (MacIntyre et al. 2015), from which it was concluded:

> the results caution against the use of cloth masks. This is an important finding to inform occupational health and safety. Moisture retention, reuse of cloth masks and poor filtration may result in increased risk of infection. Further research is needed to inform the widespread use of cloth masks globally. However, as a precautionary measure, cloth masks should not be recommended for Health Care Workers, particularly in high-risk situations, and guidelines need to be updated.

Even so, given the recent interest in determining how the general public might protect themselves and others in daily life during a pandemic, the effectiveness of cloth masks continues to be of interest (Jain et al. 2020). A randomised clinical trial was undertaken in 2019, this time to compare medical masks with N95 respirators as protection against influenza virus (Radonovich et al. 2019, 824–833) from which it was concluded that: *Among outpatient health care personnel, N95 respirators vs medical masks as worn by participants in this trial resulted in no significant difference in the incidence of laboratory-confirmed influenza.*

It may come as a surprise, but there is no indication that wearing a mask or a respirator is beneficial in preventing infection across many situations. Even so, mask-wearing has become the required routine, and

(i) for those working in operating theatres to wear *surgical masks*
(ii) for those working in environments where there are patients suffering from respiratory infections to wear *respirators*

It would be tempting to believe that a fresh set of issues would not now arise either from the application of new technology or the emergence of new types of pathogen requiring new types of medical textile, but in fact there remains considerable development work to ensure that medical practitioners and healthcare workers are protected as they work. After all, given the continual evolution of resistant strains of pathogens and modern-day international travel habits, the growing likelihood of repeated epidemic/pandemic outbreaks raises the stakes for the development of new and more widely effective barrier textiles.

2.2.6 Radiation Protection

Considerations about practitioner safety sometimes lagged behind those focused on care of the patient. In other cases, lack of understanding of technology has led to serious injury/illness amongst medical practitioners and other healthcare professionals, perhaps also to patients (see Figure 2.11). It is interesting to see the presence of a birdcage being given precedence over hygiene in the electrical department at the turn of the 19th century in the Middlesex Hospital, London; the bird was presumably placed there in an effort to try to keep the young patients calm.

Following the beginnings of the use of X-rays in 1895 to assist diagnosis of pathology, it took time for the link between radiation and its effect on cell mutations to be understood. It is sad, but fitting in some ways, that the original researchers all succumbed to radiation-induced conditions, Marie Curie having died in 1934 of aplastic anaemia, Irene of leukaemia in 1956, and Frederic succumbing to liver disease in 1958 (Howell 2016, 341–349). The electrical treatment and X-ray room in 1915 shown in Figure 2.12 is cleaner, more clinical, and somewhat more reassuring in appearance than the electrical department in the Middlesex Hospital with the birdcage, but that does not necessarily mean that it was safe; there is no evidence

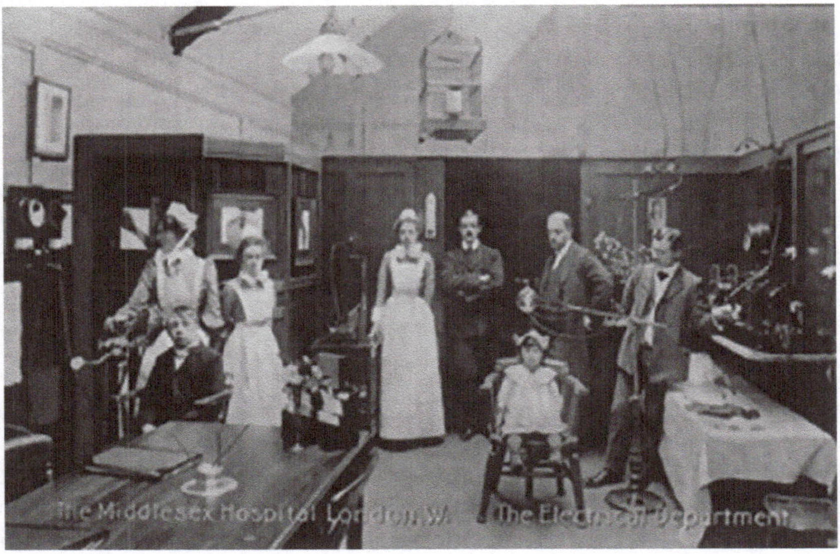

FIGURE 2.11 The Middlesex Hospital, London: the Electrical Department, ca 1900. (Reproduced by kind permission of the US National Library of Medicine.)

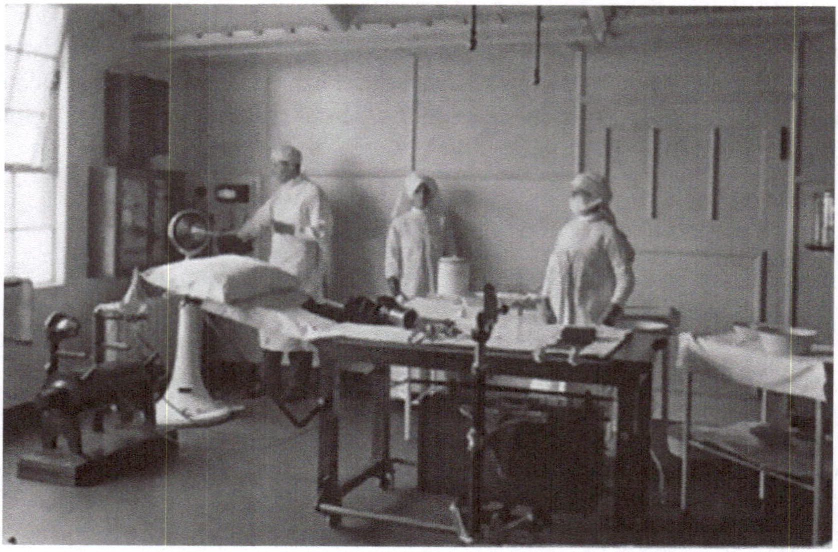

FIGURE 2.12 King George Military Hospital, Electrical Treatment and X-Ray Room, 1915. (Reproduced by kind permission of the US National Library of Medicine.)

there of any protective lead apron, for example. In fact, it was not until 1925 that best practice guided all radiographers to wear a protective lead apron.

The wearing of such aprons with an interior lining layer of lead (0.5 mm) during radiographic work has become routine. Even so, there have been concerns that their design and fit has not been improved over time to offer better protection to those wearing them (White 2003, 371), particularly to reduce the increased risk of breast cancer in the case of female radiographers as revealed by the U.S. Radiologic Technologist Health Study 1983–1998 (Sigurdson et al. 2003, 1983–1998). There has been a response in terms of non-lead, radiation-shielding apparel that can be better-tailored for improved cover for female staff members and can yield better ergonomic fit (Pulford and Ferguson 2016, 1610–1616). Other techniques have been used to reduce radiation to healthcare professionals, such as reducing the dose delivered by the equipment, hence lead aprons are not now compulsory for all procedures.

2.2.7 Uniform Wear

Figures 2.3, 2.4, 2.5, and 2.6 with nurses working in operating theatres in the early 1900s do show some move towards the need for suitable wear when involved in surgery, more so in the case of the Islington and King George Hospitals where the female headdress was more likely to be as effective as surgeons' caps than those seen in the images for the New Haven and Johns Hopkins Hospitals a few years earlier. When not in the operating room, the items worn on the head by nurses were designed more to identify the individuals as nurses than for hygiene purposes, and it could look strangely decorative, at least to our eyes (see Figure 2.13).

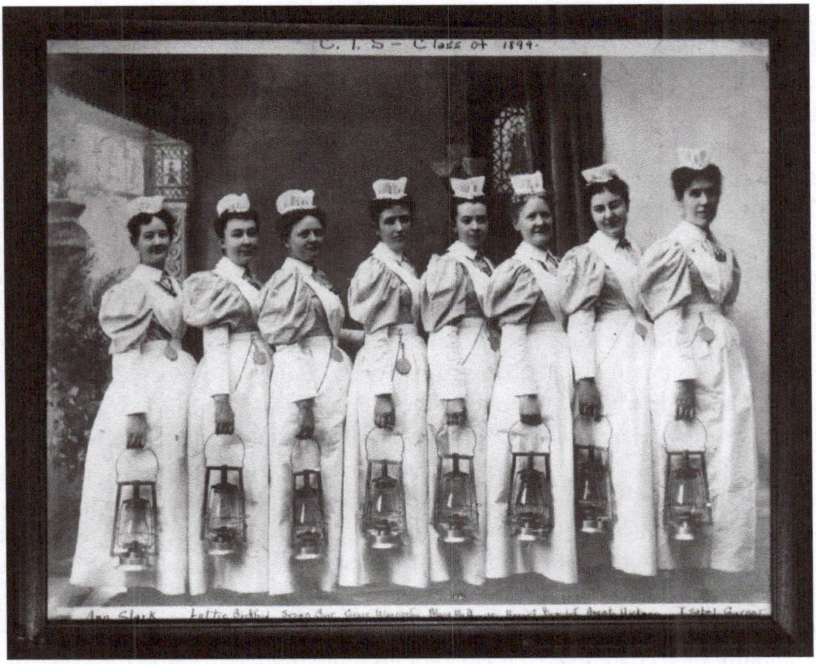

FIGURE 2.13 Connecticut Training School for Nurses, Class of 1899. (Reproduced by kind permission of the Medical Historical Library, Harvey Cushing/John Hay Whitney Medical Library, Yale University.)

2.3 REPAIRING THE PATIENT

2.3.1 Sutures

The history of the use of sutures in the medical field in the Middle East dates back over 4,000 years when fibres of the flax plant were used to close or cover wounds in ancient Egypt and much of the initial work on the development of more sophisticated sutures in the Middle East was thought to have been carried out in India (Mackenzie 1973). The most significant steps forward in somewhat more recent times have been suggested (Muffly et al. 2010, 107–112) to be:

(i) Cornelius Celsus (25 BCE–50 AD), the Roman medical author, introducing the use of suture ligatures to achieve haemostasis
(ii) sutures in the form of silk filaments or cut strips of fine linen fabric being promoted as superior to cauterisation by the French military surgeon Ambroise Paré (1510–1590)
(iii) the English surgeon Joseph Lister (1827–1912) establishing the benefits of sterilisation of sutures (see Section 2.1.2 for more detail)

The first internal use of sutures in Western medicine is credited to the French physicists Lapuyade and Sicre, who used metal wires to set a broken humerus, in Toulouse in 1775. Today, interest has grown in the application of *biodegradable* metal sutures made from alloys of iron, magnesium, and zinc. They are used predominantly for vascular stent or osteosynthesis applications, but could have wider applications, because although they would have to compete with biodegradable polymers for soft-tissue sutures, biodegradable metal sutures are thought to have the potential to replace stainless steel and titanium alloys for hard-tissue sutures (Seitz et al. 2015, 1915–1936).

By the 1930s, the absorbable sterile catgut (made from the cleaned and sterilised intestinal tube walls, mostly of sheep) and non-absorbable silk dominated the suture market (Abhari et al. 2017, 410–421). After World War II, the development of nylon, polyester, and polypropylene led to these synthetic fibre-forming polymers becoming the dominant non-absorbable suture types (Barrows 1986, 223–257). Their emergence also stimulated the Food & Drug Administration in the USA to require manufacturers to seek pre-market approval for all new sutures, and this has remained the case since 1976. Absorbable polymer sutures such as catgut are an attractive proposition, because no additional surgical intervention is required for their removal, and synthetic absorbable polymer (SAP) sutures even more so, because their properties can be more readily tailored to meet the specific preferences of the surgeons; SAP sutures made from polyglycolic acid were introduced in 1972 under the name Dexon® (Davis & Geck, Danbury, CT, USA) and were the first of the type, but followed rapidly by a coated version Dexon Plus® and the low-friction type, Dexon II® (Muffly et al. 2010, 107–112).

2.3.2 Artificial Tendons/Ligaments

High tensile strength, abrasion resistance, and no immune reaction would be the key properties of an ideal material for artificial ligaments (Chen et al. 2015, 15–26), so it would be tempting to believe that textile materials with their inherent tensile strength and flexibility would be prime candidates for direct replacement of ligaments/tendons. Indeed, an effort was made at the beginning of World War I to achieve this using silver wire as the graft and later (in 1918) to repair the ligament with silk, which failed after three months. There was then a very long delay before experimentation with new, higher-performance materials could be undertaken. It was not until the mid-1980s, by which time the use of synthetic polymer textile fibres and filaments for other medical applications had been taking place for some years, that the U.S. Food & Drug Administration (FDA) approved the use of the Gore-Tex cruciate ligament prosthesis in anterior cruciate ligament reconstruction (1986), followed by the 3M Kennedy ligament augmentation device (1987) and the Stryker Dacron ligament prosthesis (1988). Other popular products adopted in Europe and Asia were the Leeds–Keio ligament and the LARS. These artificial ligaments made of carbon fibre, polyethylene terephthalate (PET), and polytetrafluoroethylene (PTFE) can be divided into four types:

(i) permanent type
(ii) scaffold type

(iii) ligament augmentation device (LAD) type
(iv) permanent scaffold type

Dacron and carbon-fibre ligaments were abandoned in early clinical usage because of the occurrence of complications (such as severe synovitis after the implantation of those prostheses), and despite encouraging results, to begin with, from the Gore-Tex and the LAD ligaments, from the early 1990s on, poor longer-term outcomes brought an end to the use of artificial ligaments. Even so, in 2000, Guidoin and colleagues analysed polymer fibre-based replacements for the anterior cruciate ligament (Guidoin et al. 2000), suggesting that three key elements played a part in the artificial ligament failure:

(i) inadequate fibre abrasion resistance against osseous surfaces
(ii) flexural and rotational fatigue of the fibres
(iii) loss of integrity of the textile structure due to unpredictable tissue infiltration during healing

Whereas commercial research and development into textile fabric materials for prosthesis production was discontinued, artificial ligaments were available out in the field and studies of ligament reconstruction using prostheses continued to be undertaken and reported. LARS, due to its mechanical properties, biocompatibility, and particular woven structure, showed good performance, low post-operative complication rates and enabled early rehabilitation. Evidence from clinical studies showed that following refinement, the Leeds–Keio ligament could also be used safely and its derivative, Neoligaments, became available for tendon/ligament deficiencies of knees, ankles, and shoulders (Chen et al. 2015, 15–26).

2.3.3 Scaffolds and Tissue Engineering

The first reference to the regeneration of tissue, replacement of the impaired structure, and restoration of the normal bodily function as '*Tissue Engineering*' is thought to have occurred in 1991 (Vacanti 2006, 569–576). Tissue engineering is a four-step process:

(i) selection of the seed cell
(ii) biomaterial scaffold fabrication
(iii) growth factor adaptation
(iv) conditioning

Textile materials can play the key role in biomaterial scaffold fabrication. With the development of electrospun nanofibres composed of bio-absorbable polymers in the early years of the 21st century, as shown for example by Xu et al., scaffolds can be formed with sufficient strength and integrity to act as temporary replacements for many types of original tissue whilst new tissue forms on and around the scaffold (Xu et al. 2004, 1160–1168). The rate of absorption of the supporting polymer needs to be carefully selected to enable it to continue to provide support for sufficient time, whilst the very high surface area of the electrospun fibres and conveniently small pore sizes between fibres can provide important assistance to new tissue growth.

2.3.4 Hernia trusses

Hernia trusses are a mechanical support that assists in supporting the hernia. They are 'a bandage by which ruptures are restrained from lapsing' (Bynum and Bynum 2017, 1289), and have been used for at least 200 years, with reports of Sir Astley Cooper using a truss successfully; in the 1820s, he wore a truss whilst a medical student for his own hernia (Hutchison and Rayan 2011, 316–320).

2.3.5 Mesh

Support from a truss may not be an effective or appropriate treatment for a hernia in many cases. Synthetic polymer mesh placed over the defect can repair a hernia without the need to undertake extensive tissue dissection to release enough tissue to perform a tension-free repair with sutures, hence the interest in mesh. The 'father of modern-day abdominal surgery,' the Austrian surgeon Theodore Billroth (1829–1894) is cited as envisioning current practice in the use of mesh in hernia repair, saying, 'If we could artificially produce tissue of the density and toughness of fascia and tendon, the secret of the radical cure of the hernia repair would be discovered' (Skandalakis el al. 2002). However, even in the latter part of his era (the late 19th century), attempts to use materials for this purpose were plagued by infection, encapsulation, rejection, and high levels of recurrence, leading to this concept falling out of favour.

Discovery and development of synthetic fibre-forming polymers such as nylon, polyester, polyacrylonitrile, and polypropylene, and plastics such as high-density polyethylene (HDPE) and polytetrafluoroethylene (PTFE) over the period from the late 1930s and through the 1950s, interested Francis Usher. Dr Usher believed these materials could be used to address previous concerns about the use of mesh, but observed many downsides with several of them, such as rigidity, brittleness, foreign-body reaction, and loss of tensile strength. After reading about a new polyolefin material called Marlex® developed by Phillips Petroleum, Bartlesville, OK, USA, which addressed these shortcomings (the high-density polyethylene polymer, HDPE), he worked to produce a Marlex® HDPE woven mesh. His studies to improve this mesh quickly led him to develop a knitted Marlex® polypropylene mesh (Usher 1961), which was more flexible, could be autoclaved, had firm edges, did not fray, and was rapidly incorporated into the healing tissue (as opposed to being encapsulated, where the body forms a granulomatous capsule around the material). The original work with Marlex® HDPE woven mesh was published in 1959 (Usher 1959), but it was not until 1984 when Lichtenstein, through the technique commonly referred to as 'tension-free hernia repair,' popularised its use (Lichtenstein et al. 1989). In groin hernias, mesh repair reduces the risk of hernia recurrence compared to non-mesh repair (2% vs 5%) (EU Hernia Trialists Collaboration 2003) and reduces post-operative pain, resulting in a shorter hospital stay and quicker return to normal activity (Lockhart et al. 2018). The risk of hernia recurrence is also reduced in mesh repair of parastomal hernias and laparoscopic repair of inguinal hernias (Jones et al. 2018). In 2002, the European Union Hernia Trialist Collaboration Group evaluated 58 randomised control trials to conclude, unanimously, that the use of mesh was superior to other techniques, especially highlighting reduced recurrence and post-operative pain (EU Hernia Trialists Collaboration 2002). Today the use of mesh has virtually replaced sutured techniques for hernia repair across the developed world and may now be made from PTFE, polypropylene, or polyester. Polypropylene and polyester can be made in the form of microporous meshes that allow a good integration in the abdominal wall through colonisation of the prosthesis by collagen fibres from the host. Polypropylene absorbs little, if any, moisture, and for mesh, it is usually knitted or woven whereas polyester is most often woven. As was the case with sutures and stents, meshes have taken advantage most recently from the development of synthetic absorbable polymers, in this case to create resorbable meshes. Meshes derived from porcine or bovine tissue have also been used and provide an ideal scaffold for tissue penetration, but because of their expense they are usually reserved for abdominal wall reconstruction.

Mesh repair of hernias has not been without its problems. In groin hernias, a Cochrane review showed that wound infection and seroma (collection of fluid) rates were higher than in hernia repairs without mesh (Lockhart et al. 2018). Whilst permanent mesh for vaginal prolapse was associated with a higher rate of de novo stress incontinence and bladder injury (Maher et al. 2016), it also appeared in reports about vaginal mesh erosion and chronic pain. In 2011, transvaginal permanent mesh was voluntarily withdrawn from the UK market, though lightweight transvaginal permanent mesh was still available until banned in 2018. Hitting the headlines of national newspapers in the UK in 2017, NICE in updated advice in December 2017 said that evidence on the safety of the procedure showed there were serious, but well-recognised safety concerns, and recommended that the use of mesh in prolapse should be restricted to research only (National Institute for Health and Care Excellence 2017). The pause applied to the use of vaginal mesh by NICE was extended in a further communication on 29 March 2019 which indicated that high restriction would remain in force until further notice (National Institute for Health and Care Excellence 2019). The use of vaginal mesh remains under strict regulation (The Royal College of Obstetricians and Gynaecologists 2019).

2.3.6 Stents

The first vascular grafts were introduced following experimental work undertaken by Voorhees between 1947 and 1952 at Columbia University College of Physicians and Surgeons. He had noticed in the post-mortem examination of a laboratory animal in 1947 that a coating of endocardial tissue cells had developed over a silk suture that had been left in the right ventricle of the animal's heart and considered that such build-up might be used to form a bridge over damage to an artery. Tubes cast from a variety of materials had been tried in this capacity but had always led to thrombosis, so a fibrous form of graft was about to be used for the first time. Using precision-made tubes cut and sewn from fine parachute fabric composed of Vinyon-N (PVC), and having practised on laboratory animals, Voorhees and Blackmore undertook the first successful implants in human subjects in 1952 (Blakemore and Voorhees 1954). Other types of material were also tried out including nylon 66, PTFE, polyacrylonitrile, and stainless steel, but polyester (PET) fibre showed the greatest potential, as it did not exhibit any significant degree of biodegradation, loss of strength, or adverse biological reactions, and its use in arterial grafts became widespread. It would be reassuring to think that selecting appropriate fabric structures for the polyester grafts might then have followed a more systematic approach, with at least some accent on matching the physical behaviour of the artery being repaired. However, although it seems to have been appreciated that the key characteristics needing to be addressed were porosity, flexibility, and durability, it seems that this was also carried out in a trial-and-error fashion. With no standards or guidelines to follow, this resulted in an unnecessarily wide range of different devices appearing commercially in a variety of fabric structures (braids, single jersey plain-knitted fabrics, and woven structures: plain weave and 2 × 2 twill fabrics), each exhibiting widely different properties (Pourdeyhimi 1986). Metallic stents were first introduced for the treatment of coronary artery disease in 1980 and by the 1990s the first examples had received approval by the FDA; a surge of further approvals followed from that point on. The first Bio-Absorbable Stent, the Absorb GT1 Bioresorbable Vascular Scaffold System, made by Abbott Cardiovascular (Plymouth, MN, USA) from poly (l-lactic acid) and drug-loaded to slow down the formation of scar tissue, was approved in 2016. It was intended to degrade very slowly allowing the repair to complete over a three-year period, and leaving behind four small platinum markers embedded in the wall of the artery so that later surgeons can precisely identify where the repair took place (U.S. FDA 2016). Disappointingly, despite the innovative nature of the absorbable stent and its alignment with what seemed to be the attractive move over to synthetic absorbable polymers (following a similar bio-absorbable trend as seen with sutures), production of both of the company's absorbable products was discontinued after a very short time in September 2017 on account of what was described as 'low commercial sales.'

2.4 MAINTAINING PATIENT COMFORT BY DESIGN, PROTECTION AND SUPPORT, AND PERSONAL HYGIENE

2.4.1 Patient Comfort – Hospital Ward Design

In terms of the design of hospital wards, a simple, sparsely furnished environment offers the opportunity to maintain cleanliness more easily. Figure 2.14 shows an early example (from around the end of the 19th and beginning of the 20th century) which conforms to this pattern. Despite its simplicity, its contents show a degree of sophistication with window blinds, tubular-framed furniture including a desk with a glass sheet on the desktop and beds with wheels and adjustable so as to be movable or to change patient posture, plus ventilation grills and lights at the bedhead and

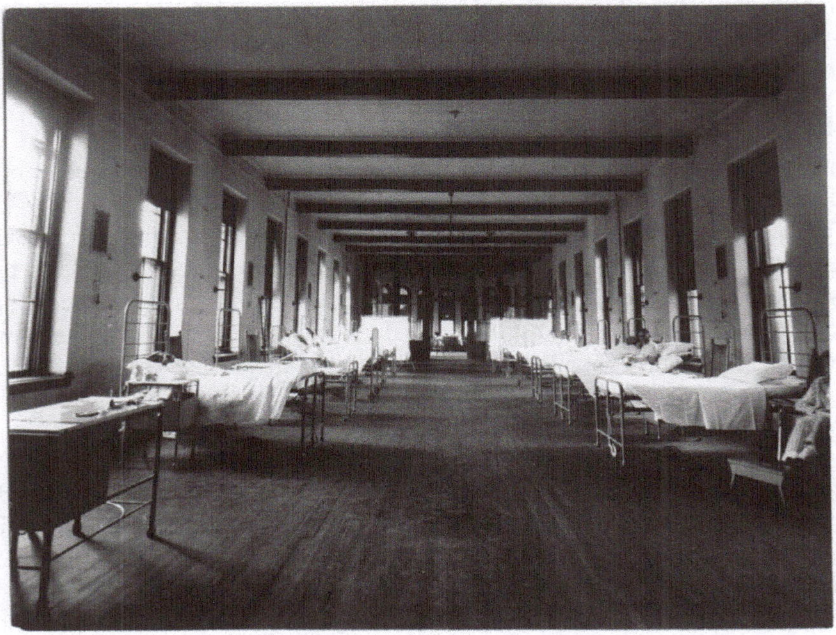

FIGURE 2.14 Ward in Gifford Wing, New Haven Hospital in Yale, Connecticut, USA, at the turn of the 19th century. (Reproduced by kind permission of the Medical Historical Library, Harvey Cushing/John Hay Whitney Medical Library, Yale University.)

circular grills beneath each bed (for heating?). The textiles present are limited to the minimum needed to function as covers and to keep the patient clean and warm. The floor-boarded floor would benefit from cleaning in this case.

2.4.2 Patient Comfort – Physical Support and Protection

2.4.2.1 Support

The intention in using scoliosis braces is to exert force in a controlled direction(s) to correct unwanted spinal curvature. Broadly speaking, they fall into two categories, rigid or flexible, and textile materials with elastomeric yarns can play a significant role as the flexible component in either type (combined with stiff elements such as metal stays in some of the rigid types). Rigid braces have been used for a long time but can cause discomfort, hence the long-time interest in the less-intrusive, mainly textile-based soft braces. The first description of the use of a soft scoliosis brace is said to have been published in 1876 (Weiss and Werkmann 2012); their overall effectiveness has been the subject of several reviews but still remains to be established.

The first medical compression garments were compression socks, invented by an engineer, Conrad Jobst in 1950, designed to exert a gradient of compression (between 15 and 20 mm Hg) intended to relieve venous pain from varicose veins and to counteract the possibility of oedema or deep-vein thrombosis. He established the company, JOBST® in Toledo, Ohio, USA, which went on to develop a range of ready-to-wear garments, consumer support stockings, plastic and reconstructive surgery garments, and anti-embolism stockings (Promedica Health Connect 2014).

2.4.2.2 Protection

Hip protectors are designed to provide some padding to protect the wearer often older individuals with difficulties maintain their balance, should they experience a fall. The intention is to prevent fracture of the hip either by absorbing or diverting the force of the fall. The first hip protector was patented in 1959 and their effectiveness has been reviewed (Cameron 2002). Hip protectors can significantly reduce the occurrence of fractures but compliance by the intended wearers is a problem; even after 60+ years, their design still requires further attention to overcome such issues.

2.4.3 Patient Comfort – Hygiene

A growing public interest in hygiene in the second half of the 19th century included the recommendation to adopt garments made from wool. The interpretation of the term 'hygiene' here was more related to health than cleanliness, involving a move away in female clothing from the fashion for tightly constricting clothing shapes to more comfortable designs; using wool in looser styles for women's everyday clothing established this health/comfort/hygiene trend and saw the award of a gold medal to Jaeger for their range of such products at the International Health Exhibition in the 1880s (Jaegar 2020). Wool can still play a role as a medical textile material today, and can be treated to render it antibacterial, as discussed in Chapters 4 and 6. Regarding a continuing aspect of feminine hygiene, for most of human history, menstruation has been associated with taboos and stigma, and the textile items intended to help were very crude. Throughout most of the 1800s, in Europe and North America, women used homemade menstrual cloths made out of flannel or woven fabric, hence the colloquial term 'on the rag.' Concerns about bacterial growth from inadequate cleaning of reusable products led to the creation of the feminine hygiene market, and from the 1850s, significant attention was turned towards this new market with patents for menstrual cups, rubber pants, and Johnson & Johnson Lister's Towels (Vostral 2008). The main issue affecting whether the products would prove successful was the taboo females had around purchasing them. The first disposable pads hit the market in 1896 and, as technology, science, and marketing have advanced, so has the range available. During World War I, it had been noticed that bagasse, the cellulose pulp fibre derived as sugarcane residue after sugar-juice extraction, absorbed more blood than woven cloth bandages. Kimberley Clark, then based at its pulp and paper mill in Wisconsin, USA, who had supplied the high-absorption bandages using that particular cellulose pulp, therefore devised its sanitary napkin (Kotex®) in 1918 from surplus high-absorption war bandages (Delaney et al. 1988; Vostral 2008). By 1921, it was the first successfully mass-marketed sanitary napkin. Efforts have been made since then to improve the performance of the napkin (and in similar ways that of disposable diapers and high-absorption bandages), by reducing the amount of material within each of these types of items whilst at the same time enhancing its absorbency.

Moving away from the idea of the fluids simply being drawn into whatever space exists within and between hydrophilic fibres such as cellulose pulp, the focus of attention turned to super-absorbent polymer hydrogels to fulfil the absorption requirement in these items. Synthetic super-absorbent polymers were developed from research conducted by the US Department of Agriculture in its search in the 1960s for materials to improve water retention in soils. Their starch-grafted acrylonitrile copolymer was capable of absorbing up to 400 times its own weight of liquid, a dramatic improvement over hydrophilic fibre (ca. 20 times) and was not subject to liquid loss on compression. Other hydrogel-forming polymer types were explored, mainly in Japan. The first sanitary napkin using super-absorbent polymers entered the market in the USA in 1978 and nappy (diaper) in Europe in 1982 swiftly followed by Japan and the USA (Matushek 2019). Modern disposable tampons were patented in 1933 (Sackren 1939, 329) and have maintained their popularity despite the link with Toxic Shock Syndrome; this challenge is considered to have served to develop the standards and textiles to what we have today (Tampax® 2020).

2.5 EXTERNAL ARTIFICIAL ORGAN SUPPORT

The concept of external artificial organ support was initiated in the 1930s with the Lindbergh-Carrel perfusion pump designed to enable blood to be oxygenated. This led to the development of the heart-lung machine, a key device for gas exchange, and revolutionising the field as it made open-heart surgery feasible. The success of the heart-lung machine used in the 1970s encouraged the development of other extracorporeal devices such as the artificial kidney and the artificial liver. The feature such devices have in common is that they are intended to be a temporary measure to support life and maintain homeostasis to enable the patient's core problem to be treated. The devices typically incorporate textiles as a key component of the filtration part(s) of the device and in the case of the Lindbergh-Carrel perfusion pump this consisted of sterilised cotton to filter the air entering the device which significantly reduced contamination.

The artificial kidney, a dialysis device, was first developed in Holland by Willem Koff in the 1940s. The requirement is for a device capable of effective dialysis of 100 to 150 litres of blood every 24 hours. The textile in these devices forms the critical component, the semi-permeable membrane. Currently these consist of hollow fibres, intended to create the high surface area required for efficient dialysis. The artificial liver, wherein the textile also plays a semi-permeable membrane type of role, has proved more difficult to achieve. Hybrid artificial liver devices developed in the 1950s by Hori, Mito, and Nosé using animal cells, continue to be the predominant useful devices with, according to Hori, much of the research being undertaken in Japan into the 2000s (Hori 1986, 211–213).

2.6 SUMMARY

Medical textiles have been designed and developed to support changes in approach to each of the key aspects of healthcare over time, namely:

(a) caring for the patient
(b) protecting patients and healthcare staff
(c) maintaining patient function, comfort, and mobility
(d) external artificial organ support

Growing understanding of pathogens and hygiene during the 1800s eventually began to be followed through by the use of surgical gowns, gloves, and masks and led to the construction of more easily cleaned and disinfected operating theatres, wards, and outpatient areas, but not routinely until the 19th century. Much of the credit for the spread of hygienic practices is ascribed to the persistence of 19th- and early-20th-century pioneers such as Lister and Halsted, but the application of medical textiles in attempts to achieve hygiene were, and continue to be, beset by tradition and habit, rather than solely by scientific evidence.

Alongside increasing demands for the need for effective protective wear, textiles forming the key components of smart garments to enable remote monitoring of patients well-being, the textiles used in devices intended to maintain patient comfort and textiles designed to support critical body functions are gaining in importance. These include items with which many people are now familiar, but also some that are of key importance but hidden from view such as implantable textiles, which are the subject of continual improvements through their modelling and subsequent refinement. The range of medical garments, devices, and equipment has widened considerably over time, and so therefore has the range of medical textiles used within them, but their introduction, adoption, and routine implementation are typically slow and stilted. The application of medical textiles is also beset by tradition and habit as illustrated by the routine of wearing the surgical mask during surgical operations, despite a growing number of trials showing that it has no significant effect on the occurrence of infection. The habit is so ingrained that it feels a sacrilege to suggest stopping wearing surgical masks for that kind of work, despite that being the logical action to take. Apart from their use for surgical operations, debate has continued about the relative effectiveness of face masks across different situations and also about their structure and composition.

Medical textiles is also a tricky field in which simply to attempt to follow trends previously blessed with positive outcomes such as the use of absorbable polymers in implantable items. For example, despite the attractiveness of the concept, there was said to be a disappointing uptake of the Absorb GT1 Bio-resorbable Vascular Scaffold System leading to its withdrawal from sales in the year following its launch (or at least that was what was stated by the company).

REFERENCES

Abhari, Roxanna E., Joana A. Martins, Hayley L. Morris, Pierre-Alexis Mouthuy, and Andrew Carr. "Synthetic sutures: Clinical evaluation and future developments." *Journal of Biomaterials Applications* 32, no. 3 (2017): 410–421.

Adams, Lu Wang, Carol A. Aschenbrenner, Timothy T. Houle, and Raymond C. Roy. "Uncovering the history of operating room attire through photographs." *Anesthesiology* 124, no. 1 (2016): 19–24.

Alexander, J. Wesley. "The contributions of infection control to a century of surgical progress." *Annals of Surgery* 201, no. 4 (1985): 423.

Barrows, T. H. "Degradable implant materials: A review of synthetic absorbable polymers and their applications." *Clinical Materials* 1, no. 4 (1986): 233–257.

Blakemore, Arthur H., and Arthur B. Voorhees Jr. "The use of tubes constructed from vinyon "N" cloth in bridging arterial defects—Experimental and clinical." *Annals of Surgery* 140, no. 3 (1954): 324.

Bynum, Bill, and Helen Bynum. "Inguinal hernia truss." *The Lancet* 389, no. 10076 (2017): 1289.

Cameron, Ian D. "Hip protectors: Prevent fractures but adherence is a problem." *British Medical Journal (Clinical Research Edition)* 324, no. 7334 (2002): 375–376.

Chen, Tianwu, Jia Jiang, and Shiyi Chen. "Status and headway of the clinical application of artificial ligaments." *Asia-Pacific Journal of Sports Medicine, Arthroscopy, Rehabilitation and Technology* 2, no. 1 (2015): 15–26.

Delaney, Janice, Mary Jane Lupton, and Emily Toth. *The Curse: A Cultural History of Menstruation*. Champaign, IL: University of Illinois Press, 1988.

Eisen, Daniel B. "Surgeon's garb and infection control: What's the evidence?" *Journal of the American Academy of Dermatology* 64, no. 5 (2011): 960-e1.

EU Hernia Trialists Collaboration. "Repair of groin hernia with synthetic mesh: Meta-analysis of randomized controlled trials." *Annals of Surgery* 235, no. 3 (2002): 322.

Forrest, Richard D. "Early history of wound treatment." *Journal of the Royal Society of Medicine* 75, no. 3 (1982): 198.

Fox, Robin Lane. *The Invention of Medicine: From Homer to Hippocrates*. City of Westminster, London: Penguin, 2020.

Guidoin, Marie-France, Yves Marois, Jacques Bejui, Nicolas Poddevin, Martin W. King, and Robert Guidoin. "Analysis of retrieved polymer fiber based replacements for the ACL." *Biomaterials* 21, no. 23 (2000): 2461–2474.

Hori, Motokazu. "Artificial liver: Present and future." *Artificial Organs* 10, no. 3 (1986): 211–213.

Howell, Joel D. "Early clinical use of the X-ray." *Transactions of the American Clinical and Climatological Association* 127 (2016): 341.

Hufnagel, Glenda Lewin. *A History of Women's Menstruation from Ancient Greece to the Twenty-First Century: Psychological, Social, Medical, Religious, and Educational Issues*. Lewiston, NY: Edwin Mellen Press, 2012.

Hutchison, Richard L., and Ghazi M. Rayan. "Astley Cooper: His life and surgical contributions." *The Journal of Hand Surgery* 36, no. 2 (2011): 316–320.

Jaegar. "British style since 1884." 2020. Accessed January 9, 2021. https://www.jaeger.co.uk/heritage.

Jain, Mehr, Sonya T. Kim, Chenchen Xu, Heidi Li, and Greg Rose. "Efficacy and use of cloth masks: A scoping review." *Cureus* 12, no. 9 (2020): e10423.

JLA. "OTEX laundry disinfection system." 2021. Accessed May 23, 2021. https://jla.com/otex/laundry.

Jones, Huw G., Michael Rees, Omar M. Aboumarzouk, Joshua Brown, James Cragg, Peter Billings, Ben Carter, and Palanichamy Chandran. "Prosthetic mesh placement for the prevention of parastomal herniation." *Cochrane Database of Systematic Reviews* 7, no. 7 (2018): CD008905.

Kean, S. "The nurse who introduced gloves to the operating room." 2020. Accessed May 23, 2021. https://www.sciencehistory.org/distillations/the-nurse-who-introduced-gloves-to-the-operating-room.

Lichtenstein, Irving L., Alex G. Shulman, Parviz K. Amid, and Michele M. Montllor. "The tension-free hernioplasty." *The American Journal of Surgery* 157, no. 2 (1989): 188–193.

Lockhart, Kathleen, Douglas Dunn, Shawn Teo, Jessica Y. Ng, Manvinder Dhillon, Edward Teo, and Mieke L. van Driel. "Mesh versus non-mesh for inguinal and femoral hernia repair." *Cochrane Database of Systematic Reviews* 9, no. 9 (2018): CD011517.

MacIntyre, C. Raina, Holly Seale, Tham Chi Dung, Nguyen Tran Hien, Phan Thi Nga, Abrar Ahmad Chughtai, Bayzidur Rahman, Dominic E. Dwyer, and Quanyi Wang. "A cluster randomised trial of cloth masks compared with medical masks in healthcare workers." *BMJ Open* 5, no. 4 (2015): e006577.

Mackenzie, David. "The history of sutures." *Medical History* 17, no. 2 (1973): 158–168.

Maher, Christopher, Benjamin Feiner, Kaven Baessler, Corina Christmann-Schmid, Nir Haya, and Jane Marjoribanks. "Transvaginal mesh or grafts compared with native tissue repair for vaginal prolapse." *Cochrane Database of Systematic Reviews* 2 (2016): CD012079.

Mast, Steven T., Jonathan D. Woolwine, and Julie Louise Gerberding. "Efficacy of gloves in reducing blood volumes transferred during simulated needlestick injury." *Journal of Infectious Diseases* 168, no. 6 (1993): 1589–1592.

Matushek, C. "History of superabsorbent polymer chemistry." 2019. Accessed June 3, 2021. https://m2polymer.com/2019/02/history-of-super-absorbent-polymer-chemistry.

Meleney, Frank L., and Franklin A. Stevens. "Postoperative haemolytic streptococcus wound infections and their relation to haemolytic streptococcus carriers among the operating personnel." *Surgery, Gynecology and Obstetrics* 43 (1926): 338–342.

Morabia, Alfredo. "Pierre-Charles-Alexandre Louis and the evaluation of bloodletting." *Journal of the Royal Society of Medicine* 99, no. 3 (2006): 158–160.

Muffly, Tyler M., Anthony P. Tizzano, and Mark D. Walters. "The history and evolution of sutures in pelvic surgery." *Journal of the Royal Society of Medicine* 104, no. 3 (2011): 107–112.

National Archives. "Smog of, December 1952, smog masks prescribed by the NHS." 2013. Accessed June 3, 2021. http://amdr.org/wp-content/uploads/2011/04/Business-Case-for-Reprocessing-for-web-1.pdf.

National Institute for Health and Care Excellence (NICE). "Extension of pause to the use of vaginal mesh." 2019. Accessed April 8, 2019. https://www.rcog.org.uk/globalassets/documents/guidelines/safety-alerts/nhs-mesh-letter-extension-of-pause-on-the-use-of-vaginal-mesh-29-march-2019.pdf.

National Institute for Health and Care Excellence (NICE). "Mesh for vaginal wall prolapse should only be used in the context of research." 2017. Accessed April 8, 2019. https://www.nice.org.uk/news/article/mesh-for-vaginal-wall-prolapse-should-only-be-used-in-the-context-of-research-says-nice.

National Institute of Occupational Safety and Health. *Guidelines for Protecting the Safety and Health of Healthcare Workers*. Washington, DC: National Institute of Occupational Safety and Health, 1988. Accessed June 3, 2021. https://www.cdc.gov/niosh/docs/88-119/pdfs/88-119.pdf?id=10.26616/NIOSHPUB88119.

Overcash, Michael. "A comparison of reusable and disposable perioperative textiles: Sustainability state-of-the-art 2012." *Anesthesia and Analgesia* 114, no. 5 (2012): 1055–1066.

Pourdeyhimi, Behnam. "Vascular grafts: Textile structures and their performance." *Textile Progress* 15, no. 3 (1986): 1–30.

Practice Greenhealth. "Greening the O.R." 2011. Accessed June 3, 2021. https://www.c4spgh.org/HCW1_Presentations/GOR_FullSet_Guidance%20Docs_Web_042711.pdf.

Promedica Health Connect. "Community Impact Team September 2014." 2014. Accessed June 3, 2021. https://promedicahealthconnect.org/news-and-community/toledo-history-meet-conrad-jobst-the-inventor/.

Pulford, Samantha, and Macarthur Fergusson. "A textile platform for non-lead radiation shielding apparel." *The Journal of the Textile Institute* 107, no. 12 (2016): 1610–1616.

Quesnel, Louis B. "The efficiency of surgical masks of varying design and composition." *Journal of British Surgery* 62, no. 12 (1975): 936–940.

Radonovich, Lewis J., Michael S. Simberkoff, Mary T. Bessesen, Alexandria C. Brown, Derek AT Cummings, Charlotte A. Gaydos, Jenna G. Los et al. "N95 respirators vs medical masks for preventing influenza among health care personnel: A randomized clinical trial." *The Journal of the American Medical Association* 322, no. 9 (2019): 824–833.

Rankin, J. Scott. "William Stewart Halsted: A lecture by Dr. Peter D. Olch." *Annals of Surgery* 243, no. 3 (2006): 418.

Sackren, H. S. "Vaginal tampons for menstrual absorption." *Clinical Medicine and Surgery* 46 (1939): 327–329.

Seitz, Jan-Marten, Martin Durisin, Jeremy Goldman, and Jaroslaw W. Drelich. "Recent advances in biodegradable metals for medical sutures: A critical review." *Advanced Healthcare Materials* 4, no. 13 (2015): 1915–1936.

Sigurdson, Alice J., Michele Morin Doody, R. Sowmya Rao, D. Michal Freedman, Bruce H. Alexander, Michael Hauptmann, Aparna K. Mohan et al. "Cancer incidence in the US radiologic technologists health study, 1983–1998." *Cancer* 97, no. 12 (2003): 3080–3089.

Skandalakis, J. E., Gene L. Colborn, L. J. Skandalakis, and D. A. McClusky. "Historic aspects of groin hernia repair." In *Nyhus and Condon's Hernia* (5th ed.), edited by Fitzgibbons, R. J., Greenburg, A. G., and Lloyd M. Nyhus, L. M., 39. Philadelphia, PA: Lippincott Williams & Wilkins, 2002.

Spirling, L. I., and I. R. Daniels. "Historical perspectives on health: William Stewart Halsted-surgeon extraordinaire: A story of 'drugs, gloves and romance'." *The Journal of the Royal Society for the Promotion of Health* 122, no. 2 (2002): 122–124.

Strasser, Bruno J., and Thomas Schlich. "A history of the medical mask and the rise of throw-away culture." *The Lancet* 396, no. 10243 (2020): 19–20.

Sun, G. "Disposable and reusable medical textiles." In *Textiles for Hygiene and Infection Control*, 125–135. Cambridge, UK: Woodhead Publishing, 2011.

Tampax®. "Tampax tampon ingredients: What are tampons made of?" 2020. Accessed December 31, 2020. https://tampax.com/en-us/tampon-truths/what-tampons-are-made-of/.

The Royal College of Obstetricians and Gynaecologists. "RCOG/BSUG response to NICE guidance on stress urinary incontinence and pelvic organ prolapse." 2019. Accessed June 3, 2021. https://www.rcog.org.uk/en/news/rcogbsug-response-to-nice-guidance-on-stress-urinary-incontinence-and-pelvic-organ-prolapse/

US FDA. "FDA approves first absorbable stent for coronary artery disease." (July 05, 2016) Accessed March 14, 2021. https://www.fda.gov/news-events/press-announcements/fda-approves-first-absorbable-stent-coronary-artery-disease.

Usher, Francis C. "Knitted Marlex mesh: An improved marlex prosthesis for repairing hernias and other tissue defects." *AMA Archives of Surgery* 82, no. 5 (1961): 771–773.

Usher, Francis C., John G. Fries, John L. Ochsner, and L. L. D. Tuttle. "Marlex mesh, a new plastic mesh for replacing tissue defects: II. Clinical studies." *AMA Archives of Surgery* 78, no. 1 (1959): 138–145.

Vacanti, Charles A. "The history of tissue engineering." *Journal of Cellular and Molecular Medicine* 10, no. 3 (2006): 569–576.

Vachon, M. "Japan's love affair with the surgical mask explained and popular face masks to purchase." 2020. Accessed September 9, 2020. https://www.tsunagujapan.com/japan-mask-culture-explained/.

Vincent, Marina, and Peggy Edwards. "Disposable surgical face masks for preventing surgical wound infection in clean surgery." *Cochrane Database of Systematic Reviews* 4 (2016): CD002929.

Vostral, Sharra L. *Under Wraps: A History of Menstrual Hygiene Technology*. Lexington, MA: Lexington Books, 2008.

Walton, J. R. "A new controversy in respiratory equipment management: Reusables versus disposed disposables versus reused disposables." *Respiratory Care* 31, no. 3 (1986): 213–217.

Weiss, Hans-Rudolf, and Mario Werkmann. "Soft braces in the treatment of Adolescent Idiopathic Scoliosis (AIS)–Review of the literature and description of a new approach." *Scoliosis* 7, no. 1 (2012): 1–11.

World Medical Association. "WMA declaration of Geneva." 2017. Accessed February 10, 2019. https://www.wma.net/policies-post/wma-declaration-of-geneva/.

Xu, Chengyu, Ryuji Inai, Masaya Kotaki, and Seeram Ramakrishna. "Electrospun nanofiber fabrication as synthetic extracellular matrix and its potential for vascular tissue engineering." *Tissue Engineering* 10, no. 7–8 (2004): 1160–1168.

Zajaczkowski, Thaddaeus. "Johann Anton von Mikulicz-Radecki (1850–1905)—a pioneer of gastroscopy and modern surgery: His credit to urology." *World Journal of Urology* 26, no. 1 (2008): 75–86.

Zins, Howard M. "Environmental, cost and product issues related to reusable healthcare textiles." *Research Journal of Textile and Apparel* 10, no. 4 (2006): 73–80.

3 Textile Materials for Healthcare and Medical Applications

3.1 INTRODUCTION

Chapter 3 provides the basis for understanding the nature of textile materials in general, the characteristics that all textiles have in common such as their flexibility, their ability to recover from deformation, their permeability, and their amenability to adjustment/engineering of their properties to meet the demands of a wide range of applications. The focus of attention here is on the properties conferred by fibre characteristics, yarn characteristics, and fabric construction on the finished item rather than on the polymer from which the fibres are made.

3.2 RANGE OF APPLICATIONS

A wide range of medical textiles are important to medicine and healthcare, and that range continues to grow. Wang (2016) neatly classified the areas within which medical textiles are applied as:

- implantable materials, e.g., sutures, grafts, scaffolds
- non-implantable materials, e.g., wound dressings, pressure garments
- healthcare/hygiene roles, e.g., clothing, disposable products such as wipes
- extracorporeal devices, e.g., artificial kidney, liver, pancreas
- intelligent medical and healthcare textiles

To which we would add

- Furnishing fabrics and textiles in fixtures and fittings in healthcare establishments
- Components of devices for environmental hygiene control

DOI: 10.1201/9781003170570-3

3.3 PROPERTIES SOUGHT FROM TEXTILES FOR MEDICAL AND HEALTHCARE APPLICATIONS

Special requirements may be placed on textiles intended for medical and healthcare use and their nature will depend upon the function that the textile is intended to perform (Wang 2016, 132). Generally speaking, implantable textiles should be non-toxic and biocompatible, hypoallergenic, and non-carcinogenic. For items making use of synthetic absorbable polymers (SA polymers; see Section 4.7), stability of the product is important, particularly because degradation rates need to be reliably uniform to allow the item to provide the expected support or controlled release of entrapped drugs for the necessary length of time, and the degradation products need to be non-toxic and must not accumulate in body tissues. Where the main purpose of the medical textile is mechanical, the textile may need to be biologically inert, but biologically active materials can also have a function in this type of role, for example, in delivering a drug to a target organ at a controlled rate.

Useful characteristics for the textile to possess in particular applications are as follows:

- strength, e.g., an implantable scaffold or suture
- flexibility, e.g., a vascular graft
- air permeability, e.g., a wound dressing
- moisture absorption and permeability, e.g., a wound dressing
- environmentally acceptable production, recycling, and disposal plus whatever would be the appropriate launderability/sterilisability to enable re-useability rather than being in the form of a single-use disposable, e.g., scrubs, gowns, aprons, surgical masks, filter face-piece masks/respirators, wipes, diapers, and incontinence underpads for bedding and furniture

The last point is there in recognition that it would be wrong to continue to think that medical textiles should be immune from economic or environmental considerations. The production and disposal of products should at the very least be in line with current guidance, either national or international, depending upon whether the target market is local or global. Implantable textiles and those used in potentially infective circumstances need to be sterile and the sterilisation process must not alter the mechanical properties, the chemical composition of the textile, or its biological function (if any). For example, artificial joints sometimes contain components made from polyethylene; sterilisation of these is possible by various methods, each of which have their own advantages and disadvantages; for example, sterilisation with high-dose irradiation produces a highly cross-linked polyethylene with better wear resistance but decreased fatigue resistance compared to standard high-density polyethylene (Miller et al. 2012) (see Chapter 4, Section 4.6.3).

3.4 FIBRES, YARNS, AND FABRICS

Natural fibres, typically collected in the form of short tufts, are described as staple fibre. Only silk exists naturally in filament form, whereas synthetic polymer fibres, or those manufactured from natural polymers such as cellulose extracted from plants, are extruded in the form of continuous filaments to begin with, so they can be used in either filament form, or cut or broken into short lengths. Cutting or breaking allows the synthetic polymer materials to fulfil the roles traditionally occupied by staple fibres. For medical or healthcare applications, textiles may be used in staple fibre form, either neatly arranged side by side as in some types of high-performance filters for liquids, in a web with fibres arranged randomly as in many non-woven fabrics, in a soft, open, absorbent mass such as in 'cotton wool,' in the yarns used to make woven fabrics for uniforms or sheeting, or in filament form for certain implants such as braided sutures or artificial tendons.

3.4.1 Fibres and Filaments

Typically, natural fibre diameters range between ca 20 and 100 µm at the coarser end of the scale, such as the stiffer types of animal hairs and human hair, through to ca 15–30 µm for merino wool, 6.5–11 µm for individual silk filaments (brins), and 8–20µm for Egyptian cotton. Changes in fibre diameter exert dramatic effects on fibre rigidity. With widths greater than ca 150mm, the materials are more bristle-like than fibre-like, whereas finer diameter fibres are characteristically soft and flexible The great flexibility of finer fibres and filaments arises because a fibre's rigidity to bending is proportional to the fibre radius to the power four (for a perfectly circular elastic fibre), so each time its radius is reduced by a factor of 2, bending rigidity is reduced by a factor of 16.

Synthetic polymer man-made fibres or natural polymer man-made fibres, of similar dimensions to those encountered in natural fibres, are first prepared as filaments by dissolving or melting the polymer, then pumping the resulting viscous fluid through the fine holes in a spinneret (50 to 110 in a spinneret disc for making conventional yarns). The emerging filaments harden either on evaporation of the solvent used to dissolve the polymer (in the case of solvent spinning), coagulation in a bath which removes the agent holding the polymer in solution (in the case of wet-spinning), or by cooling (in the case of melt spinning). Whichever spinning method is used, the emergent filaments are not immediately ready to be used as continuous filaments, because the polymer chains from which they have been formed are in a jumbled, glassy state. The polymer chains need to be aligned or caused to form crystalline regions in order to become stiff enough to perform elastically, at least to the small deformations they will normally experience in most textile applications. To achieve the necessary degree of alignment, the newly formed filaments are drawn (extended by up to five times their original length) after extrusion to bring about some alignment of the polymer chains. The result is one of partial crystallisation. Some sections of polymer chain will align sufficiently well with adjacent chains in some places along the length of the drawn filament to form microscopic crystallites and it is their presence together with sections of straightened, but less well-aligned, polymer chain which help to limit any further sliding of the polymer chains over one another on the application of more tension. To achieve greater effect from drawing and thereby deliver a higher-performance fibre or filament, drawing is carried out at elevated temperatures (hot drawing). Drawing brings about the required improvements in the mechanical properties of the filaments, and although it causes considerable thinning, it is the diameter of the spinneret hole which is used to determine the filament diameter, and its shape, the filament cross-sectional shape. The most-used cross-sectional shape is circular, but others such as a dumbbell shape (with polyacrylonitrile) or a trilobal shape (with nylon) may be employed to improve the handle, appearance, or rigidity of the filaments. Hollow fibres have been of interest as the central void offers the opportunity for that to be filled with a drug-containing medium which can then be delivered at a controlled rate (Ahn 1996), but there are alternative ways of achieving control over the rate of drug release from medical textile implants (each with their own particular strengths and weaknesses) such as by the creation of micropores within nanofibres, by nano-engineering (Müller et al. 2014), or by molecular imprinting (Section 5.2.4). It is usual with the synthetic polymers to incorporate a delustrant such as titanium dioxide (TiO_2) in the form of a fine powder into the molten polymer, because otherwise their filaments and fibres will be transparent; TiO_2 is now also incorporated as a nano-powder in what are described as 'self-cleaning' textile materials (see Chapter 9).

3.4.2 Microfibres and Microporous Fibres

Microfibres are very fine fibres with a width of 3–10 μm and a linear density between 0.3 and 1 dtex. In most instances, they are finer than the finest natural fibres, and therefore characteristically more flexible and softer for the reasons explained in Section 3.3.1. Moreover, they possess more external surface area than ordinary fibres, and this can assist in applications such as filtration or those requiring moisture transport by wicking such as incontinence wear. Microfibres can be prepared from 'Islands-in-the-Sea' bi-component fibres wherein the component intended to become the fibre is extruded from multiple feeds into a soluble, viscous matrix and the two unmixed components are extruded together through a spinneret of similar dimensions as would be used in the production of fine, commodity-synthetic-polymer man-made fibres. The soluble, viscous matrix in this arrangement supports and separates the very finely spaced fibre-forming strands, until the extruded combination hardens on emerging from the spinneret. The microfibres (actually, microfilaments at this stage) are then released from the support medium by dissolving that medium away; the cross section of the microfibres can be controlled to some extent by the spinneret-hole shape used to extrude the fibre-forming polymer into the support medium, and that is able to yield a variety of shapes of microfibre as shown in Figure 3.1. If the focus is on the production of the finest fibres possible by this method, the spinneret orifices must be very small (and there may be several hundreds of them in the spinneret disc, created for example by laser drilling). This does offer the possibility of making nanofibres from the exceedingly small islands (an alternative to electrospinning). If nanofibrrs are the intention, the second medium need not be a soluble matrix. If a second fibre-forming polymer is used, of similar but not identical viscosity to the first, the bi-component fibres that are formed are more easily handled than nanofibres in the processes leading up to web formation for the preparation of non-woven fabrics. The jets then used in hydro-entanglement during web formation

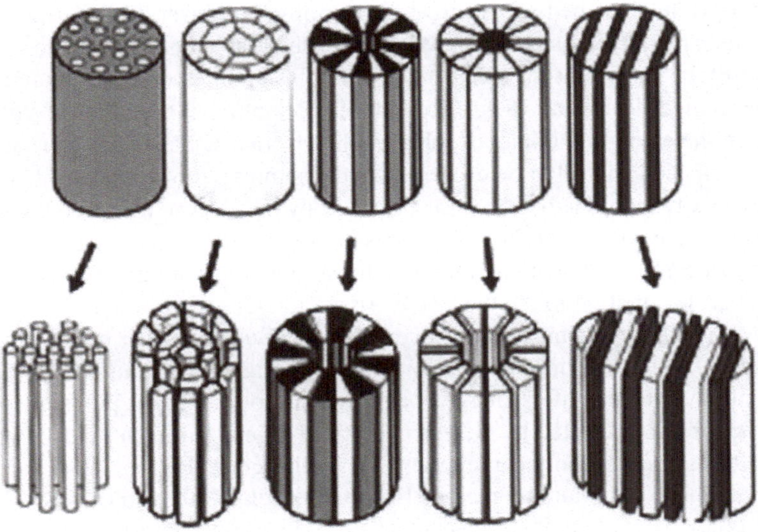

FIGURE 3.1 Microfibres created from Islands-in-the-Sea (*Textile Terms and Definitions* 2021; courtesy The Textile Institute).

are sufficiently powerful to break the components apart and create the nanofibres in situ (see Section 3.5.3).

For the production of *microporous fibres* rather than *microfibres*, it is the soluble viscous support medium which is pumped into the fibre-forming polymer before the combination is subjected to extrusion rather than the other way round. The islands formed by the soluble medium within the fibre-forming polymer can then be dissolved away, resulting in the presence of continuous micropores running along the length of the filament or fibre.

3.4.3 Nanofibres

Nanofibres are extremely fine fibres, around two orders of magnitude finer than the finest microfibres, routinely produced by electrospinning at widths between 50 and 500 nm (the term 'nanofibre' continues to be used for the larger-diameter fibres even though ISO Technical Committee 229 defines nanomaterials as 'those materials measuring less than 100 nm in at least one direction'). Finer nanofibres can be produced, but only under more specialist conditions. The idea of drawing very fine fibres out of a solution of a suitable polymer is not new, having been first filed for consideration to be patented in 1899 resulting in US Patent 692,631A being granted in 1902 to inventor John F. Cooley and described as an 'Apparatus for Electrically Dispersing Fluids' (Cooley 1902). Cooley dissolved collodion and having fed it from an orifice in a tube into a static electrically charged zone where it was subjected to convection to evaporate the solvent, he created a stream of very fine fibres. Further significant development took place in Germany in the 1930s (Formhals 1934) leading to a process he described as 'electrostatic spinning'; however, little further significant development took place until Taylor established the theory behind how a stable cone could be formed at the point the spinning solution emerged from a capillary into the applied electrostatic field (Taylor 1969). Beginning the creation of a filament, first from the emerging droplet of solution, then from a stable Taylor cone at higher voltages, enabled control to be exerted over the spinning process to enable fibres to be drawn away reproducibly from the capillary by the electric field (see Figure 3.2). Although interest in the ability of electrospinning to yield nanofibres with properties not achievable by fibres of traditional dimensions was not immediate, it did then begin to grow rapidly through the late 1990s.

In a working arrangement for producing electrospun yarns, the polymer solution is pumped through a syringe needle connected to a high-voltage direct-current electricity supply, which confers charge of a particular polarity to the polymer solution. Once the repulsion created by the electrostatic charge is sufficient to overcome the surface tension of the polymer solution, the Taylor cone (Figure 3.2) is formed at the point where the solution emerges from the needle. Although either a spray or filament may be emitted from the apex of the Taylor cone, adjusting the voltage to the right level will create a filament rather than droplets. As it heads towards the earthed collector, the newly forming filament undergoes a chaotic whirling around described in Figure 3.3 as 'whipping instability,' which helps to thin down the filament as it loses solvent and begins to harden. The newly forming filament nevertheless continues to be attracted, by its opposite charge, towards the collector, which, if it is rotated and translated as shown in Figure 3.3, may enable the filaments to be collected in the form of a yarn rather than simply deposited as a web (Sill and von Recum 2008).

Electrospinning can be used to produce fibres with widths from the sub-micrometre range to just a few nanometres across. Their great flexibility arises because fibre rigidity to bending is proportional to the fibre radius to the power four (for a perfectly circular elastic fibre), so each time its radius is reduced by a factor of 2, bending rigidity is reduced by a factor of 16 as explained in Section 3.1.1. Electroactive biomaterials such as polyaniline, polypyrrole, and polythiophenes are of particular interest not only for high-performance filtration enhancement but also for flexible

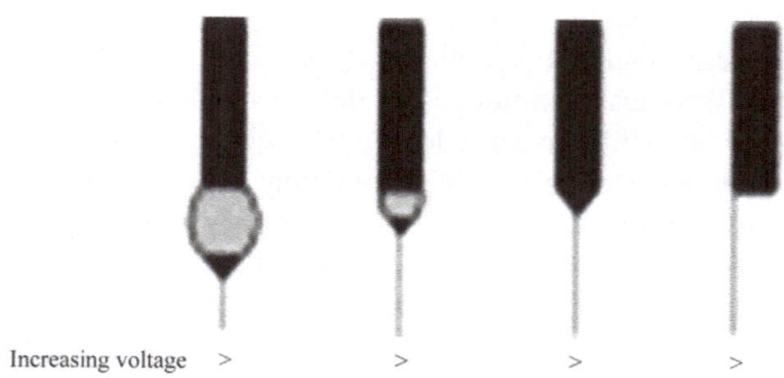

FIGURE 3.2 The effect of varying the applied voltage on the formation of the Taylor cone (Sill and von Recum 2008; reproduced by permission from Elsevier).

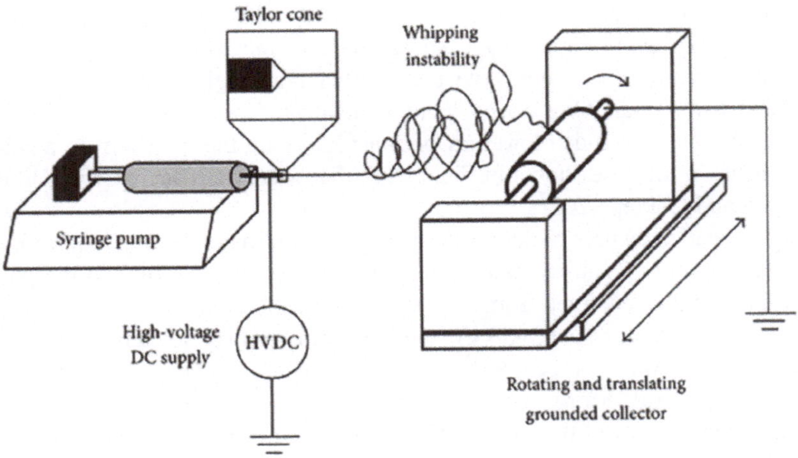

FIGURE 3.3 Schematic diagram of an electrospinning system (Sill and von Recum 2008; reproduced by permission from Elsevier).

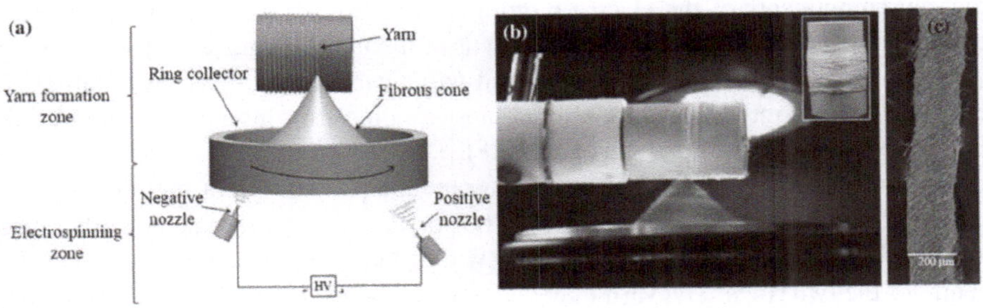

FIGURE 3.4 Direct electrospinning of nanofibre yarn. (a) Schematic; (b) Actual showing collected yarn on spool in inset; and (c) Scanning electron micrograph of 200μm-wide yarn made from nanofibres (Shuakat and Lin 2016; by permission of Taylor & Francis).

sensor and actuator structures in smart electronic wearables, and it is the great flexibility of the electrically conductive or piezoelectric nanofibrous forms of the electroactive polymers such as PEDOT or PVDF (see Chapter 4, Section 4.9) that renders them such attractive materials to incorporate.

Appropriate choice of the spinning arrangement, such as multiple jets and a rotating collector (Shuakat and Lin 2016), can enable the production of very neat electrospun nanofibre yarns rather than fibre just being collected in fibre bundles or as nanofibre webs, and such yarns are of particular interest because whilst they are ultrafine and highly flexible, they have sufficient integrity and strength to be woven or they can be knitted or braided. The spinning arrangement used by Shuakat and Lin can be seen in Figure 3.4 to consist of two nozzles oppositely charged by a DC electrical supply directing the emerging filaments towards a rotating ring. The ring controls the filament path into a cone shape between the ring and the bobbin rather than allowing it to whip around as was illustrated in Figure 3.3, and the scanning electron micrograph in Figure 3.4 (c) shows the resultant 200-μm yarn composed of many neatly arranged nanofibres twisted together at an angle close to 45°.

When woven, nanofibre yarns yield equivalent fabrics not only with lower areal density but also much lower air permeability than those woven from conventional yarns; in the case shown in Figure 3.5, they were both acrylic (PAN) fabrics (Mülayim and Göktepe 2021).

For applications where a more orderly alignment of nanofibres is required, near-field electrospinning can be used. The electrode is set much closer to the point at which the polymer emerges from the jet and the applied voltage reduced to 100–600 V rather than the usual 5–50 kV, the idea being to take advantage of the more stable zone close to the jet, before the newly forming filament begins to whip around in the electric field. More orderly arrangements of emergent nanofibre bundles have also been achieved by a modified two-jet electrospinning arrangement using 6–13 kV but also placing a neutral pointed metal rod along the yarn path from a disc (instead of the cone in Figure 3.4) close to the point at which the fibres leave the disc. The idea is to exert even more control in what would otherwise become the whipping zone than would be achieved solely by a ring collector. The distances at which the key components of the electrospinning system are set (nozzles, disc, and rod) can be adjusted to optimise the arrangement of the nano-filaments in the emerging yarn (Wu et al. 2016). Such well-arranged yarns can be assembled by small-scale circular weaving into three-dimensional fabrics suitable for insertion as a graft (see Figures 3.6, 3.7, and 3.8) (Joseph et al. 2018).

As can be seen from the schematic diagram and photograph of the robotic miniature weaving machine, it consists of two rotatable discs with nano-yarn bobbins arranged in two outer rings. The circular woven fabric is formed on the rod at the centre of the two rings. The yarn intended to form the weft (and therefore run across the emerging woven tube) is fed between the two discs directly from the side so it is the yarns intended to form the warp which are fed from the bobbins on the outer rings. The bobbins can be moved between the two discs from one side or the other before they arrive at the weft supply so that they interlace with it in the

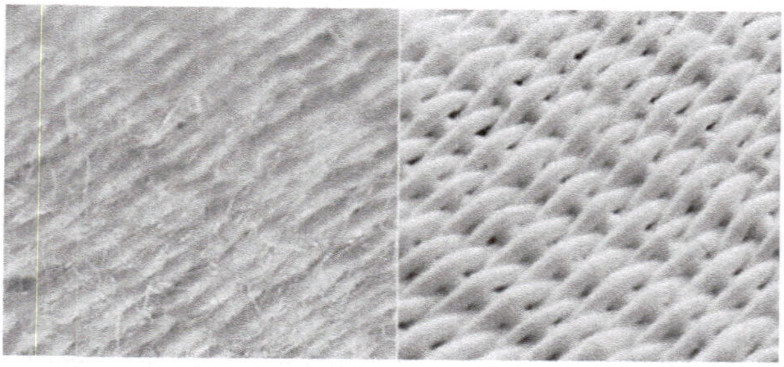

FIGURE 3.5 Woven PAN nanofabric (left) compared with conventional PAN woven fabric (right), both recorded at 10× magnification and showing larger pore sizes in the conventional fabric. (Adapted from Mülayim and Göktepe (2021); by permission of Taylor & Francis.)

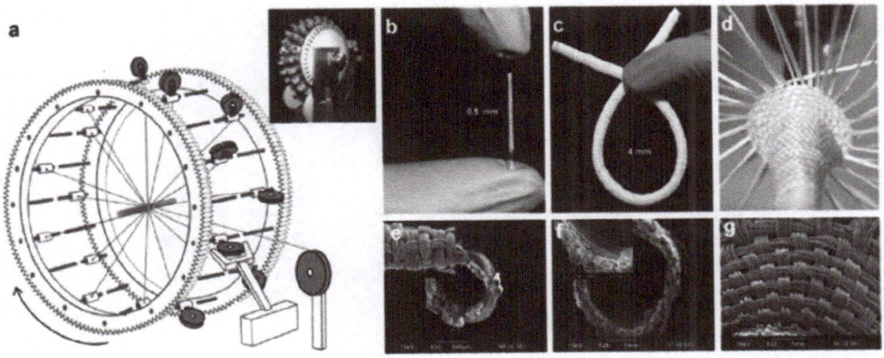

FIGURE 3.6 Fabrication of 3D woven nanotextiles. (a) Schematic of the automated weaving system (nanoweaver) showing continuous tubular woven fabric forming on the rod at the centre of the two rotating disks, with inset image of the robotic system; (b), (e) Optical and SEM images of the smallest woven fabric (0.5 mm) inside a capillary tube; the inset SEM image shows its lateral view; (c), (f) A 4-mm flexible woven tube and inset SEM image showing the cross-sectional view of the inner surface; and (d), (g) Undesirable architectures caused by inadequate yarn tension. (Reprinted/adapted with permission from Joseph et al. (2018). Copyright © 2018 American Chemical Society.)

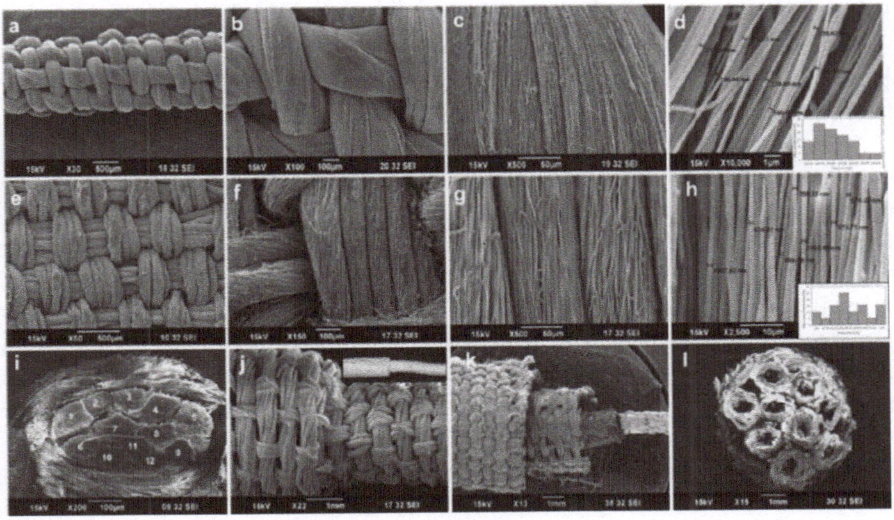

FIGURE 3.7 Hierarchical multi-scale nanotextiles. SEM images of conduits fabricated using yarns constituted of well-oriented fibres. (a–d) PCL-collagen; (e–h) PLLA; (i) Cross-sectional view showing hierarchical bundling of fibres; (j) Conduits with step change in diameter (with inset its optical image); and (k, l) Hierarchical concentric and multi-channelled structures. The red stars indicate individual conduits of same or different diameter. (Reprinted/adapted with permission from Joseph et al. (2018). Copyright © 2018 American Chemical Society.)

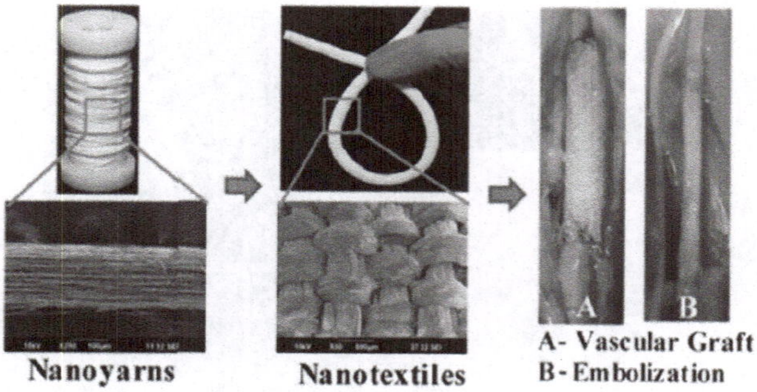

FIGURE 3.8 Nanofibre yarn converted into a circular woven tube, then inserted as a graft. (Reprinted/adapted with permission from Joseph et al. (2018). Copyright © 2018 American Chemical Society.)

desired pattern. Figure 3.6 (b) of a circular woven fabric within a capillary tube of only 0.5 mm diameter gives some illustration of the machine's capability. Given the tidiness of the fibre arrangement within the resultant yarns after doubling singles nanofibre yarns together, and the possibility of instantly changing the diameter of the woven tube along its length, means that various potentially useful tubular arrangements can be woven. For the case shown in Figure 3.7, the tubes were made from electrospun synthetic absorbable polymers consisting of either a blend of polycaprolactam with collagen (PCL-collagen) or of polylactic acid (PLLA).

The potential usefulness of woven nanofibre tubes of this type is illustrated in Figure 3.8 (Joseph et al. 2018) which shows them after having been implanted either to act as a vascular graft or as a therapeutic embolisation.

Core-spun nanofibre yarns have the advantage of the tensile properties typical of a yarn made from fibres or filaments of traditional dimensions (which is within the core), coupled with properties conferred to the exterior of the yarn by the nanofibre yarns. Appropriate choice of wrapping angle results in good adhesion of the nanofibre yarn to the conventional core and may result in improved yarn tenacity. Attractive surface properties such as moisture absorption/evaporation may be conferred to an otherwise mostly hydrophilic fibre core content. For the examples shown in the images in Figure 3.7 (Mao et al. 2021), the core fibres were mostly of a lipophilic nature and even the cotton, which was not scoured or bleached, had a waxy surface, so it did not absorb water readily. The nanofibres, however, were of polyacrylonitrile, and they conferred improved moisture management through wicking and evaporation. The terminology for core-spun nanofibre yarns can be cumbersome, so it is usefully abbreviated (Figure 3.9).

Here, just as is the case with metal–organic frameworks (MOFs) where other materials can be introduced into MOF pores and encapsulated rather than being bonded, the same notation is being used to denote a conventional fibre core encapsulated in nanofibre yarn. For an MOF the notation A@B is used to represent material A, encapsulated in the MOF material B (Sosa et al. 2018) and that type of notation is used for composite films where polymers are mixed but not combined in any other

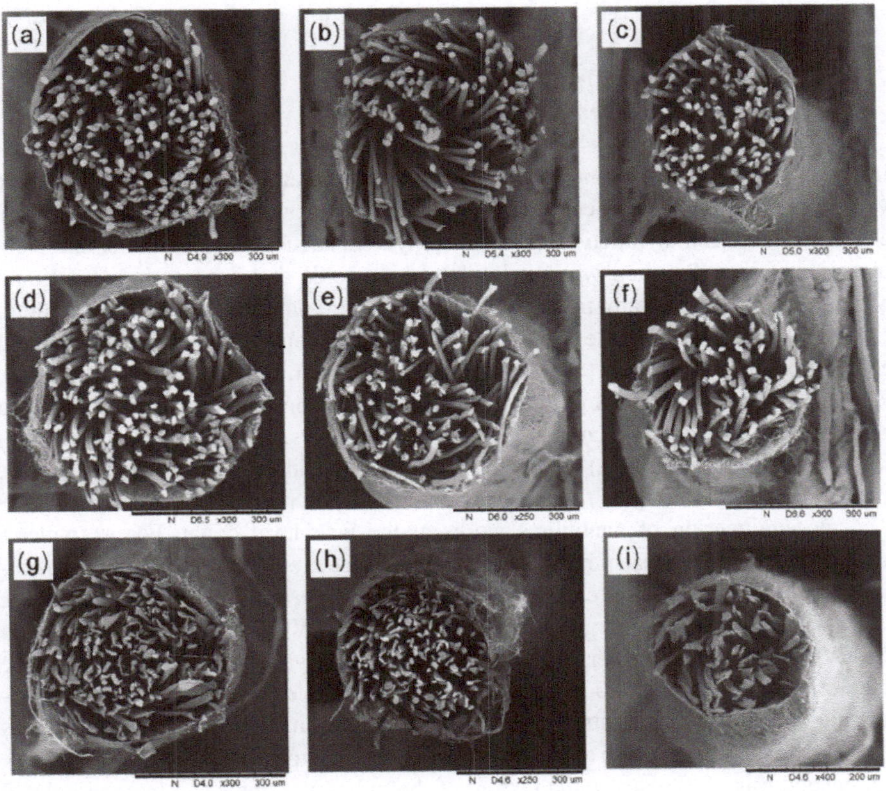

FIGURE 3.9 Hybrid core-spun yarns. Cross section SEM images of (a) 13 N_e; (b) 16 N_e; (c) 21 N_e Polyester@NFs yarn; (d) 16 N_e; (e) 21 N_e; (f) 32 N_e Acrylic@NFs yarn; (g) 16 N_e; (h) 21 N_e; and (i) 32 N_e Cotton@NFs yarn (Mao et al. 2021); image reproduced by permission of Taylor & Francis.

way, or for inorganic compounds incorporated to form a composite with a polymer but not chemically bound to it (Shi et al. 2020). Using a similar type of notation for the core-spun nanofibre yarn, acrylic@NFs represents the conventional core, acrylic in this case, encapsulated in nanofibres (NFs). In this case, various core yarns are wrapped by nanofibres and this can convey significantly different surface properties to the yarn compared with those of the core, while the core yarn provides the kind of mechanical properties consistent with those of a conventional yarn. If, however, the core were to be made from a water-soluble polymer such as polyvinyl alcohol (PVA), after being wrapped with nanofibres, the core can be dissolved away to leave a hollow fibre. The hollow fibre in this case is of traditional fibre dimensions, but the shell from which it is formed is composed of nanofibres.

To support tissue engineering, materials need to possess high porosity (over 90%) pore dimensions appropriate to the intended application depending on the application, which may range from around 10 μm to several hundreds of micrometres. The pore diameter in scaffolds should be:

- between 20 and 150 μm for liver regeneration to allow the growth of hepatocytes
- within the range of 20 to 150 μm for skin
- much larger at between 200 and 400 μm for bone

In all cases, pores must be interconnected to allow cell and tissue in-growth. A wide variety of techniques has been developed to create such scaffolds with the desired characteristics from synthetic absorbable polymers such as polyurethane, and electrospinning is well-suited when it is fibrous scaffolds that are needed (Janik and Marzec 2015). Other synthetic absorbable electrospun polymers have been explored, and Mokhtari et al. provide a long list of the candidate polymers for biomedical applications in their review of advances in electrospinning (Mokhtari et al. 2016). However, the most used SA polymers in clinical use continue to be polyesters such as the polylactides, polyglycolides, and their copolymers, namely poly (l-lactic acid) (PLLA), poly (glycolic acid) (PGA) and poly (lactic acid-co-glycolic acid) (PLGA), and the polyurethanes, plus there is growing use of polymer mixes as well.

Nano-engineering of nanofibres works at the next level down. For example, a nano-engineering approach exploited the high surface area of PVA electrospun nanofibres to support chromium catalysts for surface polymerisation of ethylene to create UHMWPE/PVA core/shell nanofibres or hollow UHMWPE nanofibres by dissolving the PVA component (Müller et al. 2014). Electrospun yarns have ultra-fine surface characteristics which help to make them suited to the role of scaffolds in tissue engineering, and ultrasonic treatment can be effective in ensuring that the nanofibrous assembly is sufficiently open to allow cellular infiltration to take place (Lee et al. 2011), but beyond this, the surfaces and texture of the individual fibres can be manipulated by various nano-engineering methods such as using high-volatility spinning solvents, humidity control in the spinning chamber, phase separation in the polymer/solvent system resulting in the formation of porous nanofibres, coaxial spinning to form hollow nanofibres, or chemical modification of the nanofibre following its formation. The example shown in Figure 3.10 is for porous polystyrene nanofibres created by phase separation of the electrospinning solution due to collecting on a cold liquid surface.

3.5 YARNS

Textile yarns are made from either:

(i) *continuous filaments*, such as those of cultivated silk or natural polymer or synthetic polymer filaments which have been extruded and drawn but not chopped or broken into staple fibre. The required number of filaments for the multi-filament yarn will be twisted sufficiently to keep the filaments together, or

(ii) *staple fibre* which has been opened and carded to completely separate the fibres and convert them into the form of a web then either:

    (a) spun directly to yield a soft yarn wherein the fibres are not well aligned (condenser-spun yarn), or

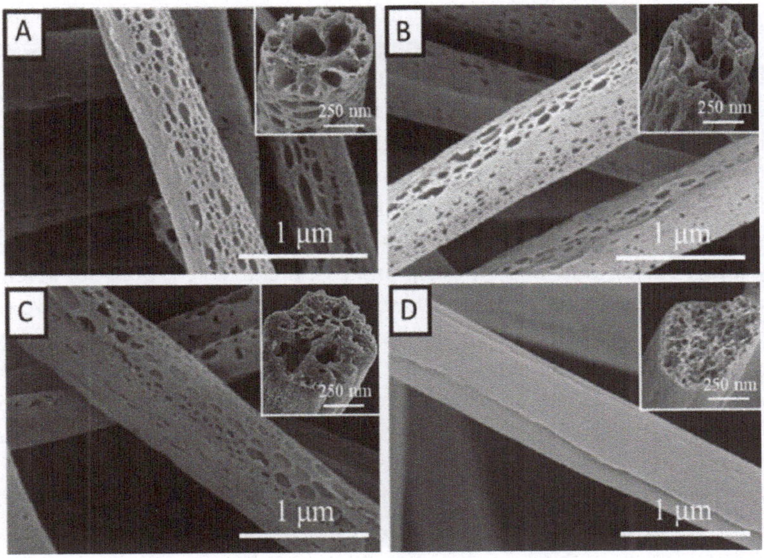

FIGURE 3.10 SEM images of porous polystyrene filaments electrospun from a solution of chlorobenzene and NN dimethylformamide at a ratio 2:1 and collected on the surface of a bath collector at different temperatures. (a) 3 °C; (b) 25 °C; (c) 40 °C; and (d) static collector (Zhu et al. 2020).

(b) combed to align fibres and remove any short ones to yield a firm yarn with fibres more neatly packed side by side. For greater evenness, strength, and to trap the fibres more firmly in place, two or more of these yarns may be twisted (folded) together. The yarn would be a twofold yarn if it was made by twisting two yarns together or a threefold yarn made by twisting three yarns together and so on. Sewing threads consist of yarns folded together for these very reasons.

Further to the classification given above, yarns are often also described according to the manufacturing method employed, but broadly speaking, the end result will conform to one of the types described above. The other important description for a yarn is its linear density (which may be thought of as a way of describing its thickness) typically given as its tex value (the direct system for expressing the yarn number or count, determined by the weight in grams of 1 kilometre of the yarn).

3.6 FABRICS

3.6.1 Woven Fabrics

Woven fabrics are widely used in hospital bedding, clothing, wound dressings, gauzes, and in some hygiene products. The yarns in woven fabrics are interlaced at right angles to one another, with the warp yarns running along the length of the fabric and the weft from side to side. Various interlacing designs can be created to satisfy a wide range of end uses requiring flat, strong sheet-like structures, particularly those which need to be inextensible in both the warp and weft directions. There is, however, a little more extensibility if tension is applied diagonally (in the bias direction) and the sheet-like structure of the woven fabric is capable of demonstrating significant flexibility (The Textile Institute 2021). While the ultimate goal of woven fabric designers is to develop a construction that has predetermined properties to fit the specific application, they also need to achieve the highest possible fabric quality and weaving efficiency (Seyam and El-Shiekh 1993); even so, given those constraints, many variables can be altered during the creation of a woven fabric to modify its mechanical performance ranging from the yarns used to the type of interlacing and the packing density of the yarns within the woven structure (Seyam and El-Shiekh 1994). However, many of the clothing and bed linen requirements can be satisfied with standard traditional woven fabrics such as plain weave or 2×2 twill woven tightly, to yield a dense sett (Figure 3.11).

In fact, *sheeting* is defined as a medium-weight, closely woven, plain weave or 2×2 twill weave fabric made from yarns of medium linear density and used primarily for bed coverings with a typical construction of either:

(i) plain weave: 25 × 23; 35 × 33 tex; K = 14.8 + 13.2, or
(ii) 2 × 2 twill weave: 24 × 28; 21 × 37 tex; K = 11.0 + 17.0

where the first sets of numbers are the numbers of threads in the warp and weft directions, and K is the cover factor for each set of threads, a measure of the density of their packing in the woven structure (The Textile Institute 2021). For institutional use, the yarns chosen are most usually combed cotton/polyester blend fabrics or the 100% polyester equivalent for ease of maintenance and durability; a condenser-spun

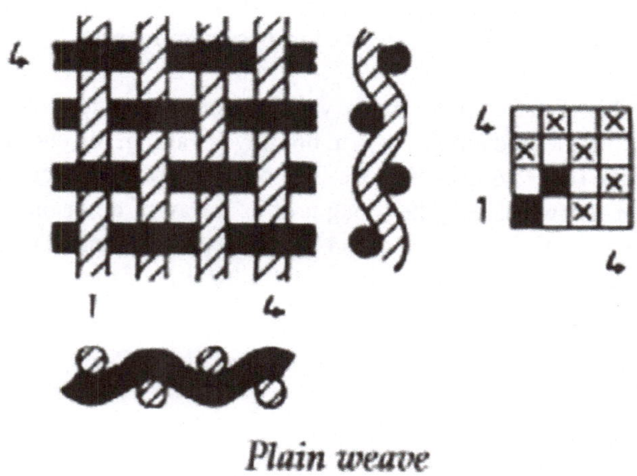

FIGURE 3.11 Plain weave structure (*Textile Terms and Definitions* 2021; courtesy The Textile Institute).

yarn may, however, be used in the weft. Typical sheeting for bed linen would have an areal density of 130 g per square metre.

3D woven fabric applications in healthcare are mostly to be found in wound dressings, implants, and in items intended for regenerative medicine (Eriksson and Sandsjo 2015, 305–340). The ability to create 3D structures out of several different yarns arranged not only on the usual x- and y-axes, but also vertically to them on the z-axis, allows for the production of different types of textiles that display a range of mechanical properties which go beyond those expected from the two-dimensional products. 3D woven textiles can be produced in multi-layer form, hollow shapes, nodal or dome structures, each of which has its own distinctive range of characteristics (Gokarneshan and Alagirusamy 2009). Two-layer structures such as warp interlock are open structures with connecting threads passing between the layers at intervals. Many such hollow structures exhibit high-energy absorption capabilities while a solid 3D structure can exhibit high dimensional stability and, therefore, substantial resistance to shear and deformation (Bilisik 2011).

3.6.2 Knitted Fabrics

Industrially, knitted fabrics are produced by one of two methods: weft knitting and warp knitting. Knitted fabrics are typically more extensible than woven fabrics, because rather than the yarns being tightly interlaced under and over one another as in woven fabrics, they consist of rows or columns of interlinked loops of yarn.

3.6.2.1 Weft-Knitted Fabrics

Weft-knitted fabrics consist of loops of yarn formed in succession one by one across the fabric, to form a horizontal row of loops interlinked to the rows above and below. The simplest type of machine-knitted, weft-knitted structure is plain knitted, often also described as stocking stitch (see Figure 3.12).

Plain weft-knitted fabrics (stocking stitch) or simple ribs can be extended to around 1.8× the original width (much further for the more corrugated of the rib structures) and to around 1.4× their original length. Their extensibility is impressive enough to enable plain knit fabrics to deform around body shapes such as in a nylon stocking fitting the shape of a leg or in tights enclosing the lower body. Rib structures, because of alternate groups of columns of stitches pulled to the face or the back, (such as two towards the face, then two to the back as in 2 × 2 rib), become corrugated with the corrugation lines running vertically up the fabric and are therefore much more extensible. However, neither plain-knitted nor weft-knitted rib structures are as extensible as the warp-knitted power nets which are particularly designed to extend and exert pressure then return completely to their original shape following each extension; power nets use elastomeric yarns in their structures to produce that effect. Even so, plain-knitted fabrics do recover reasonably well from extension if they are made from a material which itself behaves elastically towards low extensions (e.g., nylon). There will be complete return to the relaxed loop shape illustrated

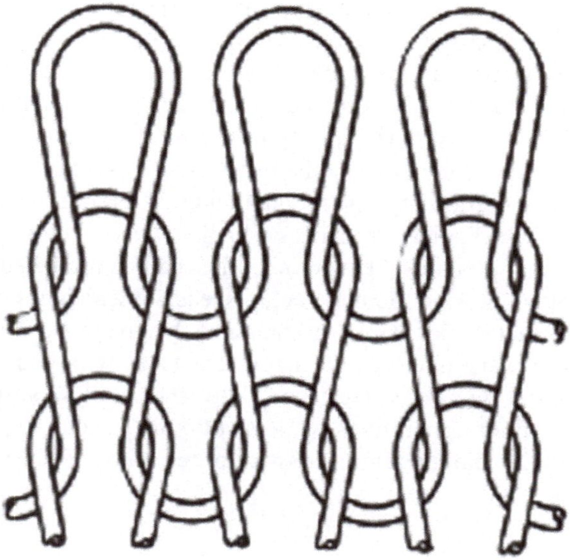

FIGURE 3.12 Plain knit/stocking stitch (*Textile Terms and Definitions* 2021; courtesy The Textile Institute).

in Figure 3.12 (and the associated fabric dimensions) on tumble drying after laundering because the agitation from a full laundry cycle brings about return of the knitted loops to positions consistent with their lowest energy state. Fortunately, in the case of wool, complete return to the relaxed loop shape takes place simply on wetting, so there is no need for the agitation, but the price to pay is that it needs to be dried flat, because the wool fibres, which easily deform when wet, will otherwise become extended.

Extensibility is a key characteristic of a knitted fabric, but the same property gives rise to its poor dimensional stability, so the sizing of a knitted article is best carried out with the plain-knitted fabric in the relaxed state. Such care is necessary most particularly in garment applications intended to exert a certain amount of pressure on part of the wearer's limb, because the relaxed state yields the size to which the item will return to after each laundering cycle. For plain-knitted wool fabrics, for example, the state of the fabric can be checked by measuring the ratio of courses to wales (the ratio should be close to 1.3 to 1 when the fabric is in the relaxed state; Munden 1959). Weft-knitted fabrics have been shown to be able to provide and sustain high levels of compression and support (Harper et al. 2010; Mikučionienė et al. 2010) and their extensibility has enabled various knitted meshes to be used for the treatment of hernias, pelvic organ prolapse, and body-wall defects. Moreover, just as is the case for weaving and warp-knitting, fabrics with two parallel faces joined by connecting threads (spacer fabrics) can be prepared by weft knitting. In addition, because of the positive effects of the open arrangement of threads in implanted weft-knitted structures on cell growth, they are being utilised as scaffolds for supporting tissue regeneration (Gokarneshan and Velumani 2018)

3.6.2.2 Warp-Knitted Fabrics

Warp-knitted fabrics are produced from a set of warp yarns that are knitted parallel to each other down the length of the fabric. Each new row of loops is drawn through the previous row of loops in the fabric such that the yarns run vertically while linking to the adjacent yarn so that each loop in the horizontal direction is made from a different thread. Some of these structures produce fabrics that are both extensible and elastic in the lengthwise direction and offer better flexibility and elasticity than that of a weft-knitted structure (Anand 2003).

The example shown in Figure 3.13 is a typical example of an Atlas fabric. The characteristic of this type of warp-knitted fabric is that one set of threads traverses in a diagonal manner, moving across a single step to the next vertical row of loops (a vertical row of loops is a wale) for every horizontal row (a horizontal row is a course) for a number of courses, then returning in the same manner to the original wale. Overall, as is the common feature of warp-knitted fabrics, the yarn path is in a vertical direction. Given the zig-zag path followed by each yarn in the Atlas fabric shown in Figure 3.13, its lengthwise extensibility will be greater the wider the diagonal traverse. Three-dimensional warp-knitted structures can be created by warp knitting that are like sandwich constructions. These spacer fabrics consist of two surface layers connected with resilient yarns whose purpose is to create and maintain the desired distance between the two layers and are similar in that respect

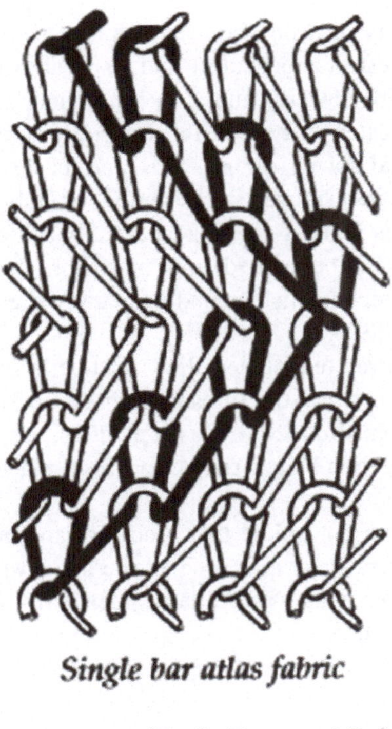

FIGURE 3.13 Warp-knitted structure (*Textile Terms and Definitions* 2021; courtesy The Textile Institute).

to spacer fabrics produced by weaving or by weft knitting. The 3D spacer-fabric structure can exhibit high porosity and allow for significant moisture transmission away from the contact layer, while also demonstrating high air permeability. The fabric is comparatively lightweight because of the open space between the layers and different materials can be used in the two layers to create different characteristics on each side of the fabric (Chen et al. 2015). In the healthcare sector, spacer fabrics are used to create artificial vessels, innovative compression bandages, and for pressure-sore management (Gokarneshan and Velumani 2018; Renkens and Kyosev 2011; Harpa et al. 2010).

3.6.3 Non-woven Fabrics

The preparation of non-woven fabrics does not require the fibres or filaments to be spun into yarns, or assembled into a fabric yarn -by yarn, as is necessary with weaving or knitting operations. When short staple fibres are being made into a non-woven fabric, it uses only the high-volume, early-stage fibre-handling processes. The first are the operations involved in opening out the tufts of fibre, then consolidating these into a thick roll of even thickness (a lap) before separating the individual fibres from one another and recombining them into the form of a web. Production of the fabric simply becomes one of layering the required number of webs together to form a sandwich of the desired thickness, then applying some method of holding them in place. The capacity therefore exists for very high production rates for non-woven fabrics and the possibility of using those fabrics to generate low-cost garments. A considerable marketing effort about safety and disposability was directed primarily at the user from the 1970s onwards and, as a consequence, non-woven fabrics have been adopted and used extensively in healthcare settings for many years in disposable PPE such as surgical gowns, drapes, caps, and masks (Rigby et al. 1997). The way in which the fibres are arranged in the non-woven fabric affects both pore size and capillary dimensions (Das et al. 2012), hence, because a wide variety of non-woven fabric structures can be created from most fibre types, they have also been widely used in the more technically demanding fields of dressings, hygiene products, and filters (Rigby et al. 1997).

By definition, non-woven techniques allow for textile fibre webs to be prepared and then assembled into layered structures wherein several layers are bonded to create a fabric (The Textile Institute 2021; Das et al. 2012), a step which can be carried out at high rates of production by a variety of processes including:

(i) wet laying, a system not unlike that used for papermaking but for longer fibres, is used to produce wipes such as eye pads, wound wipes, cleaning wipes, and surgical gowns (Ajmeri and Ajmeri 2016, 227–256);
(ii) air layering uses a current of air to disperse fibres and transport them to a perforated collection screen resulting in a soft voluminous structure, often used to produce wipes (Ajmeri and Ajmeri 2016, 227–256);
(iii) needle punching, where beds of hooked needles drive the needles through the web layers from both sides of the fabric being formed, with the hooks catching fibres and carrying them through to connect the layers together.

Needle punching has been used to produce absorbent dressing products and scaffolds for tissue engineering (Gao and Jin 2019; Kun and Chan 2018);

(iv) thermal bonding used to weld thermoplastic fibres together at their points of contact to produce materials suitable for sterile wraps and for fabrics used in compression management (Kumar 2016); and

(v) chemical bonding which has been used in the manufacture of medical masks and more recently in creating drug-encapsulated textile structures (Ajmeri and Ajmeri 2016, 227–256).

Alternatively, the fabric can be produced directly as a web utilising polymer extrusion methods, thereby eliminating the requirement for opening and rearranging fibres into webs as was required for staple fibres:

(i) melt-blowing (Gupta and Edwards 2018). The still-molten, just-forming filaments emerging from the spinneret meet a strong current of hot air pulling them away to create extremely fine fibres; such melt-blown webs are used as the centre layer to provide the high filtration performance required in surgical masks.

(ii) creation of flash-spun self-bonded microfibre (4 μm) webs (Weinberg et al. 2009) widely used as a medical and pharmaceutical sterile packaging covering material (Venugopal et al. 2019). The volatile solvent in which the polymer is dissolved is caused to evaporate very rapidly from the emerging extruded film causing its fibrillation into fine microfibres, both entangled and stuck together. One such product, used for both packaging and protective apparel and composed of high-density polyethylene (HDPE; see Chapter 4, Section 4.6.2) is Tyvek®, DuPont de Nemours Inc., Wilmington, DE, USA (Dupont 2017). The product is regarded as recyclable and when used in the form of protective apparel in the USA, the company offers a recycling service which it considers makes their disposable product a viable competitor by taking away the overall cost advantage of reusables and their associated decontamination and sterilisation by laundry services.

(iii) electrospinning for the preparation of nanofibre webs (Mokhtari et al. 2016), which have been used not only in burns and wound management (Lukanina et al. 2017), but also for filtration and as components to incorporate as one of the central layers in surgical masks.

(iv) spunbond (or spunlaid) methods (for creating webs from very long filaments; Rigby et al. 1997), used as the cover stock (outer covering) for absorbent sanitary pads (Ajmeri and Ajmeri 2016, 227–256).

(v) hydro-entanglement (or spunlace). One of the features which makes non-woven fabric manufacture so versatile is that variations in the composition of the non-woven can be made by combining layers of webs of different fibre types together. Often, this is necessary in order to take full advantage of the particular properties of certain types of web especially those where the constituent fibres or filaments are extremely fine and need support, such as for melt-blown webs and nanofibre webs, neither of which demonstrate sufficient cohesion between fibres to enable them to act as a

> self-supporting web structure. It is usually important to retain as many of the characteristics of each individual component web as possible to achieve the desired performance from the combination, so the method used to bond the layers together should not be clumsy. One method which has the right kind of characteristics to deal with a mix of fine fibre web (for its filtration abilities) and more substantial fibre web (to offer structural support) is hydro-entanglement, where high-pressure water jets directed at the layered-web arrangement supported on a perforated screen (the support surface) are used to drive fibres through to connect the layers together. As is the case for needle punching, it yields the best results if the jets are directed at the webs from both sides. The design of the support screen can be used to give a pattern to the fabric, a little like the appearance of woven fabrics designs.

Many non-woven fabrics are made for items intended for single-use items only, an approach which may be considered wasteful and gives rise to environmental concerns. However, it is encouraging to see that semi-durable non-woven items of easy-care hospital and care-home bed linen are available. One example is that of wipeable pillows with a polypropylene non-woven outer filled with polyester, which can be further protected by a thicker waterproof (wipeable but not launderable) non-woven polypropylene pillowcase (Interweave Textiles 2018). Another is a launderable non-woven composite with a super-absorbent fibre internal layer which maintains a high proportion of its original absorbency (80%) after 40 washes, an innovation which represents a major step forward not only in terms of patient care but also for the environment (SAF™ 2021). Researchers and manufacturers of non-woven fabrics would do well to learn from this particular example and focus on ensuring that in future their products are (preferably) durable to laundering (at least 50 cycles), or recyclable, or, if they must be disposable, that the constituents are biodegradable or at least compostable. This is a big challenge not only to those who have up until now focused on fuelling and profiting from the disposable trend in medical textiles, but also for those responsible for their specification and procurement (but not necessarily for the funding of the disposable habit). There are four options spelt out here in descending order of preference:

(i) durable reusable
(ii) recyclable
(iii) biodegradable
(iv) compostable

where even option (iv) would constitute improvement over many current products which still need to be sent after just a single use for incineration or landfill.

3.6.4 Braids

3.6.4.1 Types of Braid

A braid (or plait) is a narrow fabric made by interlacing three or more threads diagonally to create flat, tubular, or solid constructions (*Textile Terms and Definitions* 2021;

Kyosev 2014; Alagirusamy and Padaki 2016). A variety of braid patterns can be created by changing how the strands are interlaced as shown in Figure 3.14.

Because in a braided fabric the yarns lie at an angle to the fabric's length, the braid is extensible in the lengthwise direction, just as a woven fabric is extensible in its bias direction. The essential braid geometry is shown in Figure 3.15 (Alagirusamy and Padaki 2016). A length of flat braid can extend or contract between substantially wide limits, while remaining essentially unstressed between these limits

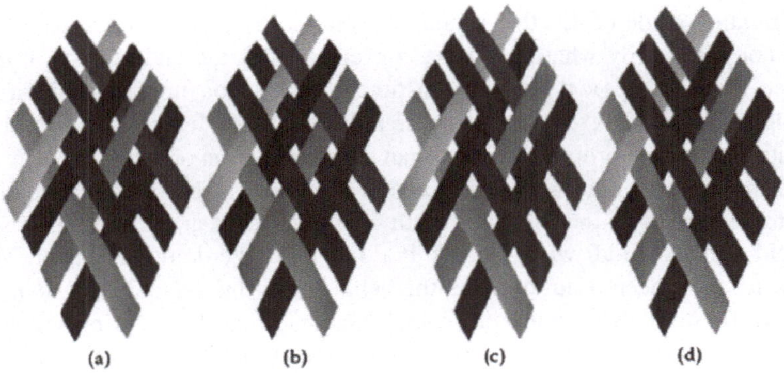

FIGURE 3.14 Braided structures: (a) Regular; (b) Diamond; (c) Basket; and (d) Hercules (Alagirusamy and Padaki 2016); reproduced by permission of Taylor & Francis.

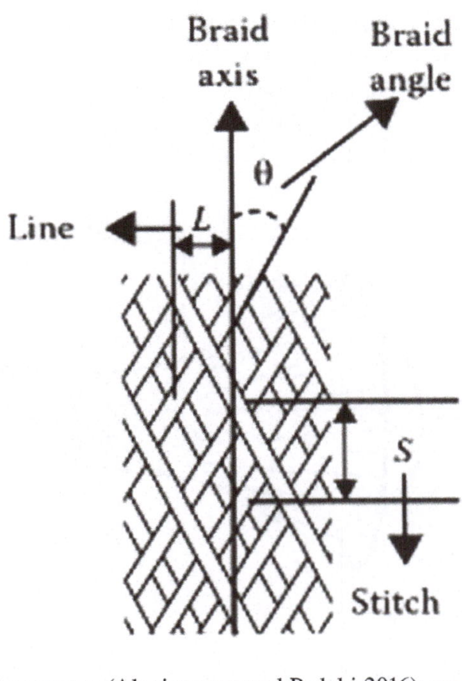

FIGURE 3.15 Braid geometry (Alagirusamy and Padaki 2016); reproduced by permission of Taylor & Francis.

(Brunnschweiler 1954) and typically will withstand a substantially greater tensile stress than one of its constituent threads (ca 1.5 times is not unusual).

3.6.4.2 Tubular Braids

Tubular braids are manufactured by braiding around a cylindrical/truncated conical rod which acts as the mandrel, as shown in Figure 3.16.

With a tubular braid for implant as a stent or embolisation, the tightness of packing of the braided yarns is a critical feature, and this can be maximised at a braiding angle of 45°, and for flat braids aimed at withstanding significant tension, it is at the same braiding angle of 45° that minimum extensibility can be achieved (although this is not necessarily what is wanted in every application and in some it may be intended to be up to 4× that of its constituent yarns). For tubular braids, a higher braiding angle provides greater resistance to kinking. The features of a braid which affect its mechanical properties, other than the composition of the yarns from which it is made, are the braid angle, the separation between the braided threads, and the compressibility of the threads (which expresses itself at high extensions when the braid tightens width wise), but the braid angle is the dominant factor. Various approaches have been used to model the behaviour of braids under tension, beginning with those of Brunnschweiler, which assumed that the braiding filaments or yarns were of circular cross section and maintained that profile, which most often they do not, but his work gave an approximation and has since provided a useful foundation for other modelling work (Brunnschweiler 1954). A number of approaches since then have successfully provided performance predictions that closely match those of actual braids under test conditions (Laurent et al. 2012; Rawal et al. 2015) and it has proved possible to include width-wise contraction for the braid under tension into the model (Saraswat et al. 2014). Because braids afford the opportunity to engineer tensile properties and include the desired degree of extensibility into the replacement structure, artificial ligaments/scaffolds have been modelled and made from multi-layered braided structures (Laurent et al. 2012; Rawal et al. 2015). The

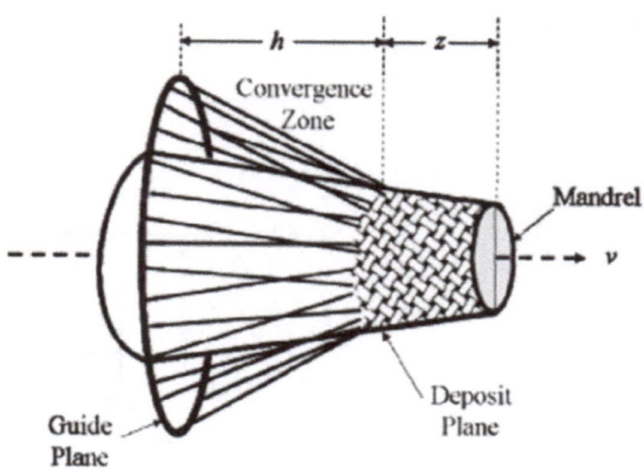

FIGURE 3.16 Tubular braid being created round a shaped mandrel (Rawal et al. 2015); image reproduced by permission of SAGE Publications.

load-bearing capacity of such scaffolds was found to be governed by the diameter of the fibres being braided and the number of layers of braid used in the scaffold, whereas the braid angle played a significant role in altering its stiffness. Braids can also be useful in other medical applications where the implant is expected to undergo repeated extension, but sutures (see Chapter 7, Section 7.2) and stents (Section 7.3) are the most common braided medical textiles. In the case of making braids suitable for stents, it is tubular braids that are sought, and these are manufactured by braiding around a cylindrical rod which acts as the mandrel, as shown in Figure 3.16. Alongside key structural features such as the braiding angle, the polymeric material used in a braided device is one of the numerous variables that affect the mechanical properties of the braid and include PET, polyamides, polypropylene, polytetrafluoroethylene and UHMWPE, biodegradable and absorbable polymers such as poly (l-lactic acid) or polyglycolide, and metal wires such as nitinol or stainless steel. The non-absorbable braids were, however, not without issues, such as bacterial proliferation aided by their surface structure, so inherently antibacterial (coated) polyamide braids have been developed (Debabi et al. 2017). For more sophisticated applications, drawn-filled-tubes or composite braids made by combining polymer filaments and wire can be used. A recent development is the incorporation of an ultrafine nichrome microwire bundle into a very fine tubular braid (100–200 μm across) using a purpose-built software operated micro-braiding machine. The braid pattern and structure is able to be precisely adjusted to meet requirements, in this case for the construction of a highly flexible, 24-channel, multi-electrode probe for electrophysiological neural recording and stimulation (Kim et al. 2019).

3.7 SUMMARY

Fibres, microfibres, and the more-recently added group, the nanofibres all have significant, complementary roles to play in medical textiles, and rather than new developments causing replacement of one for the other, at this level of organisation it is more a case of applications widening their use overall. In all cases, whether it is a filament, yarn, or fabric that is being utilised as a medical textile, flexibility is a key characteristic. Some useful fabric types such as spacer fabrics can be constructed by either weaving, weft knitting, or warp knitting, but typically the different fabric types do naturally possess quite different attractive attributes, all of which are able to be engineered and modelled to meet the demands of particular applications such as dimensional stability (woven fabrics), extensibility (knitted structures), and intermediate but controllable levels of extensibility (braided flat fabrics and tubular braided fabrics). The ease of adaptability of non-woven fabrics enables them to meet a wide range of requirements for absorption, protection, filtration, and technical performance in dressings.

Less impressive is the massive and growing contribution they make to waste by virtue of the focus on disposability. Researchers and manufacturers of non-woven fabrics would do well to change their focus and ensure that in future their products are preferably:

(i) durable to laundering (at least 50 cycles),
(ii) recyclable, or,

(iii) if the products must be disposable, that the constituents are biodegradable, or
(iv) if the products cannot be biodegradable, that they are at least safely compostable.

This is a big challenge not only to those who have up until now focused on fuelling and profiting from the disposable trend in medical textiles, but also for those responsible for their specification and procurement (but not necessarily for the funding of the disposable habit). There are four options spelt out here, each of which would bring about at least some improvement compared to current products. If manufacturers show themselves unwilling to make any such moves, it would be for governments and product procurement agencies to show their commitment to reducing the environmental burden and to take the initiative for them.

Nanofibres for medical-textile applications continue to generate substantial interest, and newer applications ranging from modification of core-spun yarn surface characteristics to improve moisture management, through to nano-engineered hollow or porous nanofibres for controlled drug release continue to be explored. The development of implantable medical textiles has often been ignored trying to match the characteristics of the environment into which the implant is going or the biological structure that it is intended to replace. It is reassuring, therefore, to see that specific ranges of micropore size have been identified which work best in tissue engineering; they vary across different tissue types and can be matched in advance by suitable adjustment of the means of nanofibre formation and assembly. Details about how nanofibres are made and how they may be modified, collected, and constructed into fabrics to fit a particular purpose, therefore, remain of particular topical importance, as does the miniaturisation of fabric construction methods to handle the matter of precise control over the conversion of nanoyarns into nanofabrics. Miniaturisation of a robotic weaving device yielding success with weaving a tubular woven stent from nanofibres which fits within a capillary tube (0.5 mm) and miniature computer-controlled braiding machine braiding with its 24-channel probe for electrophysiological recording at just the width of a human hair (100 μm) are early examples. These are exciting achievements, but perhaps it should not be a surprise that such micro-fabrics have been achieved by fabric construction methods which rely primarily on changing yarn positions such as in the interlacing yarns (weaving) or intertwining (braiding), rather than those which require significant deformation of the yarn to achieve loop formation (knitting).

REFERENCES

Ahn, Sam S. "Method of making a drug delivery system using hollow fibers." U.S. Patent 5,538,735, issued July 23, 1996.

Ajmeri, J. R., and C. J. Ajmeri. "Developments in nonwoven materials for medical applications." In *Advances in Technical Nonwovens*, edited by G. Kellie, 227–256. Cambridge, UK: Woodhead Publishing, 2016.

Alagirusamy, R., and N. V. Padaki. "An introduction to braiding." In *Braided Structures and Composites: Production, Properties, Mechanics, and Technical Applications*, edited by Rana Sohel, and Raul Fangueiro, Vol. 3. Boca Raton, FL: CRC Press, 2016.

Anand, S. "Spacers-at the technical frontier." *Knitting International* 110, no. 130 (2003): 38–41.

Anton, Formhals. "Process and apparatus for preparing artificial threads." U.S. Patent 1,975,504 issued October 2, 1934.

Bilisik, Kadir. "Multiaxis three dimensional (3D) woven fabric." In *Advances in Modern Woven Fabrics Technology*, edited by S. Vassiliadis, 79–106. London, UK: IntechOpen, 2011.

Brunnschweiler, D. "5—The structure and tensile properties of braids." *Journal of the Textile Institute Transactions* 45, no. 1 (1954): T55–T77.

Buzol Mülayim, Beyza, and Fatma Göktepe. "Analysis of polyacrylonitrile nanofiber yarn formation in electrospinning by using a conical collector and two oppositely charged nozzles." *The Journal of the Textile Institute* 112, no. 3 (2021): 494–504.

Chen, Si, Hai-ru Long, Ying-hao Liu, and Feng-chao Hu. "Mechanical properties of 3D-structure composites based on warp-knitted spacer fabrics." *Autex Research Journal* 15, no. 2 (2015): 127–137.

Cooley, John F. "Apparatus for electrically dispersing fluids." U.S. Patent 692,631 issued February 4, 1902.

Das, Dipayan, Arun Kumar Pradhan, R. Chattopadhyay, and S. N. Singh. "Composite nonwovens." *Textile Progress* 44, no. 1 (2012): 1–84.

Debbabi, Faten, Sondes Gargoubi, Mohamed Adnene Hadj Ayed, and Saber Ben Abdessalem. "Development and characterization of antibacterial braided polyamide suture coated with chitosan-citric acid biopolymer." *Journal of Biomaterials Applications* 32, no. 3 (2017): 384–398.

Dupont. "Technical reference guide for DuPont™ Transition Tyvek® 1073B, Transition Tyvek® 1059B and Tyvek® 2FS™—metric units." 2017. Accessed June 3, 2021. https://www.dupont.co.uk/knowledge/transition-tyvek-technical-reference-guide-metric-english.html.

Eriksson, Siw, and Leif Sandsjö. "Three-dimensional fabrics as medical textiles." In *Advances in 3D Textiles*, edited by Chen, X. 305–340. Cambridge, UK: Woodhead Publishing, 2015.

Gao, Yingjun, and Xiangyu Jin. "Needle-punched three-dimensional nonwoven wound dressings with density gradient from biocompatible calcium alginate fiber." *Textile Research Journal* 89, no. 14 (2019): 2776–2788.

Gokarneshan, N., and R. Alagirusamy. "Weaving of 3D fabrics: A critical appreciation of the developments." *Textile Progress* 41, no. 1 (2009): 1–58.

Gokarneshan, N., and K. Velumani. "Some significant advances in spacer fabric technology for newer areas of applications." *Journal of Textile Science and Engineering* 8, no. 339 (2018): 2.

Gupta, B. S., and J. V. Edwards. "Textile materials and structures for topical management of wounds." In *Advanced Textiles for Wound Care*, edited by S. Rajendran, 55–104. Oxford, UK: Elsevier/Woodhead Publishing, 2018.

Harpa, Rodica, Cristina Piroi, and Cezar Doru Radu. "A new approach for testing medical stockings." *Textile Research Journal* 80, no. 8 (2010): 683–695.

Interweave Textiles. "Interweave healthcare pillow protectors." 2018. Accessed March 6, 2021. https://www.interweavetextiles.com/wp-content/uploads/2018/09/pillow-protectors.pdf.

Janik, Helena, and Michalina Marzec. "A review: Fabrication of porous polyurethane scaffolds." *Materials Science and Engineering: C* 48 (2015): 586–591.

Joseph, John, Aarya G. Krishnan, Aleena M. Cherian, Balasubramoniam Rajagopalan, Rajesh Jose, Praveen Varma, Vijayakumar Maniyal, Sivanarayanan Balakrishnan, Shantikumar V. Nair, and Deepthy Menon. "Transforming nanofibers into woven nanotextiles for vascular application." *ACS Applied Materials and Interfaces* 10, no. 23 (2018): 19449–19458.

Kim, Taegyo, Kendall Schmidt, Christopher Deemie, Joanna Wycech, Hualou Liang, and Simon F. Giszter. "Highly flexible precisely braided multielectrode probes and combinatorics for future neuroprostheses." *Frontiers in Neuroscience* 13 (2019): 613.

Kumar, Bipin. "Nonwoven padding for compression management." In *Non-woven Fabrics*, edited by Han-Yong Jeon. London, UK: IntechOpen, 2016.

Kun, M., C. Chan, S. Ramakrishna, Abhilash Kulkarni, and Ketankumar Vadodaria. "Textile-based scaffolds for tissue engineering." In *Advanced Textiles for Wound Care*, edited by 329–362. Oxford, UK: Elsevier/Woodhead Publishing; Textile Institute Book Series 2018.

Kyosev, Yordan. *Braiding Technology for Textiles: Principles, Design, and Processes.* Cambridge, UK: Elsevier, 2014.

Laurent, Cédric P., Damien Durville, Didier Mainard, Jean-François Ganghoffer, and Rachid Rahouadj. "A multilayer braided scaffold for anterior cruciate ligament: Mechanical modeling at the fiber scale." *Journal of the Mechanical Behavior of Biomedical Materials* 12 (2012): 184–196.

Lee, Jung Bok, Sung In Jeong, Min Soo Bae, Dae Hyeok Yang, Dong Nyoung Heo, Chun Ho Kim, Eben Alsberg, and Il Keun Kwon. "Highly porous electrospun nanofibers enhanced by ultrasonication for improved cellular infiltration." *Tissue Engineering Part A* 17, no. 21–22 (2011): 2695–2702.

Lukanina, K. I., T. E. Grigor'ev, T. Kh Tenchurin, A. D. Shepelev, and S. N. Chvalun. "Nonwoven materials produced by electrospinning for modern medical technologies." *Fibre Chemistry* 49, no. 3 (2017): 205–216.

Mao, Ning, Hui Peng, Xiaohong Qin, and Jianyong Yu. "Contact force within electrospun nanofiber core-spun yarns and moisture management ability of their fabrics." *The Journal of The Textile Institute* (2021), published online 6 January 2021.. doi: 10.1080/00405000.2020.1869440.

Mikučionienė, Daiva, Ričardas Čiukas, and Agnė Mickevičienė. "The influence of knitting structure on mechanical properties of weft knitted fabrics." *Materials Science (Medžiagotyra)* 16, no. 3 (2010): 221–225.

Miller, Mark D., Stephen R. Thompson, and Jennifer Hart. *Review of Orthopaedics E-Book.* Amsterdam, Holland: Elsevier Health Sciences, 2012.

Mokhtari, F., M. Salehi, F. Zamani, F. Hajiani, F. Zeighami, and M. Latifi. "Advances in electrospinning: The production and application of nanofibres and nanofibrous structures." *Textile Progress* 48, no. 3 (2016): 119–219.

Müller, Georg F. J., Markus Stürzel, and Rolf Mülhaupt. "Core/shell and hollow ultra high molecular weight polyethylene nanofibers and nanoporous polyethylene prepared by mesoscopic shape replication catalysis." *Advanced Functional Materials* 24, no. 19 (2014): 2860–2864.

Munden, D. L. "26—The geometry and dimensional properties of plain-knit fabrics." *Journal of the Textile Institute Transactions* 50, no. 7 (1959): T448–T471.

Rawal, Amit, Harshvardhan Saraswat, and Apurv Sibal. "Tensile response of braided structures: A review." *Textile Research Journal* 85, no. 19 (2015): 2083–2096.

Renkens, Wilfried, and Yordan Kyosev. "Geometry modelling of warp knitted fabrics with 3D form." *Textile Research Journal* 81, no. 4 (2011): 437–443.

Rigby, A. J., S. C. Anand, and A. R. Horrocks. "Textile materials for medical and healthcare applications." *Journal of the Textile Institute* 88, no. 3 (1997): 83–93.

SAF™. "SAF™ washable superabsorbent fabrics." 2021. Accessed March 12, 2021. https://exploresaf.com/applications/hygiene.

Saraswat, Harshvardhan, Amit Rawal, and Rajendra Singh. "Tensile behaviour of multi-layered braided structures." *Journal of Materials Science* 49, no. 18 (2014): 6427–6436.

Seyam, Abdelfattah, and Aly El-Shiekh. "Mechanics of woven fabrics: Part III: Critical review of weavability limit studies." *Textile Research Journal* 63, no. 7 (1993): 371–378.

Seyam, Abdelfattah, and Aly El-Shiekh. "Mechanics of woven fabrics: Part IV: Critical review of fabric degree of tightness and its applications." *Textile Research Journal* 64, no. 11 (1994): 653–662.

Shi, Wanhui, Gaoyi Han, Yunzhen Chang, Hua Song, Wenjing Hou, and Qi Chen. "Using stretchable PPy@ PVA composites as a high-sensitivity strain sensor to monitor minute motion." *ACS Applied Materials and Interfaces* 12, no. 40 (2020): 45373–45382.

Shuakat, Muhammad Nadeem, and Tong Lin. "Direct electrospinning of nanofibre yarns using a rotating ring collector." *The Journal of the Textile Institute* 107, no. 6 (2016): 791–799.

Sill, Travis J., and Horst A. Von Recum. "Electrospinning: Applications in drug delivery and tissue engineering." *Biomaterials* 29, no. 13 (2008): 1989–2006.

Sosa, Joshua D., Timothy F. Bennett, Katherine J. Nelms, Brandon M. Liu, Roberto C. Tovar, and Yangyang Liu. "Metal–organic framework hybrid materials and their applications." *Crystals* 8, no. 8 (2018): 325.

Taylor, Geoffrey Ingram. "Electrically driven jets." *Proceedings of the Royal Society of London. A. Mathematical and Physical Sciences* 313, no. 1515 (1969): 453–475.

The Textile Institute. *Textile Terms and Definitions* (11th ed.). Edited by M. J. Denton, and P. N. Daniels. . The Textile Institute, 2021. https://www.ttandd.org/content/textile-terms-and-definitions.

Venugopal, Arun Prasad, Nicolas Bernhard, Thomas Hofbauer, and Klaus-dietmar Wagner. "Nonwoven sterile packaging." U.S. Patent Application 16/244,114, filed July 11, 2019.

Wang, Lijing, ed. *Performance Testing of Textiles: Methods, Technology and Applications*. Cambridge, UK: Woodhead Publishing, 2016.

Weinberg, Mark Gary, Gregory T. Dee, and Thomas William Harding. "Flash spun web containing sub-micron filaments and process for forming same." U.S. Patent Application 12/486,157, filed October 8, 2009.

Wu, Shaohua, Yue Zhang, Penghong Liu, and Xiaohong Qin. "Polyacrylonitrile nanofiber yarns and fabrics produced using a novel electrospinning method combined with traditional textile techniques." *Textile Research Journal* 86, no. 16 (2016): 1716–1727.

Zhu, Lei, Bilal Zaarour, and Xiangyu Jin. "Direct generation of electrospun interconnected macroporous nanofibers using a water bath as a collector." *Materials Research Express* 7, no. 1 (2020): 015082.

4 Fibre Types and the Polymers Used in Medical Textiles

4.1 INTRODUCTION

The hierarchical classification of textile fibres first places fibres into two groups, the natural fibres and the man-made fibres (The Textile Institute 2021).

The natural fibres are then placed into one of three groups:

(i) animal (protein fibres)
(ii) vegetable (cellulose fibres)
(iii) mineral (asbestos)

Man-made fibres are also placed into three groups (common representative types in each group are given in brackets):

(i) natural polymer (cellulose, cellulose ester, protein, alginate, and rubber)
(ii) synthetic polymer (polyamide, polyester, polyvinyl derivatives, polypropylene, polyethylene, aramid, polyurethane, and polyisoprene)
(iii) other (glass, metal, carbon, and ceramic)

Whilst the fibre types and polymers used in medical textiles will be discussed in a sequence broadly following the above groupings, it is worth noting that interest is being shown in the possibility of using natural fibre composites more widely because of their low environmental impact, but not much is happening on that as yet in the medical textiles area (Pickering, Efendy, and Le 2016).

4.2 NATURAL FIBRES AND FILAMENTS

4.2.1 Animal-Based: Protein Fibres

4.2.1.1 Wool

Wool fibres form the fleece that is there to protect sheep from the extremes of heat, cold, and rain. Wool and animal hairs are of similar composition; they are all keratin fibres with two distinct components:

- overlapping tile-shaped cuticular cells on the fibre surface
- long, thin cortical cells arranged lengthwise along the middle of the fibre

DOI: 10.1201/9781003170570-4

Whilst the keratin in the cortical cells contains a substantial proportion of the fibre's cysteine, each of the outer layers of the cuticular cells contains progressively more and more, and being composed of very highly cross-linked protein, the cuticular cells are therefore both physically hard and resist water penetration (Dobb, Murray, and Sikorski 1972). The cortex of the fibre in both cases is composed of the protein keratin which is typified by long helical protein chains cross-linked at regular intervals through the disulfide bonds from the amino acid cysteine. The helical protein chains confer on wool its substantial extensibility, especially when wet, and the regular cross-linkages from cysteine assist it to return to its original dimensions, again especially when wet; see, for example, the CSIRO summary of wool structure (CSIRO 2015).

Keratin can be extracted from natural sources and regenerated in the form of films, sponges, and hydrogels (Patrucco et al. 2016) and it improves the production of anti-inflammatory cytokines and decreases the quantity of pro-inflammatory cytokines (Fearing and Van Dyke 2014). Its high cystine content differentiates keratin from other structural proteins such as collagen and elastin and this influences its mechanical and chemical properties due to the inter- and intra-chain cross-links formed by the cystine disulphide bonds which give rise to a higher stability and lower solubility. The presence of ionic bonds is pH-dependent and is greatest at the isoelectric point of pH 4.9 (Shavandi et al. 2017). Keratin extracted from wool fibres can be used as scaffolding for fibroblasts and osteoblasts due to its inherent ability to facilitate cell adhesion, proliferation, and regeneration (Tachibana et al. 2002). Indeed, sheep wool has been used to prepare keratin microfibril sponges used in scaffolding (Tachibana et al. 2005; Shavandi et al. 2017). One of the key properties of the scaffolds is that the sponges demonstrated highly interconnected porosity and contain intrinsic sites of cellular regeneration that mimic the extracellular matrix (Patrucco et al. 2016).

Modification of wool fabrics with zinc oxide nanoparticles increases the UV light absorbance compared to untreated wool (Jiang, Jiang, and Cai 2018). Studies have shown that modification with graphene/titanium dioxide nanocomposites produce a fabric with antibacterial properties towards both *Staphylococcus aureus* (*S. aureus*) and *Escherichia Coli* (*E. coli*) (Shirgholami, Loghman, and Mirjalili 2016); a similar treatment is also effective on cotton fabrics (Derakhshan et al. 2018). Given the advent of antibiotic-resistant bacteria, the potential to develop dressings that outsmart resistant bacteria is particularly attractive and work undertaken by Laing's team demonstrated that socks composed primarily of wool can positively affect observable measures of skin health. In addition, merino wool socks maintained their energy-absorbing properties better than cotton socks suggesting that they may be beneficial in individuals requiring cushioned socks (Van Amber et al. 2019). This has many potential applications throughout the clinical and consumer healthcare market and is not a new concept; using animal hair in clothing began a comfort/hygiene trend in the late 1800s, particularly with the idea of moving away from the more extremely restrictive women's fashion garments of the time (Jaeger 2019).

4.2.1.2 Silk

Silk fibroin in continuous-filament form is derived from the cocoons formed by *Bombyx mori* moth grubs, with a single cocoon yielding 600–1500 m of silk. Such cultivated silk has been used as a suture material for centuries (Mackenzie 1973); for silk to be a success in this application, the filaments are often coated in wax to prevent fraying and to avoid invoking an immune response to any residual sericin. Sericin consists of warm-water-soluble glycoproteins that surround the core of two fibroin filaments as it is being spun by the silkworm (Altman et al. 2003; Chandrasekar, Sivakumar, and Kumar 2017). Typically though, cultivated silk demonstrates biocompatibility, can exhibit controllable degradation, and can be chemically modified to alter its surface properties or to immobilise growth factors (Rockwood et al. 2011). The core filament protein, fibroin, consists mainly of the amino acids glycine, alanine, and serine linked together, enabling it to adopt a highly crystalline structure in the form of β-pleated sheets of the protein chains and yields attractive mechanical properties for medical textiles. These include its toughness, with a breaking energy of 6×10^4 J/kg (Shao and Vollrath 2002); tougher than Kevlar® at 338N (DuPont 2017), the strength-to-density ratio is up to ten times higher than that of steel. It also demonstrates a high ultimate tensile strength of 0.5 GPa (Shao and Vollrath 2002); by contrast, collagen has an ultimate tensile strength of 0.2–0.85 MPa (Svensson et al. 2010, 4020–4027). A disadvantage is that silk degrades with time, the rate affected by implantation site, mechanical environment, and the way in which silk is processed. As technology has progressed, however, the ability to produce recombinant silk and to engineer silk fibroin in the form of hydrogels, sponges, nanospheres, and scaffolds have seen the uses expand into the pharmaceuticals and regenerative medicine (Wang et al. 2010; Rnjak-Kovacina et al. 2015).

There are other types of silk including those produced by spiders (Kundu et al. 2013) and they possess different mechanical properties. The Hippocratic statement of '*vis medicatrix naturae*' (the healing power of items from nature) is well known though often disregarded (Aldini, Fini, and Giardino 2008), but natural textile-based products continue to be used in current times and the progression of technology has allowed for their careful engineering to our advantage; for example, the antimicrobial properties and structure of spider webs being used in nanotechnology (Cao et al. 2013). Several different types of silk are produced by the spider, two of which are the MA silk used to form the frame of the web plus the radial connections and the Flag silk (so-called because it is produced in the spider's flagellum) used for the 'capture spiral.' The MA silk has a structure wherein lengths of crystalline pleated sheets are linked together through amorphous hydrogel regions, yielding a strong and quite a stiff filament (but not as stiff as silk from *Bombyx mori*, whilst the Flag silk consists wholly of amorphous hydrogel and exhibits rubber-like extensibility and return of up to 300% (Römer and Scheibel 2008).

Spider silk fibres not only exhibit high extensibility but also strain-hardening (an increase in the stress required to bring about further extension as a fibre is extended within the plastic region beyond the yield point). Strain-hardening is important in energy-absorbing materials, hence this particular behaviour has proved to be attractive to those involved in regenerative medicine, particularly when designing implants for use in load-bearing tissue (Lewis 1996).

The SERI Surgical Scaffold (Sofregen Inc, Framingham, MA, USA), a silk-based surgical mesh, is used in abdominal wall reconstruction and plastic surgery applications in the USA. There is published data available reporting the clinical use but no long-term data is currently available and some of the published data could not be considered to be independent (Holland et al. 2019). Externally, silk is gaining increasing interest as a hydrogel for wound dressing. It can also be sterilised; different methods cause changes in functional and mechanical properties (Siritientong, Srichana, and Aramwit 2011). Silk is already used in clothing to treat dermatological conditions including atopic dermatitis and acne vulgaris; the long, smooth filaments/few fibres ends in the fabrics made from the filament yarns minimising mechanical irritation of the skin. Processing of the silk has allowed for chemical modification and finishing treatments to achieve antibacterial properties (Holland et al. 2019).

4.2.2 Plant-Based: Cellulose Fibres

4.2.2.1 Cotton

Cotton fibre grows on the seed of a variety of plants of the genus *Gossypium* (van der Sluijs and Hunter 2016) and 95% of the world's cotton is from *G. hirsutum*, which originated in Central America. However, over two-thirds of the world's cotton grown today is genetically modified (GM) cotton, containing genes from the bacterium *B. thuringiensis*, aimed to act as an insecticide (Bt cotton) and/or genes that confer herbicide tolerance (Tausif et al. 2019). Cotton fibre is traded in more than 150 countries with around 270 million farmers living by growing cotton (Rana et al. 2015, 195–216). A natural cellulose fibre, it has 1,4-D-glucopyranose as its repeating unit along the polymer chain, a chemical structure which offers the opportunity for its polymer chains to become firmly hydrogen-bonded to one another so that some crystalline regions are formed and for moisture absorption to take place in the less well-ordered regions. Fibre length varies from approximately 10–65 mm with a diameter from 11 to 22 μm and those fibres with a length greater than 12 mm can be used in the production of non-wovens.

Cotton has a wide variety of applications given the comfort derived from the permeability of its fabrics, a property derived mainly from its twisted, hollow fibres and cotton's ability to withstand sterilisation/high temperature laundering and bleaching. Taken together, this means that within the healthcare sector, cotton is widely used in bed linen, gowns and uniforms as well as for more specialist purposes, such as baby diapers, feminine hygiene products, and nursing pads (Rupp 2009). One of the key properties of scoured and bleached cotton is its hydrophilic nature which enables fluid-absorbent textiles to be produced; care, therefore, needs to be taken in healthcare applications as it may serve as a nutrient reservoir for microbes. Contaminated fibre fragments can be lost from soiled garments into the surrounding air due to fibrillation of the cotton fibres during wear (a problem it shares with other types of cellulose fibres and filaments, and particularly with lyocell unless it has been treated to prevent such loss) (Mortimer and Péguy 1996). In attempts to counteract the contamination problem, there has been work directed towards the manufacture of antimicrobial cotton fabrics and, in particular, a focus on the production of cotton finishes with silver nanoparticles; a variety of manufacturing processes have been utilised for their application including impregnation (Zhang et al. 2009) and sonochemical deposition (Perelshtein et al. 2008). Excellent antimicrobial activity against *Escherichia coli* in vitro trials was exhibited and the inclusion of silver nanoparticles into cotton fibres improved thermal stability, which may be beneficial in the sterilisation process (Ravindra et al. 2010). Finishing cotton with nanocomposites of zinc oxide can produce a fabric that displays enhanced protection against ultraviolet light in addition to antimicrobial properties against *Staphylococcus aureus* and *Klebsiella pneumoniae* (*K. pneumoniae*) (Nadanathangam et al. 2006).

4.2.2.2 Other Cellulose Fibres: Kapok, Hemp, Flax, Sisal, Manila

Other cellulose fibres include *kapok*, a typical cellulosic fibre with a round microtube shape with smooth surface and a thin wall. The diameter is approximately 10 µm and length around 1.6 cm (Purnawati et al. 2018). It is the least dense natural fibre exhibiting lipophilic properties by virtue of a waxy cutin on the fibre surface and resistance to wetting (Mani, Rayappan, and Bisoyi 2012; Zheng et al. 2015). Conventionally, kapok has been used as stuffing for bedding and upholstery as well as for insulation against sound and heat because of its air-filled lumen (Zheng et al. 2015). It is a brittle fibre with low inter-fibre cohesion and strength and as such, cannot easily be spun like cotton fibre, although it has been successfully blended with cotton fibre to form yarns, reducing the tenacity but providing an increase in extensibility. There are few areas of general application for the fibre in medical textiles, but it is worth mentioning because kapok can be used to engineer microtubes on a large scale; essentially the kapok forms a hollow, removable form around which a synthetic polymer may be cast; experiments showed that the surface morphology and wall thickness of the microtubes were easily modulated by controlling processing conditions (Zhang et al. 2010). Coated with polyaniline, the kapok can be removed by treatment with NaOH solution to leave polyaniline microtubes suitable for use as supercapacitors, the energy-storage components in Smart Textiles (Xu et al. 2016b; Abu-thabit and Makhlouf 2016), see Chapter 11. In regenerative medicine, the ability to create a microtubule structure may be of benefit for those requiring scaffolds for cell growth. Silver nanoparticles can be combined with the fibre with good antibacterial performance in in vitro trials (Wang et al. 2015).

Flax, historically a widely utilised bast fibre derived from the stems of *Linum usitatissimum*, has been found in graves in Egypt dating back to 5000 BCE (Jones et al. 2018) and until recently was a significant fibre type across the whole of Europe, used mainly in the form of linen fabrics. Still grown in significant amounts in Eastern Europe, the growing cycle of flax is short, with just 100 days between sowing and harvesting in the Western European region (Yan, Chouw, and Jayaraman 2014). The flax fibres, produced as one of the structural components of the stems of the flax plant, are composed of cellulose in a structure that is more crystalline than that in cotton, which makes the fibres stiffer and more rigid. The fibres are extracted by partial rotting to enable removal of the outer parts of the plant stems followed by opening out and cleaning of the fibres of the stem so their structure is complex with several concentric cylinders of cells and layers of cellulose microfibrils of various lengths (Yan, Chouw, and Jayaraman 2014). Flax fibres demonstrate a non-linear stress strain curve with a transition point to a lower tangent modulus at strains between 0.3 and 0.5%. This is due to several phenomena including plastic yielding of some components of the elementary fibres, shear yielding of the bonding layer between them, and reorientation of the elementary fibres. The stiffness of flax compares well with that of glass, 55–75 GPa compared to 70–74 GPa for glass. It has a tensile strength greater than jute, at 800–1500 MPa, and also demonstrates hydrophilic properties, though such moisture absorption affects mechanical properties; as the fibre swells, stiffness and strength both decrease (Pil et al. 2016). Regarding its medical textile applications, flax is increasingly used in biocomposites, for example, as the reinforcing fibre in biocomposites for tissue engineering because of its biocompatibility. Fibroblasts are known to proliferate well on scaffolds made from flax fibres blended with polylactide or polycaprolactone (Kunert-Keil et al. 2012). In vitro trials have seen silver-nanoparticle-coated linen fabric demonstrate good antibacterial capability against both gram-positive and gram-negative bacteria (Paladini et al. 2015) which, combined with its hydrophilic properties, makes it attractive for use in wound dressings. The fibres have also been used experimentally as sutures but further work is required (Fong et al. 2015, 155–175).

Hemp has a long history of cultivation for various purposes including for the fibre from its stems, for medicine, recreational drugs, and food. It is one of the oldest fibres to have been used in textiles, having been discovered in tombs in Mesopotamia dating back to approximately 8000 BC. A bast fibre, hemp is the second most widely used natural fibre in composites, after sisal; its fibres are contained within the tissues of the stems and they impart strength and stiffness to the shrub, which is what makes them useful as a textile fibre, but one of its drawbacks is the variability between crops (Shahzad 2012). With a cellulose content of 57–77%, not dissimilar to that of flax, but with a higher lignin content of 3.7–13% compared to 2.2% for flax, hemp offers a density similar to that of flax and jute, with a tensile strength of 550–900 MPa and a Young's Modulus of 70 GPa (Li, Tabil, and Panigrahi 2007). Over 500 natural compounds have been identified in hemp; a number of these exhibit antibacterial properties which makes hemp one of the most studied of the bast fibres (Khan, Warner, and Wang 2014). The concentrations of the bioactive compounds depend upon many factors including plant tissue type, age, variety, growth conditions, harvest time, and storage conditions (Kushima, Shoyama, and Nishioka 1980; Keller et al. 2001; Ross and ElSohly 1996). Cannabinoids and the phenolic component of lignin have demonstrated antimicrobial activity against a range of bacteria and fungi, some of more clinical relevance than others (Khan, Warner, and Wang 2014). Hemp oil is already used topically for skin conditions in the consumer market and the fibres may be able to be utilised in a safe and effective way for medical dressings and bandages. In addition, given their radio-opacity, hemp fibres could prove to be a useful component in biocomposites in a wide range of prosthetics, including implantables (Namvar et al. 2014).

Sisal fibre is obtained from the leaves of *Agava sisalana* (Chand and Hashmi 1993). Native to tropical and subtropical North and South America, it is now widely grown in tropical parts of Africa, the West Indies, and the Far East (Bisanda and Ansell 1992). A plant produces approximately 250 leaves and each leaf contains 1,000–1,250 fibre bundles composed of 4% fibre, 0.75% cuticle, 8% dry matter, and 87.25% water (Mukherjee and Satyanarayana 1984). The leaf contains three types of cellulose fibres: mechanical, ribbon, and xylem. It is the mechanical fibres that are the most commercially useful and these are extracted predominantly from the periphery of the leaf by retting (partial degradation) followed by scraping or by mechanical means with decorticators (Bisanda and Ansell 1992). As for hemp, the composition of the fibre varies with age, source, growth, harvesting, and storage conditions, and figures quoted vary widely, with a cellulose content between 43 and 99% and a lignin content of 8% (Li, Mai, and Ye 2000). A fibre is between 1 and 1.5 metres in length and the diameter ranges from 100 to 300 μm (Bisanda and Ansell 1992). Mechanical properties vary between fibres; strength and stiffness depend upon the cellulose content and the angle the bands of microfibrils in the inner secondary cell wall make with the fibre axis (Chand, Satyanarayana, and Rohatgi 1986). Furthermore, tensile properties are not uniform along its fibre length: that from towards the lower part and root exhibits a low tensile strength and modulus but high fracture strain, whereas the mid portion of the fibre is stronger and stiffer. Tensile strength quoted in the literature ranges from 347 to 700 MPa and a tensile modulus of 7–22 GPa (Li, Mai, and Ye 2000). Sisal is biodegradable and recyclable and can be treated during textile finishing to adjust its functional properties in the same way as other cellulose fibres, and in the consumer healthcare market, sisal has been used to manufacture scrubbers for removing dead skin cells (Rasigha et al. 2015). Sisal may prove to be a useful natural fibre for the manufacture of surgical drapes in the near future given growing environmental legislation and requirements for safe disposal.

Manila is obtained from abaca, *Musa textilis* (Ramnath et al. 2015). The plant is closely related to the banana plant but the fruit is not for human consumption, so the abaca plant is grown only for its fibre (Faruk and Sain 2014). The fibre has one of the highest densities amongst the natural fibres at 1.5 g/cm^3. It typically has a length of 4.9 mm and a diameter of 20 μm. Tensile strength is quoted at 430–813 Mpa and a Young's Modulus of 32 GPa (Peças,et al. 2018). Interestingly, abaca fibres exhibit a strong resistance to saltwater and can be used in saline environments, a feature which may be of use in complex wound management where the wound needs to be kept moist for healing (Ramnath et al. 2015).

4.2.3 Natural-Polymer Man-Made Fibres

4.2.3.1 Protein Fibres: Casein, Collagen

Casein is a completely biodegradable natural polymer composed of the phosphoproteins extracted from raw skimmed milk by acidification (Diamond and Wormmell 1939); filaments can be wet spun by dissolving the casein in dilute sodium hydroxide solution before extruding the syrupy solution into a coagulating bath containing formaldehyde. Casein can be formed into either filaments or film and shows good heat resistance, is relatively economical to produce, and it offers a good capacity to interact with a wide variety of compounds and nutrients, for example, drugs and vitamins (Penalva et al. 2015; Semo et al. 2007). Casein filament production was first reported in the 1940s, and since then various formulations of the spinning fluid have been designed to yield filaments suitable for drug-delivery purposes (Song et al. 2010; Shapira et al. 2010), including combinations with the protein from maize – zein – in electrospun nanofibres (Wang et al. 2019); the protein chains demonstrate open and flexible conformations consisting of both hydrophilic and lipophilic segments, hence the micellar form they adopt in milk.

Collagen fibres are natural macromolecular protein assemblies that play a vital role in structures that support tensile mechanical loads in the human body/animal bodies. There are different subtypes of collagen but the most abundant form is type I collagen, the primary structural motif in tendon and ligament. The structure of collagen is complex; right-handed triple helical structures are assembled into microfibres by hydrogen bonds. Cross-linking aggregates the protein chains into a triple helix to provide stability to the molecule and then several molecules aggregate in a quarter-staggered array to form microfibrils, which further aggregate to form the fibres (Kew et al. 2011; Ramachandran 2018, 432). Collagen can be extracted from connective tissues, purified, and reconstituted into gels and scaffolds. Purified collagen remains a preferred base for ligament and tendon tissue engineering due to low antigenicity, a chemotactic surface structure for fibroblasts, biocompatibility, and proteolytic degradation pathways. Collagen-based fibres are in contemporary clinical use as sutures but cannot be used for scaffolding due to inflammatory tissue reactions (Yaltirik et al. 2003).

4.2.3.2 Cellulose Fibres: Viscose Rayon, Lyocell

Viscose rayon and its associated industry is the oldest of the currently existing man-made fibre businesses (slightly older and more extensive than that of cuprammonium rayon) with roots stretching back to the late 19th century. A fibre made from regenerated cellulose, the starting material is purified wood pulp from spruce or eucalyptus trees, but it can also be produced from parts of other plants with a high cellular cellulose content such as soy plant stems, bamboo, and sugar cane. When they are being used as the starting material, these other cellulose sources are often mentioned in promotional literature, perhaps in an attempt to make the resulting viscose rayon products sound more interesting and acceptable. In fact, the process, once the cellulose fibre pulp has been prepared, is the same as that used for wood pulp from trees. As for wood pulp, the original pulp is purified to remove lignin and undesirable colourants, then temporarily chemically modified into sodium cellulose xanthate to render it soluble in sodium hydroxide solution prior to spinning. The syrupy, so-called viscose solution is wet spun by being extruded into an acidic coagulating bath to regenerate the cellulose and yield continuous filaments of viscose rayon. The filaments are then drawn and washed before winding, and depending upon the method of manufacture and extent of drawing, different physical and mechanical properties can be provided to the resulting fibre (Woodings 2001). For example, subjecting the emerging filaments as they are being extruded to very high levels of extension causes the regenerated cellulose molecules to become better orientated along the filament axis and results in a more highly crystalline filament. This yields a somewhat stronger filament with reduced extensibility but despite the improvement, and its filament form resembling that of silk, with a breaking tenacity of 25cN/tex, elongation of 20%, and moisture absorption of 11%, the mechanical properties of the regenerated cellulose are no match for silk fibroin (Basit et al. 2018). In the case of modal viscose rayon, the method of manufacture is altered and further improvements in breaking strength and wet modulus are gained by retaining some of the original crystallinity present in the cellulose at source (The Textile Institute 2021). Viscose rayon is an inexpensive and absorbent fibre and this makes it an attractive material to use as a major component in disposable items intended for wound care, as absorbent pads, or in the base materials in advanced dressings, bandages, and gauzes (Rigby, Anand, and Horrocks 1997).

Lyocell, named in 1989, owes its genesis to the Greek word *lyein* which means 'dissolve' (Woodings 2001), and it is the generic name for a regenerated cellulosic fibre obtained by the wet spinning of cellulose from an organic cyclic polar solvent, N-methyl morpholine-N-oxide (The Textile Institute 2021; Borbély 2008; Kumar and Harnden 1999). The first commercial product, Tencel™ (Lenzing AG, Austria), was originally released by Acordis in 1988. The starting material for lyocell, as for viscose rayon, is wood pulp, but the manufacturing process used to take the cellulose into solution is different, i.e., dissolution in the organic cyclic polar solvent N-methylmorpholine-N-oxide (NMMO) hydrate under intensive shear forces coupled with simultaneous evaporation of water. The solution of cellulose in NMMO hydrate is subsequently filtered and then extruded into a water bath through fine jets. As the solvent is washed out, the fibres form into fine filaments which can be collected and a very high proportion of the solvent is able to be recycled for a further round of dissolution (Chavan and Patra 2004). The lyocell fibre possesses a high degree of orientation with a crystalline-to-amorphous ratio of approximately 9:1. This offers good wet and dry tensile strength and that makes the fibre readily washable. In addition, the fibre has good dimensional stability and its fabrics shrink less on wetting than those made from cotton and viscose rayon (Borbély 2008). However, one of the issues of lyocell is that the fibres fibrillate along their length and produce microfibres when wetted due to the highly crystalline structure of the fibre. Whilst it can be used to advantage during the production of non-woven fabrics, there has been work aimed at reducing the fibrillation because the shedding of microfibres could potentially cause harm in products implanted in the body (Mortimer and Péguy 1996). Lyocell can be blended with other fibres and it has industrial applications in wipes, medical swabs, and gauzes. For example, lyocell blended with bamboo charcoal yarn creates antimicrobial properties raising the possibility of utilising blended lyocell in hospital clothing, bedding, and surgical gowns. Hydrocell® (Integra LifeSciences Corp, Plainsboro, New Jersey, America) is based on lyocell technology and offers similar properties to calcium alginate (discussed later in this section). It forms a coherent gel in a moist environment and is utilised in wound care products (Chavan and Patra 2004).

4.2.3.3 Calcium Alginate

Calcium alginate is a polymer extracted from brown seaweed, *Phaeophyceae*, by treatment with sodium hydroxide solution, followed by wet spinning into a coagulating bath containing calcium salts or mixed calcium/sodium salts to form insoluble calcium alginate filaments (Lee and Mooney 2012). One of calcium alginate's more routine applications is its use in hospitals in the form of water-soluble alginate bags for holding 'used' (soiled) linen, a step carried out as the first layer of protection for the healthcare worker before being put in a clear plastic bag which can then be safely tagged for place of origin and date. The polymer does, however, possess several properties that make it highly suitable for wound dressings. For example, it has the ability to swell and retain water and wound exudate, thus contributing to the (preferred) moist wound environment. Furthermore, the gel-forming property allows the dressing to be removed with ease, thus reducing tissue trauma. Calcium alginate is also a natural haemostat and is non-degradable in mammals due to their lack of the enzyme alginase (Lee and Mooney 2012; Paul and Sharma 2004; Rajendran 2018). The effect of alginate fibre on wound healing was discussed in journal articles over 30 years ago; when used in dressings for both partial and full thickness wounds, the histology after 14 days confirmed not only that the alginate was well-tolerated by body fluids and cellular components but also that it was an efficient haemostatic agent (Barnett and Varley 1987).

With the advent of silver nanoparticles and interest in their biological applications, coupled with sophisticated attachment/delivery mechanisms, modifications to the alginate fibre have been trialled; researchers at Shinshu University demonstrated that even a minimum silver concentration of 1mg/g used for coating the calcium alginate fibres showed measurable antibacterial properties and that increasing the silver content could completely inhibit the growth of gram-positive *S. aureus* and gram-negative *E. coli* (Xu et al. 2016a). Zinc oxide (ZnO) is a more economical substance to use than silver and also demonstrates antimicrobial properties. In 2016, zinc oxide-sodium nanoparticles were incorporated into alginate cellulose fibres and their antibacterial properties compared to that of a blend of alginate cellulose fibres with no modification. When tested against *E. coli*, the fibres containing ZnO nanoparticles showed good antibacterial properties (Varaprasad et al. 2016). In addition to nanoparticles, commonly available drugs are being incorporated into wound dressings to promote wound healing. Simvastatin, traditionally used as a lipid-lowering drug, has been shown to be both anti-inflammatory, having the ability to promote wound healing, and a good inductor of bone growth. In 2016, Simvastatin was combined into an alginate-based composite film wound dressing. Pre-formulation studies demonstrated desirable wound-dressing properties and superior mechanical properties alongside the ability to maintain a controlled drug-release profile. The cell-viability assay demonstrated the film to be non-toxic (Rezvanian, Amin, and Ng 2016). The preparation of alginate in a gel form has allowed for the incorporation of tissue factors such as bone morphogenetic proteins. Modifying the gel to allow for sequential delivery has shown enhanced differentiation of osteoprogenitor cells in the bone marrow on testing in vitro (Lee and Mooney 2012). Given that cartilage can now be grown in vitro, the ability to regenerate bone such that it can be implanted into the human body will push forward the field of regenerative medicine.

4.2.3.4 Chitosan

Chitosan is a polycationic biopolymer derived from chitin, a major component of the outer skeletons of crustaceans, by treatment with alkali (Paul and Sharma 2004). Chitosan's polymer backbone chain is composed of randomly distributed β-linked D-glucosamine and N-acetyl-D-glucosamine residues and it is often used to modify the surface properties of cellulose fibres. Chitin and chitosan are both biocompatible materials highly suited to use in medical applications intended to treat, augment, or replace certain tissue, organs, or functional components of the human body, and recent studies suggest that chitosan and its derivatives are promising as supporting materials in tissue engineering applications (Islam et al. 2017). Chitosan possesses bacteriostatic and fungostatic properties and, like calcium alginate, is haemostatic; it also affects the function of macrophages and stimulates wound healing. Chitosan has a similar structure to cellulose and can therefore be used as a coating on cotton fabrics to provide antibacterial performance in an economical way (Rajendran 2018). For example, in one study, chitosan applied as a finishing agent to bamboo-cellulose viscose rayon demonstrated antibacterial activity against gram-positive and gram-negative bacteria and this activity remained for 30 washes (Teli and Sheikh 2012); in another, non-woven fabric made from wool/viscose rayon treated with chitosan at various concentrations by pad-dry-cure was explored to determine its potential in wound dressings. Low concentrations (0.3%) of chitosan were effective in conferring both good absorbency and antibacterial properties whilst higher concentrations led to undesirable stiffness of the dressing material (Islam, Arnold, and Padhye 2013). Chitosan has also been successfully electrospun with silk fibroin to create nanofibrous membranes that have demonstrated antibacterial activities against *E. coli* and *S. aureus* (Cai et al. 2010), whilst coating a Tencel®/cotton non-woven fabric with chitosan was shown to control evaporation and provide a barrier to microorganisms in a laboratory setting (Lou et al. 2008).

Chitosan can be manufactured into fibres, nanofibres, hydrogels, membranes, scaffolds, and sponges for use in a variety of situations, such as tissue engineering, enzyme immobilisation, drug delivery, control over the rate of absorption in synthetic absorbable sutures, and wound care. Commercially, chitosan and its derivatives are currently used in wound care in forms such as Tegasorb® and Tegaderm® (3M, Maplewood, Minnesota, USA) (Jayakumar et al. 2011). Chitosan has been demonstrated to display properties advantageous in wound dressings. The ability to blend it with other readily available fibres increases its potential applications, as was already mentioned for other fibres such as cotton and viscose rayon. For example, combining calcium alginate and chitosan has been of interest. The material formed remains biodegradable and has preferable mechanical properties to a single fibre of chitosan; in particular, it is mechanically stronger when exposed to acidic conditions (Sibajam et al. 2015). The alginate/chitosan fibres produced have a core of calcium alginate and an outer coating of chitosan (Rajendran 2018) and show acceptable tensile properties for the manufacturing of bandages. In addition, the hydrophilic nature of the fibre allowed for absorption of bodily fluids and, potentially, this phenomenon could be utilised to preferentially displace antibiotics or other molecules (Sibaja et al. 2015).

4.2.3.5 Hyaluronan/Hyaluronic Acid

Hyaluronan/Hyaluronic acid (HA) is a naturally occurring polysaccharide, an anionic unsulfated, linear glycosaminoglycan that forms part of the cell membrane. It is composed of repeating polymeric disaccharides of D-glucuronic acid and N-acetyl-D-glucosamine linked by a glucuronidic β (1→3) bond. Typically, for applications on a commercial scale, it is produced by fermenting Group C streptococci. The HA polymers occur in a great range of configurations and shapes, depending on their size, the salt concentration, pH, and the type of associated cations in the surrounding liquid. Their key characteristics are that their rate of dissolution and enzyme degradation can be controlled by chemical modifications such as the attachment of lipophilic groups and by cross-linking, and such derivatives are useful in applications requiring controlled drug release. In fact, HA and its derivatives formed by reaction with mono- and polyfunctional compounds can lead to biomedical materials with sustained drug-release capabilities such as biochemical probes, biopolymers with on-demand responsive drug release (on-off switching release by the local application of heat, light, or mechanical stress), tethered drugs for controlled release, and cross-linked hydrogels as biocompatible scaffolds for tissue engineering (Bayer 2020; Al-Khateeb and Olszewska-Czyz 2020).

4.2.4 Natural Polymer Elastomer: Rubber

Natural rubber, polyisoprene, is an important polymer used in more than 400 medical devices. The sole commercial source of natural polyisoprene is rubber that is harvested as latex from the Brazilian rubber tree, *Hevea brasiliensis* (Mooibroek and Cornish 2000). The high molecular weight of the rubber (and the consequently very long polymer chains) is coupled with high displacement and mobility in the polymer-chain sections caused by the cis arrangement in polyisoprene (a trans arrangement would allow neat packing to yield a much stiffer material), leading to high-performance properties including resilience, extremely high extensibility, elasticity, abrasion resistance, efficient heat dispersion, and impact resistance. The elastic properties/rigidity can be controlled by careful adjustment of the cross-linking process called vulcanisation to extend its use over a wider range of applications and temperatures (Mooibroek and Cornish 2000). Rubber can be combined with fibres to create fibre-reinforced rubber composites whose performance may be improved by appropriate combinations of fibre orientation, chemical treatment of the fibre and vulcanisation of the rubber (Geethamma et al. 1998) and of fibre ratio (Maya, Varughese, and Sabu 2008) to more-fully exhibit the benefits of the combined behaviour of the soft, extensible and elastic rubber matrix with the stiffness provided by the strong fibrous reinforcement. A wide variety of fibre and filament types have been explored and employed as reinforcement in rubber, not least because of their value in tyre manufacture, and these include cellulose natural fibres, natural-polymer man-made fibres such as viscose rayon and synthetic polymer fibres such as nylon and polyester (polyethylene terephthalate, PET) or, where higher performance is needed, aramid fibres such as Kevlar™, the high-performance polyester, polyethylene naphthalate (PEN – Teonex®; Teijin Ltd, Tokyo, Japan and PENTEX®, Honeywell International Inc, Virginia USA) or carbon fibre. A useful summary of combinations of reinforcement fibres, filaments and rubber is available online (VERT 2019). Whilst rubber is utilised extensively in the healthcare industry, one of the major drawbacks is IgE-mediated latex allergy caused by the presence of proteins in the latex (Mooibroek and Cornish 2000).

4.3 SYNTHETIC POLYMER FIBRES AND FILAMENTS: COMMODITY TYPES

The main commodity-type synthetic-polymer man-made fibres are nylon, polyester (PET), polypropylene, and acrylic (PAN), of which the first three are thermoplastic, i.e., they soften and become rubbery once they are heated above a particular temperature (the glass transition temperature, $T_{g,}$) and as they are heated further, at some point they will melt (see Figure 4.1). Details of the melting points and glass transition temperatures for a range of polymers are conveniently available online (Perkin Elmer, 2019). Acrylic is the exception amongst the commodity materials; the attraction between the polyacrylonitrile polymer chains is so great that it does not melt because the chains cannot be separated before the material begins to char and degrade.

4.3.1 Nylon

Nylon was the first synthetic-polymer man-made fibre to be produced commercially, and this was achieved rapidly following its discovery in 1935 by Wallace Carothers at the DuPont Experimental Station laboratory in Wilmington, Delaware, USA. DuPont brought nylon into production in late 1939 (DuPont 2021). Although never a particularly cheap fibre to make, because it was the first synthetic polymer fibre to appear on the textile market, nylon became commercialised very quickly. With women's stockings made of nylon appearing from 1940 and rapidly replacing silk in this application, it is an indication of its commercial success that the term 'nylon' became synonymous with ladies hosiery.

Nylon is a polymer made by condensation polymerisation brought about by the reaction of difunctional monomers containing equal numbers of amine and carboxylic acid groups such that amide links can be formed at both ends of each monomer residue (Ratner et al. 2013, 74–77). The reaction keeps being repeated (it is a chain reaction) continually building up the length of the molecule being formed, and that is what causes the polymer chain to be created. Nylon, the resulting synthetic linear polyamide, consists of repeating lengths of hydrocarbon chains joined together by amide links. Different nylons are classified depending on the number of carbon atoms in the sections of hydrocarbon chain between the repeating amide groups (The Textile Institute 2021); the three most important members are nylon 6.6 and

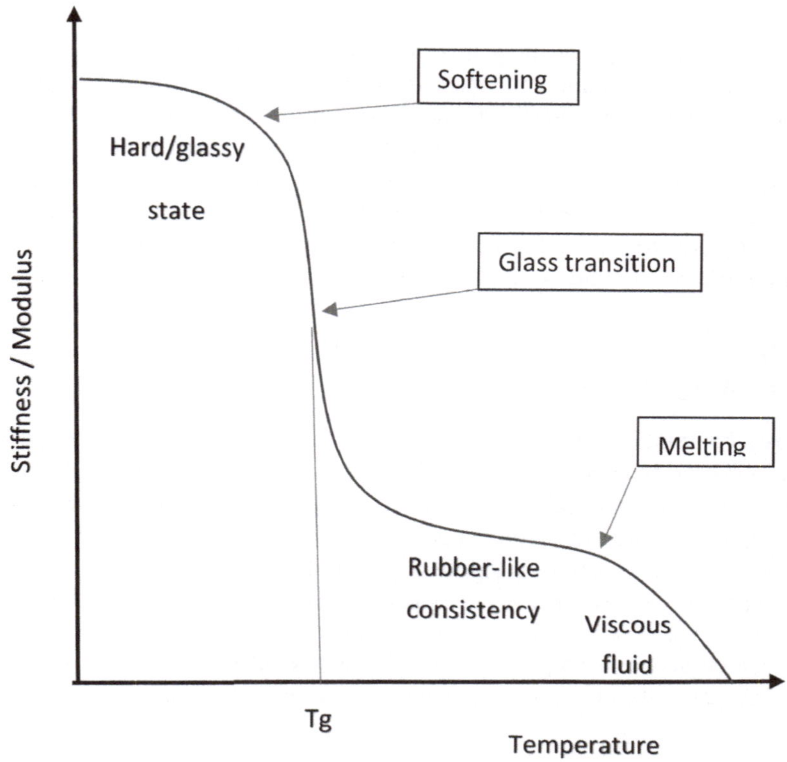

FIGURE 4.1 The effect of temperature on the stiffness and consistency of a semi-crystalline thermoplastic fibre.

nylon 6 (the most common types used in fibre or filament form) and nylon 11 (which uses castor oil as the starting point and is mainly used in resin form).

The nylon polymer is converted into filament form by melt spinning, which involves the polymer chips being melted then extruded through a spinneret into a current of air to cool and harden it to produce continuous filaments or, after a further step involving cutting or stretch-breaking, staple fibres (Bansal and Raichurkar 2016). Melt spinning of the nylon is followed by drawing of the newly formed filaments (extending the filament by four to five times its original length and thereby helping to align the polymer chains along the lengthwise direction of the filament and improve its crystallinity), a common requirement in spinning processes. Both spinning and drawing can be adjusted to alter the final filament properties to render them more suitable not only for general use but also for more demanding purposes (Morton and Hearle 2008, 1–81). In the case of tyre cord, for example, where high modulus and high strength are imperative and for demanding medical applications, higher levels of extension are required and the temperature at which the drawing is carried out may need to be raised to enable enhanced alignment of the polyamide chains to be achieved. For other applications where mixtures of polymers would work better than a single type, melt spinning as a process does allow for the incorporation of other polymers/molecules into the polymer melt if desired.

In common with other melt-spun polymers, the drawing of the nylon filaments immediately following the extrusion improves its tensile properties by bringing about a reduction in extension to break and raising the initial modulus to acceptable levels by increasing the degree of crystallinity of the filament. Typically, the tenacity of commercially produced nylon 6 and nylon 66 is 0.4–0.6 N/tex with a breaking extension of 20–30% for nylon 6.6 and 20–40% for nylon 6. Initially, as the polymer chain is grown in length, there is a linear relationship between molecular mass and tenacity, but it reaches a point where further increases in the length of the polyamide chain show little extra benefit in terms of improved tenacity and would in any case lead to too high a viscosity in the molten polymer for the extrusion stage to be successful. Apart from improving its stiffness, a higher degree of crystallinity in the nylon yarn reduces creep (the tendency of a material to slowly deform under persistent stress) which improves its dimensional stability. The elastic recovery from deformation of nylon is greater than that of many other fibres. For example, it exhibits 90% recovery from a 1% extension and 89% recovery from a 10% extension, whereas viscose rayon offers only 67% recovery from a 1% extension and a mere 23% recovery from a 10% extension (Richards 2005, 20–94).

Melting points of nylon 6.6, nylon 6, and nylon 11 are 250°C, 210°C, and 185°C, respectively, and the glass transition temperatures are also correspondingly high at 50–60°C (nylon 6.6.), 40–60°C (nylon 6), and 30–45°C (nylon 11) which makes them potentially useful in medical textiles (Polymer Properties Database 2015–2021). Given the presence of polar groups within the polyamide polymer structure, it is not surprising that nylon absorbs some moisture into its structure from the atmosphere to a level of around 4.0–4.5% under standard conditions of temperature and humidity, and on immersion in water has an absorption level of 9–10%. Moisture absorption reduces the tenacity and initial modulus and brings about a lowering of the glass transition temperature, whilst causing the extension to break to become greater. Not inherently conductive itself, the application of silver as a fabric coating to nylon can provide it with both electrical conductivity and antimicrobial properties (Marino et al. 1985). Whilst antimicrobial activity can be of benefit in preventing infection, the additional ability to connect to an electrical power supply to generate heat from the fabric produced with silver-coated nylon yarn may be of use to those in expeditions and wilderness-medicine in the form of clothing (Thilagavathi et al. 2017). There are, however, much more common applications of nylon in the healthcare field such as in support/compression stockings, hosiery, and wound dressings; in addition, nylon is quite commonly used as a non-absorbable surgical suture as well as being utilised in the form of nylon mesh membranes in regenerative medicine for cell aggregation and filtration (Pennell 2016).

4.3.2 Polyester

Polyesters are a category of polymers that contain the ester group as the linking group along their polymer chain. Although there are several other fibres and polymers within the group which are of significant interest for medical textiles, the polyester most commonly employed in commodity products is poly (ethylene terephthalate) often referred to as PET. Developed in 1940 by Whinfield and Dixon of the Calico Printers Association in the UK, PET is manufactured by the condensation polymerisation of ethylene terephthalate (itself produced by the esterification of terephthalic acid and monoethylene glycol), extruded by melt spinning, hot drawn, then used alone or in blends as a textile fibre or filament. The polymer molecules in PET are stiffened by the presence of the aromatic groups within each of the repeat units along the polymer-chain backbone, whereas aliphatic polyesters will be relatively more flexible and some of the most flexible will be elastomeric (East 2005, 95–166).

PET for medical applications involving implanting needs to be improved compared with the commodity product used in apparel, particularly in regard to it needing to possess high tenacity, high modulus, and low elongation (Rahman and Saleh 2012) and whilst PET can show enhanced properties when higher molecular weight polymer is used to improve strength and the extruded filaments are subjected to hot drawing treatments similar to those used in the production of tyre cord to fully orient the polymer, there is another higher-performance polyester, polyethylene naphthalate (PEN), coming into use. Although PEN is more expensive, it is inherently stiffer and shows better thermal performance and barrier properties to chemical agents than PET (Sakellarides 2004). For medical applications where the focus is on its ability to provide temporary support but then to be absorbed over time, the simplest linear polyester of all is polyglycolic acid (PGA), most often used in medical applications such as absorbable sutures because its hydrophilic nature leads it to become rapidly degraded (see below under Polyglycolides). It may be of interest that in plant tissue, natural polyesters composed mostly of oxygenated fatty acids can be found in cutin, where they serve as the framework for the plant cuticle, and in suberin, a waxy substance which acts as a barrier to the passage of water and solutes (Fich et al. 2016). Frequently ingested in food, they safeguard the plant cell-wall polysaccharides from degradation by colonic bacterial enzymes and are also potent in vitro absorbers of lipophilic carcinogens (Mudgil 2017, 35–59). Such properties could be of interest in medical textiles, but before these materials could be used, their allergenic potential would need to be assessed (especially given that they are natural polymers). The use of suberin in wound management, for example, may prove to be of use due to its barrier functions.

For PET, as a melt-spun synthetic polymer fibre, just as is the case with nylon, modification of the production process can allow for the manufacture of fibres with different properties and the incorporation of additional nanomaterials or molecules into the molten polymer, but this is not done so much with PET as it is with other fibre-forming polymers (see, for example, Palza 2015). PET is, however, amenable to surface treatment, for example, with copper/copper oxide nanoparticles following relatively gentle aminolysis with triethanolamine and using copper sulfate solution as the source of the metal, sodium hypophosphite as the reducing agent, and polyvinylpyrrolidone as a stabiliser. The treated fabric in this case is hydrophilic and flame-retardant with high tensile strength (Rezaie and Montazer 2017).

PET shows a very low moisture regain and as a consequence does not readily absorb finishing agents or other chemicals from aqueous solutions; it can therefore only be dyed using disperse dyes and its lipophilicity can result in staining of the fabric and fibre by oily substances both in use and in laundering. However, advantageously, polyester has a relatively high glass transition temperature at 70–80°C and melting point (260°C) and it is amenable to sterilisation. Other advantages are that fabrics made from polyester do demonstrate good resistance to extension and typically possess excellent dimensional stability plus good resistance to abrasion, but a disadvantage is that PET is thrombogenic (demonstrating a tendency to thrombosis) which needs to be considered in vascular grafts to prevent occlusion (Bide et al. 2006, 91–124), and recently, problems of lack of incorporation and scarring have been highlighted in vaginal mesh repair (BBC News 2019). Even so, PET is widely used in implant applications which include non-absorbable, braided sutures, for example, Ethibond™ (Ethicon Inc, a subsidiary of Johnson and Johnson, Belgium), in which it proffers minimal tissue reaction and has good handling and a high tensile strength (Ramachandran 2018, 433). Fracture of sutures under tension has been shown to occur at the knot (Najibi et al. 2010), and if tensile performance needs to be improved, or abrasion needs to be reduced, FiberWire® (Arthrex, Munich, Germany), with its multi-strand UHMWPE core and braided PET outer sheath, and HiFi® (Conmed Corp. Largo, Florida, USA) have been shown to be superior (Gomide et al. 2019). PET has not only been in use for many years in vascular grafts, for aneurysm and vascular repair (King et al. 1983), ligament and tendon reconstruction, in implantable mesh, and in prosthetic heart valves, but also in hygiene products such as incontinence pads. PET itself is non-conductive, so in paying attention to the requirements of home healthcare and the associated need for intelligent textile medical applications, efforts have been undertaken to create blended yarns made from polyester and stainless steel to allow electrical charges to be conducted through fabrics intended for smart garments, and trials have been undertaken by creating clothing such that physiological measurements may be recorded (Rattfalt et al. 2007). Blended with cotton, polyester is widely used in garments used within the healthcare industry, for example, in stockings, surgical gowns, caps, masks, and bedding (Qin 2015).

4.3.3 Polypropylene

Polypropylene is a thermoplastic polymer that is produced by free-radical addition polymerisation of propylene; there are three types of polypropylene wherein the degree of crystallinity varies depending on the direction in which the $-CH_3$ side groups are arranged (randomness in the direction of their arrangement along polymer chain can be controlled by the application of Ziegler/Natta catalysts during polymerisation):

(i) atactic polypropylene: irregularly arranged side groups
(ii) isotactic polypropylene: $-CH_3$ side groups arranged regularly to one side of the polymer chain

(iii) syndiotactic polypropylene: the $-CH_3$ side groups are arranged regularly but alternately first to one side of the polymer chain then to the other

Typically, it is the isotactic form which is used for filaments and fibres; the syndiotactic version is softer and finds use in medical bags and pouches.

Polypropylene in fibre or filament form possesses many useful characteristics, such as low density, low hydrophilicity, and good preservation of shape (dimensional stability) when wet, plus its fabrics exhibit high resistance to creasing and are durable to wear making them a good choice for healthcare clothing; for example, non-woven polypropylene fabric is used in the BARRIER® surgical gown (Mölnlycke, Gothenburg, Sweden). Medical applications continually increase as the polymer possesses the advantage of being able to be manufactured and sterilised by a wide range of techniques and, in fabric form, products for the healthcare industry include wipeable covering fabrics over pillows with polypropylene filling, waterproof non-woven polypropylene pillowcases, non-woven bedding covers, items of clothing, bandages, and medical dressings (Interweave Textiles Ltd. 2021; Medline Industries Ltd. 2019; B. Braun 2021). Sutures, for example, Prolene® (Ethicon Inc, a subsidiary of Johnson and Johnson, Belgium) can be manufactured from polypropylene and a considerable range of mesh products, either woven or non-woven, which can be readily cut to shape, many including polypropylene, are widely used, for example, to enhance the ease of hernia repair. The first hernia repair mesh used in 1958 was made from polypropylene. It is estimated that over 18 million hernia operations per year now involve the use of synthetic, non-degradable mesh (CORDIS 2016), and polypropylene mesh is the most widely used, but there have been both problems (for example, chronic pelvic pain) and lawsuits. Although the problems are said now to have been overcome (Drugwatch 2021), research has been undertaken at a European level with the stated aim: "to fabricate a nano-fibrous mesh with well-defined nano-topography using cellulose; human recombinant collagen, derived from transgenic tobacco plants; and biodegradable poly-ε-caprolactone or polylactic/polyglycolic acid as raw materials," to enable a move away from polypropylene to more biologically acceptable/biomaterial alternatives (Haigh, Dargaville, and Dalton 2017). The project claimed success in reaching a stage that would allow clinical trials to begin in 2020. For implants requiring fine detail (between 800 nm and 70 μm) with nanofibre support, three-dimensional digital printing methods combined with melt electrospinning, melt micro-extrusion, or laser sintering of polypropylene have been developed (Deopura and Padaki 2014, 97–114).

4.3.4 Acrylic

Acrylic (polyacrylonitrile, PAN) was first developed and marketed under the trade name Orlon by DuPont in the 1940s (DuPont 2021a). PAN fibres do not consist solely of polyacrylonitrile but are copolymers wherein over 85% of the monomer used consists of acrylonitrile and *less than* 15% is a vinyl monomer selected to improve processing and properties. For example, vinyl alcohol may be employed as the co-monomer to improve absorption. If the fibre contains *more than* 15% of a copolymer, it is described as a modacrylic (The Textile Institute 2021). The filaments are usually wet spun from aprotic solvents such as dimethyl sulfoxide into a coagulating bath, though when a higher resistance to abrasion is required, they can be dry spun. For commodity acrylic fibre products themselves, the material is used predominantly in fibre form, and tow-to-top conversion is carried out mainly by stretch-breaking of the filament tows, but it is fair to say that PAN fibres themselves have little profile at present in the medical textiles field. PAN filaments are, however, the main precursor chosen for the preparation of carbon fibres which find use in braces and artificial limbs. The internal structure of the PAN filament used can significantly affect the properties of the resultant carbon fibre and it has been shown that air-gap wet spinning can yield an improved PAN precursor with reduced numbers of voids and provide the preferred circular or close-to-circular cross-section for the carbon fibre (Wilms, Seide, and Gries 2013).

4.4 SYNTHETIC POLYMER ELASTOMERS

Although many others are possible, the most commonly used types of synthetic polymer elastomer are the segmented polyurethanes.

Spandex yarns such as Lycra® (DuPont) are segmented-polyurethane elastomers in the form of fibres, filaments, and films. Also sometimes called elastane, they are long-chain synthetic polymers that are composed of at least 85% by weight of segmented polyurethane (The Textile Institute 2021); the filaments are produced by dry spinning. Polyurethane yarns demonstrate extremely high extensibility and complete recovery from deformation, are able to be extended by up to five times the original length and return to the original length on release (rubber-like elasticity), and they also possess high tensile strength and good abrasion resistance. Another advantage is that because of their resistance to many cosmetic oils and solvents, textiles containing segmented polyurethanes can be laundered if they become contaminated with oil-based products such as emollients following contact with the skin (Shivers 1962). Spandex yarns can be manufactured as filaments, staple fibre yarns, or as composites and their excellent elastomeric performance has led to their use not only in fashion products but also in compression garments in the healthcare sector, such as the stockings used for controlling oedema (Walgreen Health Solutions 2020).

4.5 SYNTHETIC POLYMER HIGH-PERFORMANCE FIBRES AND FILAMENT MATERIALS AND OTHER SPECIALIST POLYMER STRUCTURES

4.5.1 Aramids

Aramids are a group of polyamides that are composed of aromatic groups joined together by at least 85% amide linkages through the para position or the meta position. The presence of the aromatic rings confers much greater stiffness to the aramid compared with a linear hydrocarbon chain such as those between the amide groups in nylon 66 or nylon 6. Filaments are produced by gel spinning and extruded from solutions of the aramid in strong acids or solvents. Of the many types of aramid that are known, only a few have become commercially available in filament or fibre form and they can be broadly grouped as follows: meta-aramids such as Nomex® and para-aramids such as Kevlar. There are three subgroups of that para-aramid: Kevlar 29 the high toughness type, Kevlar 49® the high-modulus type, and Kevlar 149 the ultra-high-modulus type (all DuPont, Wilmington, Delaware, USA) and there is also Twaron® (Teijin, Arnhem, Netherlands).

The p-aramid fibres have a very high tensile modulus and tensile strength, are five times stronger than steel, and lose little strength during repeated abrasion, flexing, and stretching. They also demonstrate excellent dimensional stability, which is why they are used in demanding applications such as for tyre reinforcement and in structural composites in high-performance cars. As components for improving the properties of composite structures, they are of significant help in the creation of anti-ballistic and stab-resistant items of clothing for the personal and protective equipment for police and soldiers when operating in the field (DuPont 2021b).

The m-aramid fibres are used in applications where their excellent heat resistance including low shrinkage is helpful, such as in firefighter's protective clothing, and for medical textiles this would make them ideal for heat-sterilisable items, but as yet, in the healthcare sector, aramid fibres have failed to find much of a role. Biocompatibility tests were, however, undertaken several years ago (Edwards et al. 2005, 355–365) and it was found that surface coating with m-aramids can confer improved biocompatibility and enable antimicrobial applications when m-aramid-coated fabrics are chlorinated. Such materials were demonstrated to inactivate *E. coli* and *S. aureus* through chlorine release with a 7 log reduction in 10 minutes. The original level of antimicrobial action can be restored by subsequent chlorine treatment of the coated fabric following exposure (Kim et al. 2013).

4.5.2 Ultra-High Molecular Weight Polyethylene (UHMWPE)

Ultra-high molecular weight polyethylene (UHMWPE) is a type of polyethylene in which the degree of polymerisation is extremely high, yielding long polymer chains of molecular weight between 2 and 6 million daltons. Polyethylene is produced by free-radical addition polymerisation of ethylene, a process which is carried out under high pressure (ca 2,000 atmospheres) at 200°C in the presence of some oxygen. Initiation of the polymerisation reaction occurs due to the presence of oxygen which forms very reactive peroxides under these reaction conditions. Free radicals form which produce the growing length of polymer chain as each new ethylene residue becomes attached and creates a new free radical at the chain end. Termination occurs when two of these come together, and because that is a random process, chain lengths can vary considerably. Moreover, unless branching is prevented, polymer-chain growth may not simply be linear, it may also be initiated partway along the length of the growing polymer chain. The product, when such chain branching is allowed to occur under the polymerisation conditions spelt out above, has a degree of crystallinity below 75% and is called low-density polyethylene (LDPE). When chain branching is prevented, say by the use of Ziegler-Natta catalysts at low pressure (a few atmospheres) and a reduced temperature of 60°C, the polymer chains are linear and their packing together/crystallinity is much improved, resulting in the product known as high-density polyethylene (HDPE). Typically, it is very highly crystalline (95% or above), and hence both stiffer and stronger than LDPE, but even so, HDPE is only between 3–6% denser than LDPE. A useful brief description of the various types of polyethylene is available online (United States Plastic Corp 2021).

Being a non-polar polymer, the individual macromolecular chains in polyethylene are attracted to their neighbours only by London Dispersion Forces (the weakest of the intermolecular forces) but even so, it is typically semi-crystalline (crystallites surrounded by amorphous regions) with a higher degree of crystallinity achievable when the polymer chains are unbranched. Polyethylene is known for its remarkable resistance to degradation but even so studies have been undertaken to characterise it (Restrepo-Florez, Bassi, and Thompson 2014). For example, one cause of degradation is oxidation, and ideally the storage of polyethylene products should be in an oxygen-free environment, otherwise oxygen in the surrounding atmosphere will diffuse into the polyethylene and promote oxidation. Maximum oxidation occurs 1–2 mm below the surface in what is termed the 'subsurface white band' and whilst all mechanisms for degradation are not understood in detail, it is recognised that enzymes can cause the initial oxidation of polyethylene chains. It has been suggested that metabolic pathways for degradation of hydrocarbons can be used once the size of polyethylene molecules decreases to an acceptable range for enzyme action, and because of their easier accessibility, the polymer chains in the amorphous regions are more prone to microbial attack than those in the crystalline regions. Polyethylene can also be subject to deterioration in performance caused by mechanical wear and work to combat such degradation problems has led to the development of high-performance versions of polyethylene known as:

(i) ultra-high molecular weight polyethylene (UHMWPE)
(ii) highly cross-linked polyethylene (HXLPE)

UHMWPE is prepared by polymerisation of ethylene in the presence of a zirconium-based metallocene catalyst which enables the creation of very long polymer chains with a degree of polymerisation of 100,000 to 250,000 compared with a value around 80,000 for HDPE. It is converted into filament form by gel spinning. This involves preparing a very dilute gel which is carefully heated to the point where the polymer chains become almost completely separated, then extruding through a spinneret, being drawn in the air, then passed into a cooling water bath to harden. HXLPE is most often prepared by exposing UHMWPE to gamma radiation giving rise to polymer-chain cleavage and C and H free-radical formation followed by:

(i) recombination along the polymer-chain backbone limiting the level of chain cleavage,
(ii) combination between polymer chains leading to the desired cross-linking, and

(iii) entrapped free radicals which, over time, react with oxygen to form peroxy free radicals, which then establish a damaging chain of events by creating further free radicals able to react with oxygen.

The crosslinks that have been introduced into the polyethylene prove beneficial by acting as molecular constraints and help to improve its mechanical properties (Chakrabarty et al. 2015). A high degree of resistance to the penetration of free radicals into the polyethylene is important because, in the presence of oxygen, they cause it to degrade. The melting point of polyethylene is 135°C and raising the temperature of the polyethylene towards this point causes the polymer chains to become separated and that allows relatively easy access for free radicals to all parts of the polymer chains. Below the melting point but above the glass transition temperature, the polymer chains in the crystalline regions remain rigid and well-packed together, restricting access by free radicals, but those in the less well-ordered regions are mobile, so some degradation (a reduced level) can still occur. Annealing by heating to just below the melting point, increases the degree of crystallinity and raises the softening point, which preserve the desirable mechanical properties to a higher temperature, but leads to less efficient removal of free radicals. Melting and then reforming of the HXLPE does enable the elimination of free radicals, but there have also been searches for quenching methods, and Vitamin E doping has proved successful in improving oxidative stability, resistance to wear and fatigue beyond that achievable by melting and reforming (Oral and Muratoglu 2007). UHMWPE is used as a bearing surface in joint arthroplasty. In this form, it is semi-crystalline with the polymer exhibiting a degree of crystallisation of around 50% and the human body temperature is:

- well above the UHMWPE's glass transition temperature (quoted figures vary, from as low as –160 to –80°C compared with the values for PE at –110 to –120°C (Khalil et al. 2019), but it is the figure of –80°C for UHMWPE that makes more sense as it is expected to be higher than for PE because of restricted freedom of movement owing to fewer polymer chain ends) (Ries and Pruitt 2005),
- but also well below the polymer's melting point (132.7°C) (Ahmad et al. 2013; Rochaa et al. 2017).

The polymer therefore exhibits both the rigidity expected in solids and some mobility in the non-crystalline chain segments (attributes more characteristic of a liquid). When the UHMWPE is cross-linked, it is useful in the liners of joint replacements as it has better wear characteristics than polyethylene (Oral and Muratoglu 2007) and also it has been shown to perform excellently well when incorporated together with polycaprolactone in a partially absorbable suture for tendon and ligament repair (Zhang et al. 2020).

4.5.3 Cross-Linked Polyethylene

Cross-linked polyethylene (PEX, XPE, or XLPE) is high-density polyethylene within which covalent bonds have been formed either by chemical modification through attachment of silanes, by heating in the presence of peroxide cross-linking agents, or by irradiation with an electron beam to interconnect its polymer chains to form three-dimensional polymers with high molecular weights and improved physical properties. The molecular structure that is formed by cross-linking provides greater resistance to stress cracking, improved toughness, stiffness, and chemical resistance compared to the HDPE used as the precursor, and the likelihood of such improvements may be improved by increasing crystallinity in the precursor prior to cross-linking. Improvements in both tensile strength (50% increase) and Young's Modulus (36% increase) were reported in UHMWPE fibres by virtue of cross-linking compaction at elevated temperatures in the presence of peroxide (Ratner, Weinberg, and Marom 2003). It is certainly a high-performance fibre but there are concerns that highly cross-linked polyethylene (HXLPE), made by forming cross-linkages in UHMWPE, may be too unforgiving to the host in some medical applications, although these observations related to liners made from HXLPE rather than when it was in filament form (Chakrabarty et al. 2015).

4.5.4 Dendritic Polymers

Highly branched (dendritic) polymers have a centre formed by what was originally a multifunctional compound which has made a link with each of the polymer-chain branches spreading out from the centre. The dendritic structure is characterised by a surface of functional groups (either those of the amine end group of the growing polymer chain or an acidic agent attached to the amine group). Other groups could be used in place of an amine group. Voids exist between the branches and the structure is built up in layers (see Figure 4.2).

The voids between branches have the capacity to hold molecules within the structure, molecules that are not part of the structure itself. Each new layer of polymer is called a generation and addition of further generations can be undertaken to determine the optimum number required to retain a particular size or shape of molecule within the structure. The dendritic structure in such an arrangement can be considered to be the 'host,' and the molecules held within its structure the 'guest' molecules. There is the possibility for a range of molecules such as fragrances, drugs,

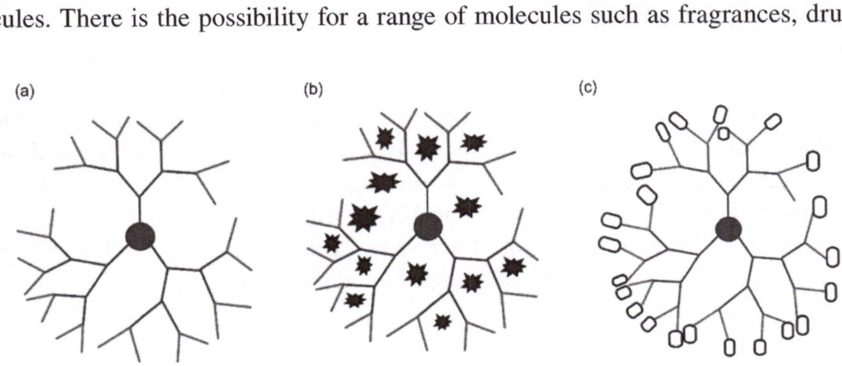

FIGURE 4.2 Dendritic structure: (a) 3rd generation structure; (b) 3rd generation structure loaded with entrapped guest molecules; and (c) 3rd generation structure with guest molecules attached to the surface (Akbari and Ryzard, 2019). With kind permission of Taylor & Francis.

or antibiotics to be held as guests which can be slowly released over time, or the items being held might be antimicrobial agents such as silver nanoparticles (Xu et al. 2016a; Akbari and Ryzard 2019).

4.6 SYNTHETIC ABSORBABLE POLYMERS (SA POLYMERS)

The idea behind synthetic absorbable or SA polymers is to create implants such as sutures, meshes, and stents to provide support for the limited amount of time over which healing takes place, and in some cases also to act as a reservoir of a drug such as an antibiotic, which may be needed to be steadily released over the healing period and thereby reduce the chance of post-operative infection. In sutures, the SA polymer replaces the natural absorbable catgut with a readily sterilisable alternative.

4.6.1 Aliphatic Polyesters

Owing to the absence of a stiffening aromatic group within the polymer-chain backbone, the aliphatic polyester polymer chains lack much of the inherent rigidity possessed by those in the commodity polymer, polyethylene terephthalate (PET), and as a consequence, their glass transition temperature (Tg) is typically lower, as is the melting point (Tm). Even so, whilst some physical properties are affected, given the appropriate choice of application, they can perform well and also possess several advantages over their aromatic counterpart. Comparing PLA, poly(l-lactic acid), for example, with PET, the Tg is reduced from 70–80°C for PET down to 55–60°C for PLA, and whereas the Tm for PET is 245–265°C, the Tm falls to 130–180°C for PLA. Whilst the lower glass transition temperature might render aliphatic polyesters less useful in the kind of traditional applications occupied by PET, such as sheeting and drapes, it is high enough for them to perform well at body temperature when they are used in implants, and they are relatively straightforward to be made into nanofibres by being electrospun. Also, despite its tensile strength and its elongation to break (6%) being less than that of PET (typically over 12%), as is its resistance to abrasion, PLA performs very well in most implant applications except for those demanding outstanding tensile behaviour. Its major advantages over PET are that it is biocompatible in most implant environments and completely biodegradable.

Several FDA-approved aliphatic polyesters are commercially available and possess attractive characteristics such as being biodegradable, biocompatible, and bioresorbable into the human body (because they are readily hydrolysable), and that makes them suitable for biomedical applications, particularly in the form of carriers for controlled drug release (Urbánek et al. 2019). Often, but not always, the aliphatic polyesters are used in the form of electrospun yarns and fabrics (Mokhtari et al. 2016, 152–154). Examples of the FDA-approved aliphatic polyesters are:

- polycaprolactone (PCL)
- poly(glycolic acid) (PGA), otherwise known as polyglycolide
- poly(l-lactic acid) (PLA)
- poly(lactic-co-glycolic acid) (PLGA)

The copolymer PLGA is of particular interest because its rate of degradation and hence of drug delivery can be adjusted by varying the ratios of lactic to glycolic acid in the reaction mixture prior to polymerisation (Pan and Ding 2012), despite neither the degradation rates nor the mechanical properties being linearly related to the copolymer composition (Mokhtari et al. 2016, 152–154). Taking poly(glycolic) acid (PGA) as an example of an aliphatic polyester, it is a biodegradable, linear, thermoplastic polymer with a Tg of 37°C, a melting point of 225°C, tensile strength of 1GPa, and a Young's Modulus of 4–14 GPa whilst its elongation at break is 30–40% (Odent, Raquez, and Dubois 2015, 235–274). For medical applications, PGA has been extruded into filaments, pins, or rods, injection moulded or shaped by compression moulding, and although fibre-reinforced composites have been used to strengthen the mechanical properties of items made with this polymer (Garvin and Feschuk 2005), polylactide-polyglycolide (PLPG) antibiotic implants was a development undertaken because the mechanical strength of the first-generation screws made from PGA was insufficient for orthopaedic applications. However, the creation of a fibre-reinforced composite in which the polymer matrix was reinforced with suture fibres of the same material also improved the strength of the rods and screws in this case (Böstman 1991). Having been introduced as the first synthetic absorbable suture in the 1970s as Dexon® (now produced by Medtronic, Dublin, Ireland), the PGA in many products is coated with another polymer to improve its ease of use in forming stitches and its passage through tissue (Chu 2013, 231–273). Components coated with antibiotic-impregnated polymer have been manufactured to allow for antibiotic delivery in cases of osteomyelitis (bone infection); they are used for absorbable sutures, screws, and implants, for example, to provide aperture fixation in anterior cruciate ligament reconstruction, and additionally, in cell scaffolding. Beyond the main four biocompatible and biodegradable aliphatic polyesters, Urbánek et al. (2019) draw attention to the attractive features of poly (alkylene succinate)-based polyesters; they are free of cytotoxic degradation products potential and could prove to be useful in the development of drug delivery structures because copolymerisation of alkylene succinates with fatty acids such as di-linoleic acid can yield a series of more lipophilic biodegradable polymers. The alkylene succinate–fatty acid copolymers can be fine-tuned by careful choice of fatty acid to bring about the desired polymer–drug interactions to control drug delivery (Urbánek et al. 2019). Another polyester type used in tissue engineering is the cross-linkable polypropylene fumarates, in this case not in fibre or yarn form, but as a biodegradable drug delivery component in composites intended to support bone regrowth. As is the case with the aliphatic polyesters and polyurethanes (see below), they may be used alone or in admixtures with other absorbable polymers such as collagen.

4.6.2 Polyurethanes

Just as it is useful in some cases to be able to construct implants from absorbable thermoplastic polymers with mechanical properties not unlike their non-absorbable counterparts, so it is useful to have the option to employ absorbable elastomeric materials to fulfil the requirement for rubber-like elasticity in implants within the central nervous system, in vascular tissue engineering, and in wound care. The synthetic absorbable polymer (SAP) requirement for thermoplastics is largely satisfied by the aliphatic polyesters, whereas for implants required to demonstrate elastomeric performance it is the segmented polyurethanes that fulfil the need (Pivec et al. 2017).

Polyurethanes for medical use are synthesised from three distinct bifunctional components: the diisocyanate, the polyol, and the chain extender (a diamine or diol). The bifunctionality of each of the three components means that during polymerisation, they become linked end to end to form linear polymer chains. The resulting long polyurethane polymer chains consist of segments with very different behaviours. The already existing polyether segment derived from the bifunctional polyol is highly mobile, whereas the newly formed segment built up by the repeated reaction of diisocyanate and bifunctional chain extender is rigid and/or tightly held in position by intermolecular bonding. It is the highly mobile sections of polyether chain continuously forming and reforming loops and contorted structures which provide the high extensibility, because those segments can be straightened out on extending the material. The polymer chains in the rigid sections are held firmly together, usually by hydrogen bonding and the attraction between other polar groups, so they cannot easily slip over one another, even when the material is extended to several times its own length.

There is such a wide range of possibilities for new compositions and associated new properties that it is said that segmented polyurethanes can have their performance 'tuned' to meet the needs of a particular application. Some of them behave as thermoplastics and others as elastomers and they are suitable for use in fibre form, or as flexible or rigid foams. It is the different behaviours of each of the segment types under tension and on release that lead to the outstanding elastomeric performance of the polyurethanes, whilst haemo-compatibility has been shown to depend on the relative proportions of rigid and flexible segments, with higher thrombogenicity being shown by polyurethanes with higher contents of rigid chain segments (Vermette et al. 2001). The mobile segments of the chain most often consist of polyether oligomer. In searching for starting materials from more environmentally acceptable sources than petroleum, polyols and polycarbonates derived from plants have been explored. Each type has its own particular attraction; whereas the polyether-polyurethanes typically possess the best mechanical properties because of the greater flexibility of the polyether segments, the polycarbonate-polyurethanes are more bio-stable due to the absence of sensitive ester and ether links in the flexible segments (Pivec et al. 2017).

Porous polyurethane scaffolds can be electrospun to mimic the extracellular matrix as it exists naturally and provide physical support of a type suitable for central nervous system tissue engineering (Carlberg et al. 2009) Electrospun polyurethane/graphene oxide tubular scaffolds have been explored for use in vascular tissue engineering (Jing. et al. 2015) whilst a novel composite scaffold fabricated from electrospun polyurethane with grapeseed oil, honey, and propolis exhibited improved performance in bone-tissue engineering (Chao, Mani, and Jaganathan 2018).

4.7 SUPER-ABSORBENT POLYMERS

The development of super-absorbent polymers was stimulated by demands made for safe, highly absorbent components to incorporate into female hygiene products, babies' disposable nappies (diapers), and incontinence products both to reduce the amount of material in each item and to improve their performance. Traditional absorbents such as wood pulp, bagasse pulp, and cotton linters can demonstrate absorption of up to 20 times the fibre weight (often somewhat less) but super-absorbent polymers are in a different league, as they can absorb water to become hydrogels and take in up to 400 times their own weight and some claim 1,000 times (much more than an ordinary hydrogel which is typically able to absorb its own weight in water). A further benefit is that the high-capacity hydrogel does not lose the absorbed liquid on squeezing. Incorporating super-absorbent polymers in granular form into absorbent products can lead to problems such as escape of granules and a slow rate of absorption into the interior of the grains, so the preference now is for fine super-absorbent fibres of around 30 μm even though they are more expensive. There is less possibility of fine particles being generated from super-absorbent fibres and of those escaping from the interior of the product than with a granular absorbent, and the other key reason is one of improved performance. Super-absorbent fibres absorb the moisture between the fibres first, before it penetrates into their interiors, and this occurs rapidly (in about 15 seconds), that quick response being a major advantage for an incontinence product.

Super-absorbent polymers consist of hydrophilic long-chain polymers cross-linked at well-spaced intervals so that whilst they can freely attract and become attached to water molecules, they cannot fully separate and enter into solution. They can be categorised in a similar manner to surfactants, i.e., on the basis of the presence, absence, type, and arrangement of electrical charges located on the cross-linked polymer chains, as non-ionic, anionic, cationic, or amphoteric including zwitterionic (polybetaines). Most commercially available super-absorbent-polymers hydrogels are anionic.

As regards their chemical composition, super-absorbent polymers can be made from:

(i) starch-PAN graft copolymers (the earliest types) or hydrolysed cellulose
(ii) polyacrylonitrile (PAN)
(iii) cross-linked polyacrylates and polyacrylamides
(iv) cross-linked copolymers of maleic anhydride

There was some interest in biodegradable high-amylopectin (waxy) starch-based super-absorbents created by blending the base material with synthetic super-absorbents and fibres (Thibodeau et al. 2014), leading to so-called SNAPs (safe and natural absorbent polymers) but the most conventional type of super-absorbent polymers is the anionic acrylics that consist of an open co-polymeric network based on partially neutralised acrylic acid or acrylamide.

The super-absorbent polymers used today are most usually the sodium salts of cross-linked acrylic homo-polymers (Matushek 2019), but a more sophisticated cross-linked acrylic terpolymer, prepared in part-neutralised form as its sodium salt and with its polymer-chain network held together by (infrequent but effective) ester links, may offer better overall performance. Converted into the form of 10 dtex fibres, it can be used as a component in the central non-woven layer of laminate fabrics, especially in applications such as diapers and incontinence products, absorbing 200× its own weight of water or 60× its own weight of saline solution and exhibiting good durability to laundering (50 cycles) (SAF 2021).

4.8 ELECTROACTIVE POLYMER FIBRES

There are four main categories of electroactive biomaterials: conductive polymers, piezoelectric polymers, photovoltaic materials, and electrets.

4.8.1 Conductive Polymers

Conductive polymers show electrical conductivity typically less than most metals, but not dissimilar to that of semiconductors. The major advantage of conductive polymers over metals is that they can offer the type of flexibility and recovery from deformation expected from a textile material. However, because these types of polymer are highly insoluble, it is necessary to add a dopant (a charge carrier) such as dodecylbenzene sulfonic acid to enable spinning of the polymers into filaments not only to make the resultant fibres/filaments less stiff and more manageable, but also because the retained dopant is essential in providing an enormous boost in electrical conductivity. Smaller dopants such as chloride ions are more readily lost from the fibres, and that action can be used to both assist and control drug delivery from the fibre. The most widely researched conductive polymers are polyaniline (PANI), poly-pyrrole (PPy), and polythiophene (Pth). More usually, it is its derivative, poly (3,4-ethylenedioxythiophene) (PEDOT), that is used because it possesses better all-round properties than Pth including improved chemical, electrical, environmental, and thermal stabilities and better electrical conductivity. All three conductive polymers exhibit good biocompatibility, hence their use in biosensors, neural implants, drug delivery devices, and in tissue engineering scaffolds, particularly in the form of nanofibres (Maiti, Das, and Sen 2017; Balint, Cassidy, and Cartmel 2014; see also Chapter 11).

4.8.2 Piezoelectric Polymers

Piezoelectric polymers become electrically polarised in response to the application of mechanical stress, and the reverse is also true, they will deform on the application of an electric charge. Such responses are rapid and the power requirements to achieve them are small, so this makes them attractive for the generation of electrical signals in sensors, and also as nano-generators in the case of electrospun versions of the piezoelectric polymer. There are subsets of piezoelectric materials, some of which may demonstrate pyroelectric properties (by responding to changes in temperature by emitting an electric signal) and others, ferroelectric polymers, whose polarisation can be reversed by the application of an electric field. PVDF, poly (vinylidene fluoride), falls into the last category and it is currently the most important piezoelectric polymer with the highest electromechanical response over a broad temperature range of all known synthetic polymers; the fact that having been electrospun to yield nanofibres, it can be adjusted to match its surface properties to that of the host environment whilst retaining its piezoelectric properties (Mokhtari et al. 2016), makes it an attractive material to employ in nanofibrous-textile-based bone bio-implants (Mirzaei et al. 2019). Piezoelectric textiles are also of interest for their antimicrobial action, which has been found for PLA (Ando et al. 2019) and Murata Manufacturing and Teijin Frontier in Japan have established a joint venture, Pieclex Co. Ltd., to exploit this property of PLA in items such as sportswear and underwear (Innovation in Textiles 2020). Given that antimicrobial treatments for surgical gowns, other medical textile PPE, and uniforms have been found to be largely ineffective in reducing the chances of the transfer of pathogens from contaminated items, perhaps piezoelectric materials should be further explored to determine whether they might be better able to yield the desired antimicrobial performance.

4.8.3 Photovoltaic Materials

The development of straightforward methods for producing photovoltaic fibres useable in textiles remains aspirational. The interest exists because they would create the possibility of fully integrated and flexible solar cells for powering active electronics in textiles (of use, for example, in 'intelligent' garments intended to provide continual feedback of physiological data from the wearer). Conventional photovoltaic cells use rigid silicon wafers, so these do not have the ability to be fully integrated or to meet the flexibility requirements. Currently, it is still necessary to resort to one of two alternatives, either to coat the fibre in yarns the successive layers of semi-conductor needed to make a sandwich device on top of conductive thin metal and conductive polymer layers prior to fabric manufacture, or to coat the fabric with those types of layers. Wilson and Mather were able to maintain reasonable flexibility achieve relatively good performance (10% efficiency) and through coating calendered polyester fabric with three layers of silicon/hydrogen alloy above a thin layer of aluminium on top of a coating of the intrinsically conductive polymer poly(3,4-ethylenedioxythiophene) polystyrene sulfonate (PEDOT:PSS) (Wilson and Mather 2019). Even so, it is expected that photovoltaic fibres would need to perform better than this.

4.8.4 Electrets

Electrets are polymers that have been caused to adopt a substantial semi-permanent electric charge either by corona charging or triboelectric charging. The polymer acts as a dielectric, hence if the polymer contains little if any moisture, this will help the retention of the charge by the polymer. Polypropylene fibres, because of their very low electrical conductivity and extremely low regain values at most humidity levels, are therefore very good at retaining electrical charge; hence they are widely deployed as electrets in filters. Electret filters are used in high-efficiency filtration because their effect is additive to the usual mechanical means of particle capture. They have the additional ability to trap airborne particles through coulombic attraction of charged particles and/or induced polarisation (dielectrophoresis) of uncharged particles, and by virtue of the resultant deflection of the particles, they are captured at the surface of the electret (Romay, Liu, and Chae 1998). Such performance is of particular importance in filters required to remove particles whose size coincides with that where mechanical capture is least effective, i.e., for particles with sizes within the range of 0.1–0.4 µm, a size range within which many aerosols and viruses lie. The presence of the electret significantly boosts performance in the filter in terms of collection of these particle or aerosol sizes.

4.9 OTHER MATERIALS

4.9.1 Carbon Fibres

Carbon fibres (fibres that contain at least 90% weight carbon) are manufactured by thermally treating a precursor fibre in an inert atmosphere in a process termed carbonisation. The precursor most used is PAN followed by pitch (less than 10% of the precursors used); graphite fibres, produced by heating to a graphitising temperature of around 2,500°C and containing at least 99% weight carbon, are much more unusual. The precursor PAN fibres in filament form are subjected to thermo-stabilisation at 200–400°C (a process that causes cross-linking in the precursor polymer prior to carbonisation), followed by carbonisation in an inert atmosphere at around 1,000°C. Flaws within the fibre fine structure greatly influence the tensile strength of the fibres as does the temperature used for carbonisation (due to effects at an atomic level on bonding) (Jones and Duncan 1971) and also the (beneficial) existence of an air gap during wet spinning of the PAN precursor (Wilms, Seide, and Gries 2013).

Carbon fibres are able to provide lightweight fabrics that can demonstrate high strength, flexibility, and fatigue resistance and they may be classified as either general purpose or high performance; the fibre may be cut short or kept as continuous filaments, and may be highly crystalline, amorphous, or partly crystalline, structural variations which affect their tensile properties – a high modulus of elasticity is demonstrated if the crystalline carbon layers within the fibre structure lie parallel to the fibre axis (Bajpai 2017, 17–23). For PAN-based carbon fibres, the conditions of temperature/time and tension applied during stabilisation during the heat treatment prior to carbonisation have important influences, caused, it is suggested, by their effects on crystallisation. Prolonging the duration of heat pre-treatment improved both tensile strength and modulus for carbon fibres produced by low-temperature carbonisation (800°C rather than the more usual 1300–1500°C) whereas increasing applied tension improved their tensile strength only up to a particular limit (15 mg per filament in the reported work), above which it deteriorated (Yun et al. 2009).

Carbon fibres can be manufactured into a range of textile structures as well as being incorporated into composites. In the healthcare sector, they have a structural role in orthotics, artificial limbs, braces, and medical equipment, often as the lightweight reinforcement for composites (Verdonk et al. 2012). Related nanomaterials such as carbon nanotubes have potential in drug delivery and in radiation therapy by targeted cellular internalisation and hence may revolutionise some aspects of medical care, though their safety profile in nanotube form needs to be fully elucidated (Jafar et al. 2016). It is possible to cause carbon nanotubes to become interlocked and aligned into single continuous-filament form which is expected to enhance their applicability by seamlessly connecting the nano- to the micro- and macro levels (Yadav et al. 2017; Rodiles et al. 2019).

4.9.2 Glass

Glass is a non-crystalline (amorphous) solid. Additives in the manufacturing process can be used to create bioactive glasses, and there are several types available based upon silicates, phosphate, and borate (Jones 2013). Bioactive glass is a brittle type of material that demonstrates a unique set of properties such as the ability to degrade at a controllable rate and convert to a hydroxyapatite-like structure (Rahaman et al. 2011; Baino, Fiorilli, and Vitale-Brovarone 2016). Bioactive sol-gel glasses were first synthesised in the 1990s. They have been used in regenerative medicine for osseous growth. In addition to creating a structure that mimics the trabecular architecture of cancellous bone, the sol preparation can be foamed to create a porous structure to more closely mimic certain biological materials. In addition to bone tissue engineering, bioactive glass has applications in wound dressings, ocular implants, and clinical imaging (Baino, Fiorilli, and Vitale-Brovarone 2016). Other glass compounds can be created into yarns that can be manufactured into fabrics, the bio-resorbable compounds being particularly attractive for the prospect of development of medical devices (Zhu et al. 2018). The original Bioglass® was created into a middle ear prosthesis and 10-year follow-up studies demonstrated that 4 out of 21 had failed but that the others maintained their original function (Jones 2013).

4.10 SUMMARY

The variety of fibre types and polymers employed in medical textiles has been significantly extended in recent years, not least because electrospun nanofibres have grown in importance and a wide range of bioabsorbable materials have been found to provide good performance in nanofibrous form as temporary support scaffolds for tissue repair and engineering. There is considerable focus on adjusting the composition of synthetic absorbable polymers to yield very specific kinds of performance; for example, in terms of drug delivery, alongside the usual temporary physical support, where to achieve this may be particularly challenging using a single polymer, and it has been proved possible to blend polymers to gain the desired behaviour. In other cases, the accent in the development of the fibres has been on improving their performance and making their use more economic, more environmentally acceptable, and more convenient, and in this respect, particular mention should be made to durable, launderable, super-absorbent fibres for incontinence wear and wound care. There is a continuing need for more attention to be paid across a wider range of personal protective items of clothing and hygiene products on designing reusable products rather than assuming it is only safe to use disposables. Alongside the performance of the polymer/fibre in the item itself, guiding principles in research and development into medical textile fibres and polymers should always be on:

- focusing design and development resources on the creation of reusable medical textile items for all high-volume applications, and
- deploying single-use medical textile items in low-volume applications only.

REFERENCES

Abu-Thabit, Nedal Y., and Abdel Salam Hamdy Makhlouf. "Smart textile supercapacitors coated with conducting polymers for energy storage applications." In *Industrial Applications for Intelligent Polymers and Coatings*, 437–477. Cham: Springer, 2016.

Ahmad, Mazatusziha, Mat Uzir Wahit, Mohammed Rafiq Abdul Kadir, Khairul Zaman Mohd Dahlan, and Mohammad Jawaid. "Thermal and mechanical properties of ultra-high molecular weight polyethylene/high-density polyethylene/polyethylene glycol blends." *Journal of Polymer Engineering* 33, no. 7 (2013): 599–614.

Akbari, Somaye, and Ryszard Michal Kozłowski. "A review of application of amine-terminated dendritic Materials in textile engineering." *The Journal of the Textile Institute* 110, no. 3 (2019): 460–467.

Aldini, Nicolò Nicoli, Milena Fini, and Roberto Giardino. "From Hippocrates to tissue engineering: Surgical strategies in wound treatment." *World Journal of Surgery* 32, no. 9 (2008): 2114–2121.

Al-Khateeb, Rami, and Iwona Olszewska-Czyz. "Biological molecules in dental applications: Hyaluronic acid as a companion biomaterial for diverse dental applications." *Heliyon* 6, no. 4 (2020): e03722.

Altman, Gregory H., Frank Diaz, Caroline Jakuba, Tara Calabro, Rebecca L. Horan, Jingsong Chen, Helen Lu, John Richmond, and David L. Kaplan. "Silk-based biomaterials." *Biomaterials* 24, no. 3 (2003): 401–416.

Ando, Masamichi, Daiji Tamakura, Takafumi Inoue, Kenichiro Takumi, Tetsuya Yamanaga, Ryo Todo, Koichi Hosoya, and Osamu Onishi. "Electric antibacterial effect of piezoelectric poly (lactic acid) fabric." *Japanese Journal of Applied Physics* 58 (2019): SLLD09.

Baino, Francesco, Sonia Fiorilli, and Chiara Vitale-Brovarone. "Bioactive glass-based materials with hierarchical porosity for medical applications: Review of recent advances." *Acta Biomaterialia* 42 (2016): 18–32.

Bajpai, Pratima. *Carbon Fibre from Lignin*. Singapore: Springer, 2017.

Balint, Richard, Nigel J. Cassidy, and Sarah H. Cartmell. "Conductive polymers: Towards a smart biomaterial for tissue engineering." *Acta Biomaterialia* 10, no. 6 (2014): 2341–2353.

Bansal, Sahas, and Pramod Raichurkar. "Review on the manufacturing processes of polyester-PET and nylon-6 filament yarn." *International Journal on Textile Engineering and Processes* 2, no. 3 (2016): 23–28.

Barnett, S. E., and S. J. Varley. "The effects of calcium alginate on wound healing." *Annals of the Royal College of Surgeons of England* 69, no. 4 (1987): 153.

Basit, Abdul, Wasif Latif, Sajjad Ahmad Baig, Abdur Rehman, Muhammad Hashim, and Muhammad Zia Ur Rehman. "The mechanical and comfort properties of viscose with cotton and regenerated fibers blended woven fabrics." *Materials Science* 24, no. 2 (2018): 230–235.

Bayer, Ilker S. "Hyaluronic acid and controlled release: A review." *Molecules* 25, no. 11 (2020): 2649.

BBC NEWS. "Vaginal mesh ban can be lifted with changes, NICE says." 2019. Accessed April 2, 2019. https://www.bbc.co.uk/news/health-47735253.

B.Braun. "Askina® 2 layer-system." 2021. Accessed May 8, 2021. https://www.bbraun.com/en/products/b1/askina-2-layer-system.html.

Bide, Martin, Matthew Phaneuf, Philip Brown, Geraldine McGonigle, and Frank LoGerfo. "Modification of polyester for medical uses." In *Modified Fibers with Medical and Specialty Applications*, 91–124. Dordrecht: Springer, 2006.

Bisanda, E. T. N., and Martin P. Ansell. "Properties of sisal-CNSL composites." *Journal of Materials Science* 27, no. 6 (1992): 1690–1700.

Borbély, Éva. "Lyocell, the new generation of regenerated cellulose." *Acta Polytechnica Hungarica* 5, no. 3 (2008): 11–18.

Böstman, O. M. "Absorbable implants for the fixation of fractures." *Journal of Bone and Joint Science* 73, no. 1 (1991): 148–153.

Cai, Zeng-xiao, Xiu-mei Mo, Kui-hua Zhang, Lin-peng Fan, An-lin Yin, Chuang-long He, and Hong-sheng Wang. "Fabrication of chitosan/silk fibroin composite nanofibers for wound-dressing applications." *International Journal of Molecular Sciences* 11, no. 9 (2010): 3529–3539.

Cao, Xinwang, Xianfeng Wang, Bin Ding, Jianyong Yu, and Gang Sun. "Novel spider-web-like nanoporous networks based on jute cellulose nanowhiskers." *Carbohydrate Polymers* 92, no. 2 (2013): 2041–2047.

Carlberg, Björn, Mathilda Zetterström Axell, Ulf Nannmark, Johan Liu, and H. Georg Kuhn. "Electrospun polyurethane scaffolds for proliferation and neuronal differentiation of human embryonic stem cells." *Biomedical Materials* 4, no. 4 (2009): 045004.

Chakrabarty, Gautam, Mayank Vashishtha, and Daniel Leeder. "Polyethylene in knee arthroplasty: A review." *Journal of Clinical Orthopaedics and Trauma* 6, no. 2 (2015): 108–112.

Chand, Navin, and S. A. R. Hashmi. "Mechanical properties of sisal fibre at elevated temperatures." *Journal of Materials Science* 28, no. 24 (1993): 6724–6728.

Chand, Navin, K. G. Satyanarayana, and P. K. Rohatgi. "Mechanical characteristics of sunhemp fibres." *Indian Journal of Textile Research* 11 (1986): 86–89.

Chandrasekhar, Harshinee. "Comparison of influence of vicryl and silk suture materials on wound healing after third molar surgery-A review." *Journal of Pharmaceutical Sciences and Research* 9, no. 12 (2017): 2426–2428.

Chavan, R. B., and A. K. Patra. "Development and processing of lyocell." *Indian Journal of Fibre and Textile Research* 29 (2004): 483–492.

Chao, Cui Yan, Mohan Prasath Mani, and Saravana Kumar Jaganathan. "Engineering electrospun multicomponent polyurethane scaffolding platform comprising grapeseed oil and honey/propolis for bone tissue regeneration." *PLoS One*13, no. 10 (2018): e0205699.

Chu, C. 2013 "Materials for absorbable and non-absorbable medical implants." In *Biotextiles as Medical Implants*, edited by King, M. W., Gupta, B. S., and Guidoin, R., 231–273. Cambridge, UK: Woodhead Publishing/The Textile Institute.

CORDIS. "Green nano-mesh; final report summary - Green nano-mesh (targeting hernia operation using sustainable resources and green nanotechnologies. An integrated Pan European approach)." 2016. Accessed January 27, 2020. https://cordis.europa.eu/project/id/263289/reporting.

CSIRO. "The chemical & physical structure of merino wool." 2015. Accessed June 3, 2021. https://csiropedia.csiro.au/wp-content/uploads/2015/01/6229343.pdf.

Deopura, B. L., and N. V. Padaki. *Textiles and Fashion; Materials, Design and Technology.* Edited by R. Sinclair. Oxford, UK: Elsevier/Woodhead, 2014; The Textile Institute Book Series, 97–114.

Derakhshan, Seyed Javad, Loghman Karimi, Salar Zohoori, Abolfazl Davodiroknabadi, and Lida Lessani. "Antibacterial and self-cleaning properties of cotton fabric treated with TiO_2/Pt." *Indian Journal of Fibre & Textile Research (IJFTR)* 43, no. 3 (2018): 344–351.

Drugwatch. "Polypropylene mesh." 2021. Accessed April 9, 2021. https://www.drugwatch.com/hernia-mesh/polypropylene/ Polypropylene Mesh.

Diamond, Claude, and Robert Louis Wormmell. "The manufacture and properties of "casein fibre"." *Journal of the Textile Institute Proceedings* 30, no. 7 (1939): 224–228.

Dobb, M. G., R. Murray, and J. Sikorski. "Specific labelling of thiol groups in mammalian keratin suitable for electron microscope studies." *Journal of Microscopy* 96, no. 3 (1972): 285–299.

DuPont. "History." 2021a. Accessed April 9, 2021. https://www.dupont.com/about/our-history.html.

DuPont. "Kevlar." 2021b. Accessed June 3, 2021 https://www.dupont.com/brands/kevlar.html.

DuPont. "Kevlar Aramid fibre technical guide." 2017. Accessed June 3, 2021. https://www.dupont.com/content/dam/dupont/amer/us/en/safety/public/documents/en/Kevlar_Technical_Guide_0319.pdf.

East, A. J. *Synthetic Fibres; Nylon, Polyester, Acrylic, Polyolefin*. Edited by McIntyre. Cambridge, UK: Woodhead/ Boca Raton, FL: CRC Press, and The Textile Institute, 2005, 95–166.

Edwards, S. L., S. J. Russell, E. Ingham, J. B. Matthews, and W. Mitchell. "Nonwoven scaffolds of improved design for the tissue engineering of the anterior cruciate ligament." In *Medical Textiles and Biomaterials for Healthcare*, Ist edition, edited by Anand, S.C. et al., 355–365 Cambridge, UK: Woodhead Publishing/The Textile Institute, 2005.

Faruk, Omar, and Mohini Sain, eds. *Biofiber Reinforcements in Composite Materials*. no. 51. Elsevier, 2014.

Fearing, Bailey V., and Mark E. Van Dyke. "In vitro response of macrophage polarization to a keratin biomaterial." *Acta Biomaterialia* 10, no. 7 (2014): 3136–3144.

Fich, Eric A., Nicholas A. Segerson, and Jocelyn KC Rose. "The plant polyester cutin: Biosynthesis, structure, and biological roles." *Annual Review of Plant Biology* 67 (2016): 207–233.

Fong, T. C., N. Saba, C. K. Liew, R. De Silva, M. Enamul Hoque, and K. L. Goh. "Yarn flax fibres for polymer-coated sutures and hand layup polymer composite laminates." In *Manufacturing of Natural Fibre Reinforced Polymer Composites*, 155–175. Cham: Springer, 2015.

Garvin, Kevin, and Connie Feschuk. "Polylactide-polyglycolide antibiotic implants." *Clinical Orthopaedics and Related Research®* 437 (2005): 105–110.

Geethamma, V. G., K. Thomas Mathew, R. Lakshminarayanan, and Sabu Thomas. "Composite of short coir fibres and natural rubber: Effect of chemical modification, loading and orientation of fibre." *Polymer* 39, no. 6–7 (1998): 1483–1491.

Gomide, Leandro Cardoso, Dagoberto de Oliveira Campos, Cleudmar Amaral Araújo, Gabriela Lima Menegaz, Rafael Silva Cardoso, and Sérgio Crosara Saad Júnior. "Mechanical study of the properties of sutures used in orthopedics surgeries." *Revista brasileira de ortopedia* 54, no. 3 (2019): 247–252.

Haigh, Jodie N., Tim R. Dargaville, and Paul D. Dalton. "Additive manufacturing with polypropylene microfibers." *Materials Science and Engineering: C*, 77 (2017): 883–887.

Holland, Chris, Keiji Numata, Jelena Rnjak-Kovacina, and F. Philipp Seib. "The biomedical use of silk: Past, present, future." *Advanced Healthcare Materials* 8, no. 1 (2019): 1800465.

Innovation in Textiles. "Smart textiles: Japanese develop piezoelectric fabric with antimicrobial performance." 2020. Accessed June 3, 2021. https://www.innovationintextiles.com/japanese-develop-piezoelectric-fabric-with-antimicrobial-performance/.

Interweave Textiles Ltd. "Dri-shield wipe clean polypropylene pillow." 2021. Accessed June 3, 2021. https://www.interweavetextiles.com/product/bedding/pillows-duvets/pillows/wipe-clean-polypropylene-pillow/

Islam, Saniyat, Lyndon Arnold, and Rajiv Padhye. "Application of chitosan on wool-viscose nonwoven for wound dressing." *Journal of Biobased Materials and Bioenergy* 7, no. 4 (2013): 439–443.

Islam, S., M. A. Rahman Bhuiyan, and M. N. Islam. "Chitin and chitosan: Structure, properties and applications in biomedical engineering." *Journal of Polymers and the Environment* 25, no. 3 (2017): 854–866.

Jaeger. "British style since 1884." 2019. Accessed April 7, 2019. https://www.jaeger.co.uk/heritage.

Jafar, Ali, Yaqoub Alshatti, and Ali Ahmad. "Carbon nanotube toxicity: The smallest biggest debate in medical care." *Cogent Medicine* 3, no. 1 (2016): 1217970.

Jayakumar, R., M. Prabaharan, P. T. Sudheesh Kumar, S. V. Nair, and H. Tamura. "Biomaterials based on chitin and chitosan in wound dressing applications." *Biotechnology Advances* 29, no. 3 (2011): 322–337.

Jiang, Jinhuan, Jiang Pi, and Jiye Cai. "The advancing of zinc oxide nanoparticles for biomedical applications." *Bioinorganic Chemistry and Applications* 2018 (2018).

Jing, Xin, Hao-Yang Mi, Max R. Salick, Travis M. Cordie, Xiang-Fang Peng, and Lih-Sheng Turng. "Electrospinning thermoplastic polyurethane/graphene oxide scaffolds for small diameter vascular graft applications." *Materials Science and Engineering: C* 49 (2015): 40–50.

Jones, B. F., and R. G. Duncan. "The effect of fibre diameter on the mechanical properties of graphite fibres manufactured from polyacrylonitrile and rayon." *Journal of Materials Science* 6, no. 4 (1971): 289–293.

Jones, Julian R. "Review of bioactive glass: From Hench to hybrids." *Acta Biomaterialia* 9, no. 1 (2013): 4457–4486.

Jones, Jana, Thomas F. G. Higham, David Chivall, Raffaella Bianucci, Gemma L. Kay, Mark J. Pallen, Ron Oldfield, Federica Ugliano, and Stephen A. Buckley. "A prehistoric Egyptian mummy: Evidence for an 'embalming recipe' and the evolution of early formative funerary treatments." *Journal of Archaeological Science* 100 (2018): 191–200.

Keller, A., M. Leupin, V. Mediavilla, and E. Wintermantel. "Influence of the growth stage of industrial hemp on chemical and physical properties of the fibres." *Industrial Crops and Products* 13, no. 1 (2001): 35–48.

Kew, S. J., J. H. Gwynne, D. Enea, M. Abu-Rub, A. Pandit, D. Zeugolis, R. A. Brooks, N. Rushton, S. M. Best, and R. E. Cameron. "Regeneration and repair of tendon and ligament tissue using collagen fibre biomaterials." *Acta Biomaterialia* 7, no. 9 (2011): 3237–3247.

Khalil, Yas, Neil Hopkinson, Adam Kowalski, and John Patrick Anthony Fairclough. "Characterisation of UHMWPE polymer powder for laser sintering." *Materials* 12, no. 21 (2019): 3496.

Khan, Belas Ahmed, Philip Warner, and Hao Wang. "Antibacterial properties of hemp and other natural fibre plants: A review." *BioResources* 9, no. 2 (2014): 3642–3659.

Kim, Sam Soo, Kyu Yul Ryoo, Jinsuk Lim, Byungjoo Seo, and Jaewoong Lee. "Cellulose fibers coated with m-aramid for medical applications." *Fibers and Polymers* 14, no. 3 (2013): 409–414.

King, M. W., R. G. Guidoin, K. R. Gunasekera, and C. Gosselin. "Designing polyester vascular prostheses for the future." *Medical Progress through Technology* 9, no. 4 (1983): 217–226.

Kumar, Akhil, and Alix Harnden. "Cellulase enzymes in wet processing of lyocell and its blends." *Textile Chemist & Colorist & American Dyestuff Reporter* 1, no. 1 (1999).

Kundu, Banani, Rangam Rajkhowa, Subhas C. Kundu, and Xungai Wang. "Silk fibroin biomaterials for tissue regenerations." *Advanced Drug Delivery Reviews* 65, no. 4 (2013): 457–470.

Kunert-Keil, Christiane, Tomasz Gredes, Annelie Meyer, Magdalena Wróbel-Kwiatkowska, Marzena Dominiak, and Tomasz Gedrange. "The survival and proliferation of fibroblasts on biocomposites containing genetically modified flax fibers: An in vitro study." *Annals of Anatomy-Anatomischer Anzeiger* 194, no. 6 (2012): 513–517.

Kushima, Hirofumi, Yukihiro Shoyama, and Itsuo Nishioka. "Cannabis. Xii. Variations of cannabinoid contents in several strains of Cannabis sativa L. with leaf-age, season and sex." *Chemical and Pharmaceutical Bulletin* 28, no. 2 (1980): 594–598.

Lee, Kuen Yong, and David J. Mooney. "Alginate: Properties and biomedical applications." *Progress in Polymer Science* 37, no. 1 (2012): 106–126.

Lewis, Ricki. "Unraveling the weave of spider silk." *Bioscience* 46, no. 9 (1996): 636–638.

Li, Xue, Lope G. Tabil, and Satyanarayan Panigrahi. "Chemical treatments of natural fiber for use in natural fiber-reinforced composites: A review." *Journal of Polymers and the Environment* 15, no. 1 (2007): 25–33.

Li, Yan, Yiu-Wing Mai, and Lin Ye. "Sisal fibre and its composites: A review of recent developments." *Composites Science and Technology* 60, no. 11 (2000): 2037–2055.

Lou, Ching-Wen, Ching-Wen Lin, Yueh-Sheng Chen, Chun-Hsu Yao, Zen-Shoung Lin, Chieh-Yu Chao, and Jia-Horng Lin. "Properties evaluation of tencel/cotton nonwoven fabric coated with chitosan for wound dressing." *Textile Research Journal* 78, no. 3 (2008): 248–253.

Mackenzie, David. "The history of sutures." *Medical History* 17, no. 2 (1973): 158–168.

Mani, Ganesh Kumar, John Bosco Balaguru Rayappan, and Dillip Kumar Bisoyi. "Synthesis and characterization of kapok fibers and its composites." *Journal of Applied Sciences* 12, no. 16 (2012): 1661–1665.

Maiti, Syamal, Dipayan Das, and Kushal Sen. "Flexible non-metallic electro-conductive textiles." *Textile Progress* 49, no. 1 (2017): 1–52.

Marino, Andrew A., Visit Malakanok, James A. Albright, Edwin A. Deitch, and Robert D. Specian. "Electrochemical properties of silver-nylon fabrics." *Journal of the Electrochemical Society* 132, no. 1 (1985): 68.

Matushek, C. "History of super absorbent polymer chemistry." 2019. Accessed February 21, 2019. https://m2polymer.com/2019/02/history-of-super-absorbent-polymer-chemistry.

Maya, John, Jacob, K. T. Varughese, and Sabu Thomas. "Green composites from natural fibers and natural rubber: Effect of fiber ratio on mechanical and swelling characteristics." *Journal of Natural Fibers* 5, no. 1 (2008): 47–60.

Medline Industries Ltd. "Single-use spun bond polypropylene surgical cap without elastic." 2019. Acessed June 3rd, 2021. https://www.medline.eu/uk/single-use-spunbond-polypropylene-surgical-cap-without-elastic

Mirzaei, Ali, Abbas Shapouri Moghadam, Mohamad Foad Abazari, Fatemeh Nejati, Sepehr Torabinejad, Mohamad Kaabi, Seyed Ehsan Enderami et al. "Comparison of osteogenic differentiation potential of induced pluripotent stem cells on 2D and 3D polyvinylidene fluoride scaffolds." *Journal of Cellular Physiology* 234, no. 10 (2019): 17854–17862.

Mokhtari, F., M. Salehi, F. Zamani, F. Hajiani, F. Zeighami, and M. Latifi. "Advances in electrospinning: The production and application of nanofibres and nanofibrous structures." *Textile Progress* 48, no. 3 (2016): 119–219.

Mooibroek, H., and K. Cornish. "Alternative sources of natural rubber." *Applied Microbiology and Biotechnology* 53, no. 4 (2000): 355–365.

Morris, H., and R. Murray. "Medical textiles." *Textile Progress* 52, no. 1–2 (2020): 1–127.

Mortimer, S. A., and A. A. Péguy . "Methods for reducing the tendency of lyocell fibers to fibrillate." *Journal of Applied Polymer Science* 60, no. 3 (1996): 305–316.

Morton, W. E., and J. W. S. Hearle . *Physical Properties of Textile Fibres* (4th ed.). Oxford, UK: Elsevier/Woodhead; The Textile Institute, 2008, 1–81.

Mudgil, Deepak. "The interaction between insoluble and soluble fiber." In *Dietary Fiber for the Prevention of Cardiovascular Disease*, 35–59. Academic Press, 2017.

Mukherjee, P. S., and K. G. Satyanarayana. "Structure and properties of some vegetable fibres." *Journal of Materials Science* 19, no. 12 (1984): 3925–3934.

Nadanathangam, Vigneshwaran, Sampath Kumar, A. A. Kathe, P. V. Varadarajan, and Virendra Prasad. "Functional finishing of cotton fabrics using zinc oxide–soluble starch nanocomposites." *Nanotechnology* 17, no. 20 (2006): 5087.

Najibi, S., R. Banglmeier, J. M. Matta, and Moritz Tannast. "Material properties of common suture materials in orthopaedic surgery." *The Iowa Orthopaedic Journal* 30 (2010): 84.

Namvar, Farideh, Mohamad Jawaid, Paridah Md Tanir, Rosfarizan Mohamad, Susan Azizi, Alireza Khodavandi, Heshu Sulaiman Rahman, and Majid Dehghan Nayeri. "Potential use of plant fibres and their composites for biomedical applications." *BioResources* 9, no. 3 (2014): 5688–5706.

Odent, J., Raquez, J. -M. and Dubois, P. 2015. "Highly toughened polylactide-based materials through melt-blending techniques." In *Biodegradable Polyesters*, Ist edition, edited by Fakirov, 235–274. Wiley, 2015.

Oral, Ebru, and Orhun K. Muratoglu. "Radiation cross-linking in ultra-high molecular weight polyethylene for orthopaedic applications." *Nuclear Instruments and Methods in Physics Research Section B: Beam Interactions with Materials and Atoms* 265, no. 1 (2007): 18–22.

Paladini, Federica, R. A. Picca, M. C. Sportelli, N. Cioffi, A. Sannino, and M. Pollini. "Surface chemical and biological characterization of flax fabrics modified with silver nanoparticles for biomedical applications." *Materials Science and Engineering: C* 52 (2015): 1–10.

Palza, Humberto. "Antimicrobial polymers with metal nanoparticles." *International Journal of Molecular Sciences* 16, no. 1 (2015): 2099–2116.

Pan, Zhen, and Jiandong Ding. "Poly (lactide-co-glycolide) porous scaffolds for tissue engineering and regenerative medicine." *Interface Focus* 2, no. 3 (2012): 366–377.

Patrucco, A., F. Cristofaro, M. Simionati, M. Zoccola, G. Bruni, L. Fassina, L. Visai et al. "Wool fibril sponges with perspective biomedical applications." *Materials Science and Engineering: C* 61 (2016): 42–50.

Paul, Willi, and Chandra P. Sharma. "Chitosan and alginate wound dressings: A short review." *Trends in Biomaterials & Artificial Organs* 18, no. 1 (2004): 18–23.

Peças, Paulo, Hugo Carvalho, Hafiz Salman, and Marco Leite. "Natural fibre composites and their applications: A review." *Journal of Composites Science* 2, no. 4 (2018): 66.

Perelshtein, Ilana, Guy Applerot, Nina Perkas, Geoffrey Guibert, Serguei Mikhailov, and Aharon Gedanken. "Sonochemical coating of silver nanoparticles on textile fabrics (nylon, polyester and cotton) and their antibacterial activity." *Nanotechnology* 19, no. 24 (2008): 245705.

Penalva, Rebeca, Irene Esparza, Maite Agüeros, Carlos J. Gonzalez-Navarro, Carolina Gonzalez-Ferrero, and Juan M. Irache. "Casein nanoparticles as carriers for the oral delivery of folic acid." *Food Hydrocolloids* 44 (2015): 399–406.

Pennell, Marissa Noelani. "Cell aggregate dissociation and filtration through the use of nylon woven mesh membranes." PhD diss., UC Irvine, 2016.

Perkin Elmer. "MPTG and structure of common polymers." 2019. Accessed June 26, 2019. https://www.perkinelmer.co.uk/CMSResources/Images/44-74863TCH_MPTGAndStructureOfCommonPolymers.pdf.

Pickering, Kim L., MG Aruan Efendy, and Tan Minh Le. "A review of recent developments in natural fibre composites and their mechanical performance." *Composites Part A: Applied Science and Manufacturing* 83 (2016): 98–112.

Pil, Lut, Farida Bensadoun, Julie Pariset, and Ignaas Verpoest. "Why are designers fascinated by flax and hemp fibre composites?" *Composites Part A: Applied Science and Manufacturing* 83 (2016): 193–205.

Pivec, T. et al. 2017 "Polyurethanes for medical use." *Tekstilec* 60, no. 3: 182–197.

Polymer Properties Database. "Thermophysical properties." 2015–2021. Accessed June 26, 2019. http://polymerdatabase.com/home.html.

Purnawati, Renny, Fauzi Febrianto, I. Wistara, Siti Nikmatin, Wahyu Hidayat, Seunghwan Lee, and Namhun Kim. "Physical and chemical properties of Kapok (Ceiba pentandra) and Balsa (Ochroma pyramidale) fibers." *Journal of the Korean Wood Science and Technology* 46, no. 4 (2018): 393–401.

Qin, Yimin, ed. *Medical Textile Materials*. Cambridge, UK: Woodhead Publishing, 2015.

Rahaman, Mohamed N., Delbert E. Day, B. Sonny Bal, Qiang Fu, Steven B. Jung, Lynda F. Bonewald, and Antoni P. Tomsia. "Bioactive glass in tissue engineering." *Acta Biomaterialia* 7, no. 6 (2011): 2355–2373.

Rahman, Mashiur, and H. E. D. M. Saleh. *Degradation of Polyesters in Medical Applications*. London, UK: IntechOpen, 2012.

Rajendran, Subbiyan, ed. *Advanced Textiles for Wound Care*. Cambridge, UK: Woodhead Publishing, 2018.

Ramachandran, Manoj, ed. *Basic Orthopaedic Sciences*. CRC Press, 2018.

Rana, S., S. Karunamoorthy, S. Parveen, and R. Fangueiro. "Life cycle assessment of cotton textiles and clothing." In *Handbook of Life Cycle Assessment (LCA) of Textiles and Clothing*, 195–216. Cambridge, UK: Woodhead Publishing, 2015.

Rasigha, T. et al. 2015 "Disposable natural scrubber from sisal and bamboo fibres." *International Journal of Engineering Research and Applications* 5, no. 11 part 3: 8–11.

Ratner, Buddy D., Allan S. Hoffman, Frederick J. Schoen, and Jack E. Lemons, eds. *Biomaterials Science: An Introduction to Materials in Medicine*. Amsterdam: Elsevier, 2013, 74–77.

Ratner, Stanislav, Amotz Weinberg, and Gad Marom. "Neat UHMWPE filament wound composites by crosslinking compaction." *Advanced Composites Letters* 12, no. 5 (2003): 096369350301200503.

Rattfält, Linda, Maria Lindén, Peter Hult, Lena Berglin, and Per Ask. "Electrical characteristics of conductive yarns and textile electrodes for medical applications." *Medical & Biological Engineering & Computing* 45, no. 12 (2007): 1251–1257.

Ravindra, S., Y. Murali Mohan, N. Narayana Reddy, and K. Mohana Raju. "Fabrication of antibacterial cotton fibres loaded with silver nanoparticles via "Green Approach"." *Colloids and Surfaces A: Physicochemical and Engineering Aspects* 367, no. 1–3 (2010): 31–40.

Restrepo-Flórez, Juan-Manuel, Amarjeet Bassi, and Michael R. Thompson. "Microbial degradation and deterioration of polyethylene–A review." *International Biodeterioration & Biodegradation* 88 (2014): 83–90.

Rezaie, Ali Bashiri, and Majid Montazer. "Polyester modification through synthesis of copper nanoparticles in presence of triethanolamine optimized with response surface methodology." *Fibers and Polymers* 18, no. 3 (2017): 434–444.

Rezvanian, Masoud, Mohd Cairul Iqbal Mohd Amin, and Shiow-Fern Ng. "Development and physicochemical characterization of alginate composite film loaded with simvastatin as a potential wound dressing." *Carbohydrate Polymers* 137 (2016): 295–304.

Richards A. F. "Synthetic Fibres; nylon, polyester, acrylic, polyolefin." Edited by McIntyre, J.E., 20–94. Cambridge, UK: Woodhead Publishing/Boca Raton, FL: CRC Press and The Textile Institute, 2005.

Ries, Michael D., and Lisa Pruitt. “Effect of cross-linking on the microstructure and mechanical properties of ultra-high molecular weight polyethylene.” *Clinical Orthopaedics and Related Research®* 440 (2005): 149–156.

Rigby, A. J., S. C. Anand, and A. R. Horrocks. “Textile materials for medical and healthcare applications.” *Journal of the Textile Institute* 88, no. 3 (1997): 83–93.

Rnjak-Kovacina, Jelena, Lindsay S. Wray, Kelly A. Burke, Tess Torregrosa, Julianne M. Golinski, Wenwen Huang, and David L. Kaplan. “Lyophilized silk sponges: A versatile biomaterial platform for soft tissue engineering.” *ACS Biomaterials Science & Engineering* 1, no. 4 (2015): 260–270.

Rocha, Marisa Cristina Guimarães, Lorena Rodrigues da Costa Moraes, and Norberto Cella. “Thermal and mechanical properties of vinyltrimethoxysilane (VTMOS) crosslinked high molecular weight polyethylene (HMWPE).” *Materials Research* 20, no. 5 (2017): 1332–1339.

Rockwood, Danielle N., Rucsanda C. Preda, Tuna Yücel, Xiaoqin Wang, Michael L. Lovett, and David L. Kaplan. “Materials fabrication from Bombyx mori silk fibroin.” *Nature Protocols* 6, no. 10 (2011): 1612.

Rodiles, X., V. Reguero, M. Vila, B. Alemán, L. Arévalo, F. Fresno, V. A. de la Peña O’Shea, and J. J. Vilatela. “Carbon nanotube synthesis and spinning as macroscopic fibers assisted by the ceramic reactor tube.” *Scientific Reports* 9, no. 1 (2019): 1–10.

Romay, Francisco J., Benjamin Y. H. Liu, and Soo-Jae Chae. “Experimental study of electrostatic capture mechanisms in commercial electret filters.” *Aerosol Science and Technology* 28, no. 3 (1998): 224–234.

Römer, Lin, and Thomas Scheibel. “The elaborate structure of spider silk: Structure and function of a natural high performance fiber.” *Prion* 2, no. 4 (2008): 154–161.

Ross, Samir A., and Mahmoud A. ElSohly. “The volatile oil composition of fresh and air-dried buds of Cannabis sativa.” *Journal of Natural Products* 59, no. 1 (1996): 49–51.

Rupp, Jurg. *Nonwovens Made of Cotton*. Textile World, Billian Publishing Inc., 2009.

SAF. “SAF FABRIC.” 2021. Accessed June 3, 2021. http://exploresaf.bluestorm.design/product-range.

Sakellarides, S. L. “Polyethylene napthalate (PEN).” In *Encylopedia of Polymer Science and Technology*, 4th edition, edited by Mark, H. F. Wiley, 2004.

Semo, Efrat, Ellina Kesselman, Dganit Danino, and Yoav D. Livney. “Casein micelle as a natural nano-capsular vehicle for nutraceuticals.” *Food Hydrocolloids* 21, no. 5–6 (2007): 936–942.

Shahzad, Asim. “Hemp fiber and its composites–A review.” *Journal of Composite Materials* 46, no. 8 (2012): 973–986.

Shao, Zhengzhong, and Fritz Vollrath. “Surprising strength of silkworm silk.” *Nature* 418, no. 6899 (2002): 741–741.

Shapira, Alina, Yehuda G. Assaraf, Dikla Epstein, and Yoav D. Livney. “Beta-casein nanoparticles as an oral delivery system for chemotherapeutic drugs: Impact of drug structure and properties on co-assembly.” *Pharmaceutical Research* 27, no. 10 (2010): 2175–2186.

Shavandi, Amin, Tiago H. Silva, Adnan A. Bekhit, and Alaa El-Din A. Bekhit. “Keratin: Dissolution, extraction and biomedical application.” *Biomaterials Science* 5, no. 9 (2017): 1699–1735.

Shirgholami, Mohammad Ali, Loghman Karimi, and Mohammad Mirjalili. “Multifunctional modification of wool fabric using graphene/TiO_2 nanocomposite.” *Fibers and Polymers* 17, no. 2 (2016): 220–228.

Shivers, Jr Joseph Clois. “Segmented copolyetherester elastomers.” U.S. Patent 3,023,192 issued February 27, 1962.

Sibaja, Bernal, Edward Culbertson, Patrick Marshall, Ramiz Boy, Roy M. Broughton, Alejandro Aguilar Solano, Marianelly Esquivel, Jennifer Parker, Leonardo De La Fuente, and Maria L. Auad. "Preparation of alginate–chitosan fibers with potential biomedical applications." *Carbohydrate Polymers* 134 (2015): 598–608.

Siritientong, Tippawan, Teerapol Srichana, and Pornanong Aramwit. "The effect of sterilization methods on the physical properties of silk sericin scaffolds." *Aaps Pharmscitech* 12, no. 2 (2011): 771–781.

Song, Fei, Li-Ming Zhang, Jun-Fei Shi, and Nan-Nan Li. "Novel casein hydrogels: Formation, structure and controlled drug release." *Colloids and Surfaces B: Biointerfaces* 79, no. 1 (2010): 142–148.

Svensson, René B., Tue Hassenkam, Colin A. Grant, and S. Peter Magnusson. "Tensile properties of human collagen fibrils and fascicles are insensitive to environmental salts." *Biophysical Journal* 99, no. 12 (2010): 4020–4027.

Tachibana, Akira, Yasunari Furuta, Hideyuki Takeshima, Toshizumi Tanabe, and Kiyoshi Yamauchi. "Fabrication of wool keratin sponge scaffolds for long-term cell cultivation." *Journal of Biotechnology* 93, no. 2 (2002): 165–170.

Tachibana, Akira, Sumika Kaneko, Toshizumi Tanabe, and Kiyoshi Yamauchi. "Rapid fabrication of keratin–hydroxyapatite hybrid sponges toward osteoblast cultivation and differentiation." *Biomaterials* 26, no. 3 (2005): 297–302.

Tausif, Muhammad, Abdul Jabbar, Muhammad Salman Naeem, Abdul Basit, Faheem Ahmad, and Thomas Cassidy. "Cotton in the new millennium: Advances, economics, perceptions and problems." *Textile Progress* 50, no. 1 (2019): 1–66.

Teli, M. D., and Javed Sheikh. "Extraction of chitosan from shrimp shells waste and application in antibacterial finishing of bamboo rayon." *International Journal of Biological Macromolecules* 50, no. 5 (2012): 1195–1200.

The Textile Institute. "Textile terms and definitions." 2021. https://www.ttandd.org/content/textile-terms-and-definitions and 11th edition. Edited by Denton, M.J. and Daniels, P.N. The Textile Institute, 2002.

Thibodeau, Claude, David Bergeron, Isabelle Bolduc, Claude Couture, and Nicolas Nourry. "Starch networks as absorbent or superabsorbent materials and their preparation by extrusion." U.S. Patent 8,710,212 issued April 29, 2014.

Thilagavathi, G., N. Muthukumar, and T. Kannaian. "Development and characterization of electric heating fabric based on silver coated nylon yarn." *Journal of Textile Engineering & Fashion Technology* 1, no. 6 (2017): 224–226.

Urbánek, Tomáš, Eliézer Jäger, Alessandro Jäger, and Martin Hrubý. "Selectively biodegradable polyesters: Nature-inspired construction materials for future biomedical applications." *Polymers* 11, no. 6 (2019): 1061.

United States Plastic Corp. "What's the difference between LDPE, LLDPE, MDPE, HDPE, XLPE and UHMW sheeting?" 2021. Accessed June 3, 2021. https://www.usplastic.com/knowledgebase/article.aspx?contentkey=508

van der Sluijs, M. H. J., and Lawrance Hunter. "A review on the formation, causes, measurement, implications and reduction of neps during cotton processing." *Textile Progress* 48, no. 4 (2016): 221–323.

Van Amber, Rebecca, Raechel M. Laing, Cheryl A. Wilson, Linda A. Dunn, and Tim Jowett. "Effect of sock type on foot health." *Textile Research Journal* 89, no. 18 (2019): 3871–3881.

Varaprasad, Kokkarachedu, Gownolla Malegowd Raghavendra, Tippabattini Jayaramudu, and Jongchul Seo. "Nano zinc oxide–sodium alginate antibacterial cellulose fibres." *Carbohydrate Polymers* 135 (2016): 349–355.

Verdonk, René, Lieven De Wilde, and Johan Berte. "Orthopedic arm and shoulder brace." U.S. Patent 8,142,379 issued March 27, 2012.

Vermette, Patrick, Hans J. Griesser, Gaétan Laroche, and Robert Guidoin. *Biomedical Applications of Polyurethanes*. Georgetown, TX: Landes Bioscience, 2001.

VERT (Virtual Education for Rubber Technology). "Reinforcing materials in rubber products." 2019. Accessed May 20, 2019. http://laroverket.com/wp-content/uploads/2015/03/reinforcing_materials.pdf.

Ramnath, Vijaya B., V. M. B. Manickavasagam, C. Elanchezhian, A. Rajendra Prasad, C. Kavin, B. Karthik Subramanian, and V. Rahul. "Investigation of tensile properties of manila fibre reinforced composite." In *Applied Mechanics and Materials*, vol. 766, 96–99. Trans Tech Publications Ltd, 2015.

Walgreen Health Solutions. "Edemewear® open toe stockinettes." 2020. Accessed June 17, 2020. https://www.walgreenhealthsolutions.com/product/edema-wear-stockinettes/.

Wang, Runkai, Chul ho Shin, Siho Park, Longzhe Cui, Daeik Kim, Joon-Seok Park, and Moonhee Ryu. "Enhanced antibacterial activity of silver-coated kapok fibers through dopamine functionalization." *Water, Air, & Soil Pollution* 226, no. 1 (2015): 1–9.

Wang, Xiaoqin, Tuna Yucel, Qiang Lu, Xiao Hu, and David L. Kaplan. "Silk nanospheres and microspheres from silk/pva blend films for drug delivery." *Biomaterials* 31, no. 6 (2010): 1025–1035.

Wang, Y. H., M. Zhao, Susan Anne Barker, P. S. Belton, and D. Q. M. Craig. "A spectroscopic and thermal investigation into the relationship between composition, secondary structure and physical characteristics of electrospun zein nanofibers." *Materials Science and Engineering: C* 98 (2019): 409–418.

Wilms, Christian, Gunnar Seide, and Thomas Gries. "The relationship between process technology, structure development and fibre properties in modern carbon fibre production." *Chemical Engineering Transactions* 32 (2013): 1609–1614.

Wilson, John I. B., and Robert R. Mather. "Photovoltaic solar textiles." In *Multidisciplinary Digital Publishing Institute Proceedings*, vol. 32, no. 1, p. 4, 2019.

Woodings, Calvin, ed. *Regenerated Cellulose Fibres*. Elsevier, 2001.

Xu, Sijun, Feng Zhang, Jiangchao Song, Yuki Kishimoto, and Hideaki Morikawa. "Preparation of silver nanoparticle-coated calcium alginate fibers by hyperbranched poly (amidoamine)-mediated assembly and their antibacterial activity." *Textile Research Journal* 86, no. 8 (2016a): 878–886.

Xu, Weibing, Bin Mu, Wenbo Zhang, and Aiqin Wang. "Facile fabrication of well-defined polyaniline microtubes derived from natural kapok fibers for supercapacitors with long-term cycling stability." *RSC Advances* 6, no. 72 (2016b): 68302–68311.

Yadav, Manishkumar D., Kinshuk Dasgupta, Ashwin W. Patwardhan, and Jyeshtharaj B. Joshi. "High performance fibers from carbon nanotubes: Synthesis, characterization, and applications in composites–A review." *Industrial & Engineering Chemistry Research* 56, no. 44 (2017): 12407–12437.

Yaltirik, M., K. Dedeoglu, B. Bilgic, M. Koray, H. Ersev, H. Issever, O. Dulger, and S. Soley. "Comparison of four different suture materials in soft tissues of rats." *Oral Diseases* 9, no. 6 (2003): 284–286.

Yan, Libo, Nawawi Chouw, and Krishnan Jayaraman. "Flax fibre and its composites–A review." *Composites Part B: Engineering* 56 (2014): 296–317.

Yun, Jeong-Hyeon, Bo-Hye Kim, Kap-Seung Yang, Yun-Hyuk Bang, Sung-Ryong Kim, and Hee-Gweon Woo. "Process optimization for preparing high performance PAN-based carbon fibers." *Bulletin of the Korean Chemical Society* 30, no. 10 (2009): 2253–2258.

Zhang, Feng, Xiaolan Wu, Yuyue Chen, and Hong Lin. "Application of silver nanoparticles to cotton fabric as an antibacterial textile finish." *Fibers and Polymers* 10, no. 4 (2009): 496–501.

Zhang, Qian, Chaojing Li, Jiayan Luan, Guoping Guan, Jing Lin, Fujun Wang, and Lu Wang. "Polycaprolactone/ultra-high molecular weight polyethylene partially absorbable suture with improved mechanical performances for tendon and ligament repair." *Textile Research Journal* 90, no. 19–20 (2020): 2123–2135.

Zhang, Xiao-yan, Chun-ting Duan, Ning Zhao, Hong Xiao, Mei-wu Shi, Xiao-li Zhang, and Jian Xu. "Facile fabrication of large scale microtubes with a natural template—Kapok fiber." *Chinese Journal of Polymer Science* 28, no. 5 (2010): 841–847.

Zheng, Yian, Jintao Wang, Yongfeng Zhu, and Aiqin Wang. "Research and application of kapok fiber as an absorbing material: A mini review." *Journal of Environmental Sciences* 27 (2015): 21–32.

Zhu, Chenkai, Ifty Ahmed, Andrew Parsons, Yunqi Wang, Chao Tan, Jingsong Liu, Chris Rudd, and Xiaoling Liu. "Novel bioresorbable phosphate glass fiber textile composites for medical applications." *Polymer Composites* 39 (2018): E140–E151.

5 Medical Textiles
Finishing

5.1 INTRODUCTION

Textile finishing is the final stage in the manufacture of textile and it is crucial in defining or adjusting the properties of the finished goods. Described below are the purposes of the finishing treatments applied to a wide range of fabrics:

(i) *Removal*, such as the removal of any naturally occurring substances from the fibres, agents that have been applied to facilitate fibre or yarn processing, contaminants. Natural waxy substances and coloured contaminants such as those present on cotton fibres plus lubricants that may have been applied to fibres during yarn manufacture are removed by scouring and bleaching. Any projecting surface fibre, if that is not wanted, can be removed by flame treatment.

(ii) *Rearrangement*, such as closing up the intersections between yarn in a fabric thereby rearranging the yarns and fibres into a denser and/or more-regular arrangement with improved dimensional stability – typically achieved by compressing the fabric in some way such as passing between heavy steel rollers (calendaring) under hydraulic compression; the rollers may be heated or unheated.

(iii) *Impregnation*, such as passing the fabric in open width through a trough containing a solution of an agent intended to modify the fabric's performance, then removing the excess by squeezing the fabric between stainless steel rollers. Adjustment of the amount of the agent taken up by the fabric can be very precise.

(iv) *Exhaustion*, accomplished by immersing the fabric in a solution of an agent with an affinity for the fibre type from which the fabric is made. This approach is used in dyeing for the application of direct dyes to cotton for example, and although exhaustion may not become complete, as with impregnation, adjustment in the amount of the agent taken up by the fabric can be very precise, this time by control over the concentration of the agent in the solution to begin with and ensuring that the time of treatment is sufficient for whatever degree of exhaustion is possible to be achieved.

(v) *Surface application*, achieved, for example, by virtue of a roller with its lower edge dipping into a trough containing a solution of an agent intended to modify the fabric's performance; the amount of solution being held on the roller is precisely controlled by a doctor blade located just above the

DOI: 10.1201/9781003170570-5

surface of the liquid in the trough. The fabric passes over the top surface of the wet roller picking up the solution of the agent either just or mainly on that particular side of the fabric. Alternatively, methods such as aerosol deposition can be used, and these have been shown to be highly effective means of applying nanoparticle finishes to fabrics (Feng et al. 2016).

(vi) *Surface modification*, for example, by plasma treatment (either in air or in a controlled atmosphere of a selected gas – depending on whether improved moisture absorption or moisture-repellency is required) or through surface deposition by methods such as vapour deposition or sputtering of a metal over the fabric surface to achieve antimicrobial effects or conductivity.

(vii) *Surface coating*, achieved, for example, by 'calendar spreading' of an elastomer or thermoplastic over the surface of the fabric by having set the rollers on the calendar a definite distance apart, so that the synthetic rubber or thermoplastic mass is attenuated to a thin uniform sheet, which is then pressed into the surface to achieve firm adhesion of the coating on that side of the fabric as it passes between the rollers (The Textile Institute, 2021).

(viii) *Heat treatment*, achieved, for example, by heated calendaring in open width or by carrying through a treatment chamber where the fabric is held in open width and follows a route up and down over a series of rollers with the intention of moving the fabric rapidly but causing it to dwell for sufficient time in the hot chamber for it to be heat set in the flat, pressed shape (at a temperature above the glass-transition temperature for thermoplastic fibres) and/or to cause the intended reaction with added agents (heat fixation).

For medical textiles, finishing addresses cleanliness considerations such as scouring, bleaching, and sterilisation, whether the density of the fabric and its surface need to be adjusted to prevent fluid penetration/strike-through on splashing, and also if the intended application of the medical textile requires the fabric to be fluid repellent and antimicrobial and/or absorbent but dry to the touch, as in a wound dressing (Liu, Xin, & Choi 2012; Zhu et al. 2018). If the material is intended for use in hospital, clinic, or care home furnishings such as curtains, screens, or similar semi-permanent applications, it should be treated with flame retardant to help to improve safety in that regard.

Sometimes the polymer or the structure and texture of a fabric may confer most of the required properties on the medical textile item without the need for any finishing agent to be applied, but most usually that characteristic will need to be enhanced by judicious selection and application of a specific chemical agent during finishing (Debabi et al. 2017). By the time the fabric reaches the finishing stage, there has already been considerable investment in its creation, so in finishing there needs to be a strong accent on care and precision in its further treatment. The way in which the agent is applied to material intended to become the medical textile, by pad-dry-heat fixation, for example, is, in fact, typically capable of being very precisely controlled so that exactly the right amount of the agent needed to achieve the necessary performance is taken up by the fabric. A crucial aspect that should always be addressed following treatment, is the application of an approved or agreed test procedure to ensure that the finished medical textile demonstrates the promised performance and that in the case of the reusable types of medical textiles, i.e., textiles for applications in which high numbers of the items or garments are routinely utilised, that such performance is durable to a realistic number of hospital/commercial laundering cycles (50+). Some useful aspects of finishing for personal protective equipment were addressed in a recent review (Karim et al. 2020), so it is unfortunate that within it artistic license was practised in one of the diagrams showing silver nanoparticles above the fabric coated with nanoparticles 'attacking' pathogens.

5.2 ANTIMICROBIAL FINISHES

There has long been interest in improving the performance of textiles intended for medical use against bacteria, fungi, and viruses, not only for implanted items but also to protect both patients and healthcare professionals from their contamination and spread. Some of the important terminology concerned with cleaning, sterilising, and maintaining hygiene according to the United States Food and Drugs Administration and the Environmental Protection Agency are:

- *sterilant* – chemical germicide which achieves sterilisation
- *high-level disinfectant* – a germicide which when used according to the instructions kills all microbial pathogens except for bacterial endospores when present in large numbers
- *intermediate-level disinfectant* – a germicide which when used according to the instructions kills all microbial pathogens except for bacterial endospores
- *low-level disinfectant* – a germicide which when used according to the instructions kills most vegetative bacteria and lipid-enveloped or medium-sized viruses

The setting of appropriate levels of hygiene across the healthcare environment was addressed by Spaulding in an article entitled 'Chemical Disinfection in the Hospital' (Spaulding, 1957, 1971). Originally proposed in 1957, the Spaulding Classification has become a widely used system for selecting treatments for the disinfection and sterilisation of surfaces in relation to the risks they pose, particularly those of reusable medical/surgical devices. There are, however, concerns that the classification and the related expectations of high-, intermediate-, and low-level disinfection now need to be adjusted to better address matters such as atypical tolerance, or the resistance profiles to disinfection processes now being demonstrated by microorganisms (McDonnel & Burke 2011). Even so, keeping those caveats in mind, the Spaulding Classification does still have the capacity to help in guiding the initial selection of methods for the reprocessing of contaminated medical devices. The system classifies a medical device as critical, semi-critical, or non-critical on the basis of risk to patient safety from contamination present on a device, and prescribes three levels of germicidal activity (sterilisation, high-level disinfection, and low-level disinfection) for the three classes of medical devices (critical, semi-critical, and non-critical) as shown in Table 5.1.

TABLE 5.1
Spaulding's Classification of Medical Equipment and Devices and the Required Levels of Processing/Reprocessing

Classification	Definition	Level of Processing/Reprocessing
Critical Equipment/ Device	Equipment/Device which enters sterile tissues including the vascular system.	Cleaning followed by sterilisation.
Semi-critical Equipment/Device	Device that comes in contact with non-intact skin or mucous membranes but does not penetrate them.	Cleaning followed by high-level disinfection (as a minimum); sterilisation is preferred.
Non-critical Equipment/Device	Equipment/device that touches only intact skin and not mucous membranes, or does not directly touch the patient.	Cleaning followed by low-level disinfection (in some equipment/ device cases, cleaning alone may be acceptable).

Various types of medical textiles fall into each of these categories:

- **Critical**, therefore needs to be sterile – items such as *sutures, scaffolds, and implants*
- **Semi-critical**, also preferable sterile – *dressings, bandages*
- **Non-critical**, needing at least to be made clean and hygienic – *bed linen, pyjamas/patient coverings, pillowcases, bedcovers, uniforms, bed-screens, furnishings*

The degree of difficulty in rendering the various types of pathogen inactive is shown in Figure 5.1.

Although a pathogen may become ineffective over time or by a simple/gentle disinfection treatment, if untreated it may pose problem in terms of further contamination because of the length of time it can persist on the surface upon which it has been transferred/deposited. Times may vary substantially depending on the virus and the nature of the material upon which the virus is deposited. The persistence of coronaviruses loaded onto a variety of surfaces has been measured and the data has been brought together and reported. The viruses tested were those of MERS (Middle East respiratory syndrome), HCoV (human coronavirus), TGEV (transmissible gastroenteritis virus), MHV (mouse hepatitis virus), and SARS (severe acute respiratory syndrome). The viruses persisted on hard surfaces for times between a few hours and up to 28 days depending on virus type and the load applied; HCoV persisted for less than 8 hours on surgical gloves whilst SARS persisted for between 1 hour and 2 days on disposable surgical gowns, depending on the load applied (Kampf et al., 2020). Regarding the surfaces in the working environment rather than those on personal protective equipment and medical devices, it was suggested that laboratory trials on COVID-19 fomites overemphasised the chance of transmission from those types of hard surfaces (Goldman, 2020) and it was shown that for two different hospital

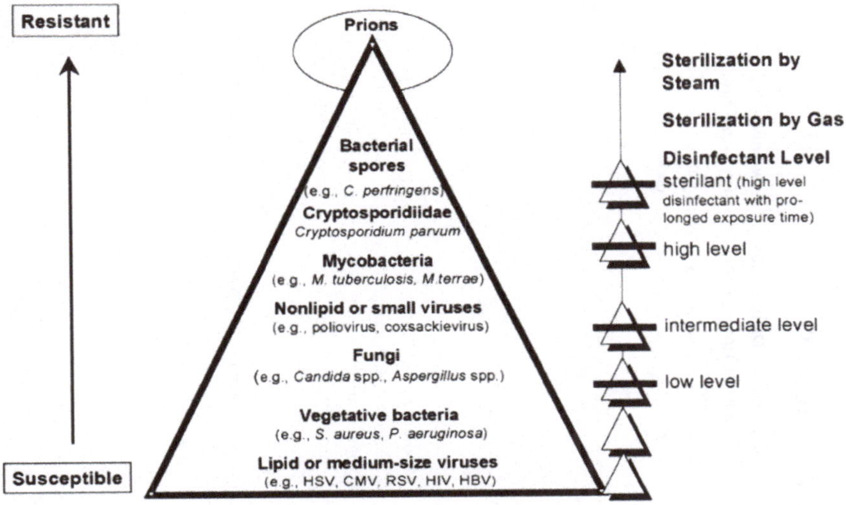

FIGURE 5.1 Relative susceptibility of various pathogens to disinfection treatments (Wendt, Frei, and Widmer 2015; reproduced with permission from John Wiley & Sons).

environments (an infectious-disease ward and emergency rooms in an Italian hospital) there was little chance in such real-life settings of environmental contamination leading to transmission of the virus if standard precautions were taken and standard cleaning operations carried out (Mondelli et al., 2021). Their conclusions were in line with the findings from trial inoculations on various surfaces, but these tests also showed that the virus persisted up to 7 days on the outer surface of a surgical mask and for a day on textile materials (Chin et al. 2020).

A range of acceptable disinfection and sterilisation treatments for use in healthcare facilities have been established by the Centers for Disease Control in the USA (CDC, 2019) as 'Methods for Disinfection and Sterilisation' in their *Guideline for Disinfection and Sterilization in Healthcare Facilities* (2008), last updated in May 2019. Table 5.2 provides details of their suggested treatments for a range of devices/materials likely to be present within a healthcare setting. There is no section in their table for textile materials, so those for smooth hard surfaces.

The details given in Table 5.2 were derived by the CDC from publications by Simmons and Rutala (Simmons 1983; Rutala, 1996, 1997, 1999). They indicate that sterilisation may take a time between 3 and 30 minutes using heat provided by steam or hot air, and that reasonably rapid sterilisation can be achieved by hydrogen peroxide gas plasma, but other treatments take some hours. Because of the presence of large numbers of intricately shaped pores in textile fibre, yarn, and fabric structures, and the need for penetration of disinfection agents, the time taken to achieve disinfection is greater for the textiles than for smooth, hard surfaces. When personal protective equipment items are in use, there is often the possibility of contamination during the early stages of wear, hence the clear need for medical textile materials to be able to be given safe and durable fluid repellent and antimicrobial treatments

TABLE 5.2
Methods for Disinfection and Sterilisation of Hard Surfaces (Centers for Disease Control, 2019)

Sterilisation Procedure	Time	High-Level Disinfection (Exposure Time 12–30 m at ≥20°C)	Intermediate Disinfection (Exposure Time ≥1 m)	Low-Level Disinfection (Exposure Time ≥1 m)
Heat sterilisation, including steam or hot air (see manufacturer's recommendations, steam sterilisation processing time from 3–30 minutes)	Manuf's recommend-ations	Glutaraldehyde-based formulations (>2% glutaraldehyde, caution should be exercised with all glutaraldehyde formulations when further in-use dilution is anticipated); glutaraldehyde (1.12%) and 1.93% phenol/phenate. One glutaraldehyde-based product has a high-level disinfection claim of 5 minutes at 35°C.	Ethyl or isopropyl alcohol (70–90%)	Ethyl or isopropyl alcohol (70–90%)
Ethylene oxide gas (see manufacturer's recommendations, generally 1–6 hours processing time plus aeration time of 8–12 hours at 50–60°C)	Manuf's recommend-ations	Ortho-phthalaldehyde (OPA) 0.55%	Sodium hypochlorite (5.25–6.15% household bleach diluted 1:500 provides >100 ppm available chlorine)	Sodium hypochlorite (5.25–6.15% household bleach diluted 1:500 provides >100 ppm available chlorine)
Hydrogen peroxide gas plasma (see manufacturer's recommendations for internal diameter and length restrictions, processing time between 45–72 minutes).	Manuf's recommend-ations	Hydrogen peroxide 7.5% (will corrode copper, zinc, and brass)	Phenolic germicidal detergent solution (follow product label for use-dilution)	Phenolic germicidal detergent solution (follow product label for use-dilution)

(Continued)

TABLE 5.2 (CONTINUED)
Methods for Disinfection and Sterilisation of Hard Surfaces (Centers for Disease Control, 2019)

Sterilisation Procedure	Time	High-Level Disinfection (Exposure Time 12–30 m at ≥20°C)	Intermediate Disinfection (Exposure Time ≥1 m)	Low-Level Disinfection (Exposure Time ≥1 m)
Glutaraldehyde-based formulations (>2% glutaraldehyde, caution should be exercised with all glutaraldehyde formulations when further in-use dilution is anticipated); glutaraldehyde (1.12%) and 1.93% phenol/phenate. One glutaraldehyde-based product has a high-level disinfection claim of 5 minutes at 35 °C.	10 h at 20–25 °C	Hydrogen peroxide (7.35%) and 0.23% peracetic acid; hydrogen peroxide 1% and peracetic acid 0.08% (will corrode metal instruments)	Iodophor germicidal detergent solution (follow product label for use-dilution)	Iodophor germicidal detergent solution (follow product label for use-dilution)
Hydrogen peroxide 7.5% (will corrode copper, zinc, and brass)	6 h	Wet pasteurisation at 70°C for 30 minutes with detergent cleaning	n/a	Quaternary ammonium germicidal detergent solution (follow product label for use-dilution)
Peracetic acid, concentration variable but 0.2% or greater is sporicidal. Peracetic acid immersion system operates at 50–56 °C	12 m at 50–56 °C	Hypochlorite, single-use chlorine generated on-site by electrolysing saline containing >650–675 active free chlorine (will corrode metal instruments)	n/a	n/a
Hydrogen peroxide (7.35%) and 0.23% peracetic acid; hydrogen peroxide 1% and peracetic acid 0.08% (will corrode metal instruments)	3–8 h	n/a	n/a	n/a

to counteract such contamination and for those fabrics and treatments to be able to withstand laundering, in order to ensure that their surfaces do not retain active pathogens.

The agents responsible for antimicrobial action in medical textiles operate on the basis of one of the following mechanisms.

(i) *Leaching* – prolonged release of the agents from the treated textile into any moisture coming into contact with the material (in much the same way as a direct dye is lost into the washing liquid on each wash) or by slow evaporation if the agent is a volatile organic compound (VOC). Microbes in the moisture (or nearby for the VOC) will be acted upon by the agent that has been released, a process often well-suited to implantable devices.

(ii) *Contact* – the agent is held in place by particular chemical groups on the fibre-forming polymer or those on a selected carrier attached to the fibre. They remain in position and have their effect only upon microbes which come into contact with the fabric.

(iii) *Photocatalytic oxidation* – as is the case with certain of the 'contact' types, the agent is held in place by a selected carrier, but in this case rather than activity being initiated by contact with a microbe, it occurs because of the energy received on exposure to light. A high amount of energy (associated with the near-UV) is necessary unless the active agent is doped, for example, with a nano-metallic additive, before application.

The research record bears out that a lot of attention has been given in recent years to the development of antimicrobial textiles. A search conducted in Pubmed®/Medline® revealed that a total of 3,197 research papers about medical textiles were published since the year 2000, over half of them (1,785) within the last 5 years; the largest sub-category over the whole period was antimicrobial textiles, accounting for 2,049 papers. Most reported methods for achieving antibacterial and antifungal activity worked on the basis of being applied as a finish to the textile material with just over 25% taking the alternative approach of incorporating the active/protective agent in the fibre-forming polymer and only a single paper reported the application of an agent and testing of the treated fabric to demonstrate its antiviral activity (Parthasarathi & Thilagavathi 2015).

Most of the surge in research outputs on the development of effective antimicrobial textiles is attributable to successes in nanoscience and technology (Mishra et al. 2014), enabling the application of nanometals such as nano silver, nano metal oxides such as zinc oxide and nano titanium dioxide, copper oxide, iron oxide, and to a lesser extent as yet, boron, zirconium oxide, graphene oxide, and carbon nanotubes (either as the active agent itself or to enhance the durability of the agent). Although the term 'nanotechnology' is used here, much of what has been achieved has depended only on nanoparticulate material being taken up by the textile rather than on ensuring that it was arranged in any particular pattern. This would not satisfy members of the Hohenstein Institutes, because they would quite rightly expect more than just the application of a nanomaterial to a textile by a traditional finishing treatment before using the term 'nanotechnology':-'Nanotechnology is dealing with production and/or processing technologies leading to systematic alignment of functional structures consisting of particles with size-dependent properties' (Beringer 2007). Currently, nanoparticles for antibacterial and antifungal activity are still being applied mainly by traditional finishing treatments with around twice as many papers focused on the finishing approach rather than incorporation of the active/protective agent in nanoparticulate form into the fibre-forming polymer itself. Where incorporation has been deployed, however, it has yielded both good antimicrobial performance and excellent durability.

Also noticeable is the emergence of chitosan as a widely used fibre pre-treatment not only to enhance uptake and adhesion of the nanoparticulate finishes but also to act as an antibacterial agent itself. Interest in nanofibre scaffolds for tissue growth, pre-treated to yield antibacterial action and more now in the form of electrospun yarns rather than as webs (Mokhtari et al. 2016), has grown steadily over just the past 10 years. Additional methods to assist in achieving antimicrobial textiles include plasma treatments applied to modify surface properties and confer anti-bacterial action itself or enhance uptake and retention of various antimicrobial finishing agents (Shahidi et al. 2014). While both successful and environmentally acceptable, and useful in preparing multifunctional finishing treatments (Irfan et al. 2019), plasma treatments have been less widely employed for those purposes than chitosan, although nitrogen-plasma treatment has been used to enhance chitosan's antibacterial effectiveness and render it rechargeable as is the case for N-halamines (Zhou & Kan 2014). Cyclodextrins may be used as an alternative to metal or metal-oxide nanoparticles; they possess a further advantage in that they also demonstrate an ability to hold and control the release of active agents, drugs, and other partly hydrophilic/partly lipophilic molecules at the fibre surface and release them at a predictable rate.

Environmental considerations can easily be overlooked. The main accent with antimicrobial treatments for textiles has to be on their effectiveness, but consideration should also be given to their environmental acceptability wherever possible. Rather than being considered as the source of potential pollutants, more attention could be given to the potential of antimicrobial-treated medical textiles to make a huge contribution to improving the ecological performance of hospitals by reducing the consumption of traditional disinfectants. For example, it is estimated that hospitals consume 2 tonnes of glutaraldehyde and 800 kg of chlorine per 1,000 beds per annum (Boillot et al. 2008) and much of this might always have to remain, but any possible reduction should be welcome. Antimicrobial-treated medical textiles could help in some ways, but the way agents are applied to a fabric needs to be carefully selected in order to achieve performance without the agents becoming significant pollutants themselves. The report from a project funded by the European Union 'COST' programme illustrates the problems that may arise if an inappropriate method of application is employed. The project was carried out to provide an assessment of the potential eco-toxicological effects of antimicrobial surface coatings. It was found that silver-based coatings were the most prevalent followed by those based on titanium, copper, zinc, chitosan, and quaternary ammonium compounds.

Although most agents were present because of their antimicrobial action, chitosan and titanium were mainly used as carriers for release-based antimicrobial ingredients such as conventional antibiotics. Published data on the eco-toxicological effects of the antimicrobial coatings was scarce but what did exist showed that silver, copper, and zinc are often released in substantial amounts (up to 100%) from such coatings into the aqueous environment, which is not surprising given that the way in which they work is by leaching from the antimicrobial-loaded textile (because leaching will also take place during laundering). Although the total amount of agent released into the environment from medical textiles applications is currently small compared with the quantities of traditional disinfectants, the review concluded that caution should be exercised in widening the use of antibacterial-coated textiles (Rosenberg et al. 2019). For these reasons we would suggest that future research and development into antimicrobial agents for medical textiles should focus on replacing those which depend on leaching metal or metal ions out onto microbes for their antimicrobial activity treatments with others which achieve both effectiveness and durability through embedment, attachment, or covalent bonding to the fibres.

Some proposed antimicrobial treatments make particular claims to being 'green' (Ravindra et al. 2010), and attention has also been given to the antibacterial properties of 'naturally-occurring antimicrobials' for the treatment of textiles, such as those derived from plant extracts (Murugesh Babu & Ravindra 2015), and others in natural dyes which arise from the presence of tannins, flavonoids, and quinonoids (Pal et al. 2016); more work needs to be done to demonstrate their effectiveness and durability under conditions which realistically reflect everyday hospital use.

5.2.1 Inorganic Antimicrobial Finishes

Copper has long been recognised as offering effective antimicrobial action following its introduction in the 18th century by the British Royal Navy as cladding for the hulls of their ships to prevent biofouling. For medical textiles, copper oxide is the favoured copper antimicrobial, but except for a few instances, there has not been a great deal of work published on copper oxide as an antimicrobial. Copper oxide microparticles of between 1.5 and 2.0 μm prepared by the controlled reduction of alkaline Cu(II)-tartaric acid complexes were applied to fabrics using a pigment dyeing binder system and a pad-dry process to yield 250–270 mg of copper per kilogram of fabric. The product exhibited excellent reduction in viability of 100% for *Staphylococcus aureus* and 84% for *Klebsiella pneumoniae* as estimated by the ASTM E2149 antimicrobial test. Although simulated wash processes reduced the copper content to between 50 and 60%, antibacterial activity remained high at 99% and 78%, respectively, indicating potential for it to become a useful, simply made antibacterial product (Turalija et al. 2015). Copper oxide has also been applied to polyester fabric in nanoparticulate form and combined with fatty acids to yield high-level antibacterial performance coupled with so-called super-hydrophobicity and low cytotoxicity (Rezaie, Montazer, & Mahmoudi 2019). Research and development into the performance and application of copper oxide as an antimicrobial agent remains lower than for zinc, silver, and titanium, but perhaps the most important outcome from research into its use has emerged from carefully designed experiments in real settings which showed that copper impregnation of textiles used alongside copper surfaces was effective in bringing about reductions in 'healthcare-associated infections' (HCAIs) in different hospital settings, namely:

- wards for chronic ventilator-dependent patients (Marcus et al. 2017)
- a long-term care brain injury ward (Lazary et al. 2014)
- an acute care community hospital setting (Sifri et al. 2016)

Copper may not always be the best choice for antibacterial fabrics, but rather than focusing on the copper treatment, what this group of outcomes should be taken to indicate is that the search for acceptable, cost-effective antimicrobial medical textiles is extremely worthwhile, because in combination with disinfected hard surfaces, they can help bring about reductions in HCAI indicators in environments where patients are most vulnerable.

Zinc-based antimicrobial finishes are broad-spectrum agents which can be effective against bacteria, fungi, and algae. The zinc finish may be applied in the form of zinc salts, nanoparticles, or zinc-containing compounds. One such compound is zinc pyrithione, which itself may be encapsulated to improve its ease of application as a finish to a textile material and to enhance safe handling, as is the case for ZPTech® products (Microban® 2021; Microban®, Huntersville, NC, USA). Of the zinc salts, the water-soluble zinc chloride is taken up by cotton, nylon, and polyester fabrics and has been shown to be more effective and durable to rubbing on polyester than colloidal zinc oxide, apparently because it causes some hydrolysis of ester groups at the fibre surface to enable it to become bonded to the fibre, whereas the colloidal zinc oxide is just deposited on the fibre surface by sedimentation (Holt et al. 2018). The durability of the antimicrobial treatment to rubbing is always important with an antimicrobial treatment for PPE or for uniform clothing as this represents one way through which contamination can easily be transferred from one healthcare worker to another, or to a patient. The treatment applied in the work of Holt et al. (2018) was intended as a residual treatment aimed at providing antimicrobial action on existing medical textile products rather than as a fabric finish and could be useful as an interim measure to apply during the remainder of existing items' lives before their replacement by items made from effective antimicrobial-finished textiles. As a residual antimicrobial treatment, zinc chloride was much more durable on the textiles than alcohol-based disinfectants, demonstrating an ability to inhibit growth for over 30 days and to withstand drying in a commercial dryer following treatment in the solution. It would of course need to be re-applied after every laundry cycle, because of its water solubility. Zinc nanoparticles applied by sonochemical means showed antibacterial activity but most of this was lost after ten laboratory wash cycles (Petkova et al. 2016), whereas zinc nanoparticles and gallic acid applied by sonochemical means and bonded to the fibre by enzymatic crosslinking of the gallic acid were attached durably to cotton and held in place sufficiently well by the adhesive generated that way to survive 60 laundry cycles and still retain 60% of its original activity (Salat et al. 2018). Zinc oxide is preferred over other zinc compounds because of its low toxicity and its high effectiveness, which is based on the release of hydrogen peroxide, and also because like other zinc compounds it is uncoloured and cost-effective to apply, and more effective against *S. aureus* because of its greater affinity to that bacterium than *E. coli*. As is also the case for certain titanium dioxide and silica nanofinishes, zinc oxide can be used to create a super-hydrophobic surface on cotton fabrics when zinc oxide nanorods are applied in combination with a silane (Xu & Cai 2008), in this case, *n*-dodecyl trimethoxysilane. An antibacterial super-hydrophobic fabric exhibiting abrasion resistance can also be prepared without recourse to the use of silanes, by doping zinc oxide nanoparticles with magnesium ions prior to spin coating (Shaban, Mohamed, & Abdallah 2018).

Of all metals employed in medical textiles for their antibacterial function, and particularly because of its effectiveness against both gram-positive and gram-negative bacteria, *silver* is by far the most widely used. It can be applied in the form of metal salts, metal wires, metal coatings, and metal nanoparticles, but the nanosilver examples have become the most prolific on account of their broad-spectrum antibacterial activity combined with durability to repeated use and to laundering. There is some likelihood of it discolouring the fabric, an effect which is of little importance in products such as men's socks or support hosiery but may be undesirable in other items; the colour formation can be eliminated by incorporating fine particles of silver sodium hydrogen zirconium phosphate instead of metallic silver. Alternatively, discolouration can be reduced to an acceptable level by lowering the addition of nanosilver, but of course, only if antibacterial effectiveness can be maintained. Such an effect has been shown to be achievable by aerosol finishing with silver nanoparticles to a loading of 10 ppm of silver (an order of magnitude less than that applied by traditional wet routes such as pad-dry-heat fixation, but effective against both gram-positive and gram-negative bacteria because 10 ppm is the point at which increases in effectiveness level off; Feng et al. 2016). The aerosol nano-finishing approach was described as low-cost, scalable, and environmentally benign and the work done up to this point accurately described as 'proof of concept,' because although it illustrated its potential, more work would need to be done to determine the treatment's durability and performance in the real-life setting. Silver nanoparticles may be applied alone and can be effective, but their durability is much improved if they are linked more firmly to the fabric. One such example employed a hyper-branched/dendritic amine-terminated polymer to entrap silver nanoparticles after which the amino-active silver nanoparticles were grafted onto oxidised cotton fabric; antibacterial activity remained high even after 50 wash cycles (Zhang et al. 2013). A simpler process of silver nanoparticle attachment combined them with carboxymethylchitosan covalently bonded to cotton through ester linkages which meant that the silver nanoparticles could be held in place by coordinate bonding with the amine groups of the carboxymethylchitosan (Xu et al. 2018). The treated fabric retains a high level of antibacterial action even after 50 wash cycles and can be applied by a one-pot process which should prove an attractive feature industrially.

Just as it is possible to prepare super-hydrophobic fabrics by treatment with zinc oxide or titanium dioxide nanoparticles and then a silane, so it is possible to achieve the same effect on cotton with silver nanoparticles produced by reduction of the silver/ammonia complex $[Ag(NH3)_2]^+$ with glucose followed by treatment with hexadecyltrimethoxysilane. Not only was the fabric superhydrophobic, but the silver nanoparticles were sufficiently densely packed to render the fabric conductive and it also exhibited high antibacterial activity against *E. coli* (Xue et al. 2012).

Of several more traditional ways by which silver can be introduced into a fabric, all of which can be effective in some way in terms of antimicrobial action, there are ones in the form of silver salts, silver wires, silver coatings, and silver nanoparticles applied as a finish or by mixing with the polymer prior to extrusion, but those made by mixing nanosilver with the polymer prior to extrusion typically show the best durability. An example was described which demonstrated the high durability to repeated laundering for items made from such fabrics for either 100 home laundry cycles or 100 cycles of the more aggressive commercial laundering by still showing high reductions in colony-forming units by both ram-positive and gram-negative bacteria as assessed by AATCC 100 test method (lower than the 99.99% achieved against the gram-positive *S. aureus*, but for the gram-negative *Klebesiella pneumoniae* still over 92.5% after the repeated commercial laundry processing.

Titanium dioxide (TiO_2) has been used as a delustrant for synthetic fibres since the 1960s because otherwise the yarns are too transparent for use in apparel wear. To accomplish this delustering function, the TiO_2 in powder form is mixed into the molten polymer before extrusion, and in the filaments/fibres that are formed it scatters incident light thereby rendering them opaque. When the titanium dioxide is in the form of nanoparticles, however, its strong interaction with light makes it useful in antibacterial and so-called self-cleaning medical textile applications. Its interaction with light is one whereby it absorbs energy and this lifts electrons up into the conductive level, where that energy can then be released and transferred to bacteria, fungal spores, or viruses, disrupting their normal functions and rendering them uninfective. The energy requirement to achieve the desired electron promotion effect for photocatalytic attack on microorganisms is high and the light required therefore has to be from the high-energy end of the electromagnetic spectrum, i.e., the near-ultraviolet region. Fortunately, in combination with silver or silicon dioxide nanoparticles, the incident energy requirement is lowered and the same effect can be achieved by light from within the visible region of the spectrum. Although there was hope that nanosilver-treated fabrics might be able to exhibit broad-spectrum antimicrobial effectiveness, including antiviral action, nothing has emerged in the literature to indicate antiviral action at a useful level, at least not by adequate testing of that or any other finishing treatment (or by incorporation of an active agent in the fibre-forming polymer) apart from one exception, which involves TiO_2 rather than silver. A nano-composite finish of nano-titanium dioxide/methylene blue was applied to a three-layer barrier fabric consisting of a PET outer layer, a microporous membrane middle layer, and an inner layer made of non-woven viscose rayon. The fabric exhibited light-activated antiviral properties (Parthasarathi & Thilagavathi 2015).

Titanium dioxide has also been applied together with a fluorosiloxane in a single-step method to yield super-hydrophobicity (contact angle with water 156°; sliding angle <10°) coupled with self-cleaning, a sought-after type of performance when coupled with antimicrobial action in protective wear for healthcare personnel

(Mitchell, Spencer, & Edmiston 2015); moreover, preliminary tests indicated that the treatment might be durable to laundering (Li et al. 2015). A much closer approximation to the multifunctional finish requirement may be that reported more recently, based on immersion of cotton fabric in a solution of TiO_2 nanoparticles and the fluoroalkylsilane, perfluorodecyltriethoxysilane (PFDTS) then removing and heating it to 120°C (Tudu, Sinhamahapatra, & Kumar 2020). The product exhibited a contact angle of 169.3° with a tilting angle of 6.3° (super-hydrophobic), durable for up to 20 laundry cycles and it exhibited antibacterial properties. It has been tested on tea, turmeric water, milk, mud water, urine, and blood and liquids of lower surface tension such as glycerol and ethylene glycol, and shown to perform well in the laboratory against being struck by droplets with varying levels of impact up to splash, so now it should be put to the test in a realistic environment as would be encountered by medical garments.

Silicon is most often applied to fabrics in the form of silicon dioxide (silica) nanoparticles in support of metallic antibacterial agents such as nanosilver and nano titanium dioxide, or in the form of silanes to achieve fluid repellency, or both silica nanoparticles and silanes. One treatment used silica to envelop silver nanoparticles to achieve a core-shell structure of silver nanoparticles as the core within a silica shell (SiO_2@ AgNPs). The SiO_2@ AgNPs were then treated with silane. The resultant product was cross-linked to the cotton fabric and exhibited antibacterial properties (Mohamed et al. 2017). Cotton fabric treated with silica nanoparticles plus a water-repellent finish exhibited super-hydrophobicity and was more economic because of the low add-on requirement (0.1%) of the water repellent (Bae et al. 2009).

5.2.2 Organic Antimicrobial Finishes

The aim with *quaternary ammonium compounds (QACs)* in recent applications has been to ensure their firm attachment to the fibre while retaining a high level of antimicrobial action. A variety of attachment mechanisms have been used. For example, a betaine was used as the finishing agent for preparing antibacterial fabrics through ester linkage between the carboxyl group of the betaine and the hydroxyl groups of the cellulose fibres of fabrics; the quaternary ammonium moiety of this compound exerted the antibacterial effect. Analyses showed that the antibacterial efficiencies of betaine-modified cotton fabrics against *E. coli* and *S. aureus* were 99.0 and 99.3%, respectively, and that the fabrics were durable to laundering with antibacterial action remaining greater than 91.5% after 20 washing cycles; cytotoxicity tests showed the modified fabrics were safe to wear (Duan et al. 2020). In other successful cases, antibacterial action and its durability was achieved with a quaternary ammonium salt plus a sulfopropylbetaine (Zhang et al. 2018, 2020), or by an isocyanate group using a dip-pad-dry application process (Gu et al. 2018), or coupled with perfluorination to yield both superhydrophobicity and antimicrobial effects (Lin et al. 2018; Song et al. 2019), or were applied in nanoparticulate form (Kim, Kim, & Rhee 2010); they may also be used in combination with N-halamines (Liang et al. 2006).

N-halamines offer another effective option. A major issue in using chlorine, bromine, or iodine as disinfectants is one of stability, but there is no such problem with their organic derivatives, the N-halamines, a diverse class of rechargeable biocides in the form of amines, amides, or imides, which can form covalent bonds with halogens (Liang et al. 2007). The oxidative halogen ion (chlorine, bromine, or iodine) in the N-halamine is stabilised but biocidal (Kocer et al. 2011). They are inexpensive and unlike many other biocides used for antimicrobial applications, N-halamines show rapid inactivation of a broad spectrum of microorganisms (gram-positive and gram-negative bacteria, yeasts, fungi, and viruses) and do not exhibit any evidence of bacterial resistance.

N-halamines can be applied as a coating by synthesising them using the sol-gel process and then applying by pad-dry-cure (Ren et al. 2008), and it is possible by careful choice of coating or by covalent attachment to surfaces that the treatment will show great durability. It did not prove necessary, for example, following epoxide tethering attachment of three different heterocyclic N-halamines to cotton, to recharge any of the three N-halamine coatings even after 50 wash cycles (Cerkez et al. 2012). Covalent attachment was achieved for cotton by reaction with methylene-bis-acrylamide and then its conversion into a non-cyclic N-halamine by dilute sodium hypochlorite solution. The agents used were inexpensive and readily available commercially, treatment was mild and did not cause damage to the cotton, it was highly effective against both gram-positive and gram-negative bacteria, and it was rechargeable. Antimicrobial testing showed that the treated cotton inactivated 5.78×10^7 CFU/mL of *S. aureus* and 7.58×10^8 CFU/mL of the serotype of *E. Coli* named *E. coli* O157:H7 completely within 1 minute of contact, and following 50 wash cycles, although the remaining oxidative chlorine fell from 0.43 to 0.06%, it was able to be recovered to 0.30% via a simple re-chlorination using dilute NaOCl (Tian et al. 2017). Similarly, good results have been achieved by UV-photo-initiated thiolene click chemistry to apply the halamine precursor (Ma et al. 2019a; Wen et al. 2020).

Considering N-halamines as a group, the long-term nature of their halogen stability and antimicrobial functionality does depend on their chemical composition, but they have been successfully grafted onto cellulose, polyester, and polyamide fibres, and the mechanism of action of stable N-halamines involving direct contact of the N-halamine with the bacterial cell during which process the oxidative halogen is transferred to the microbial cell rather than dissociating into free oxidative chlorine before its transfer, is highly effective. Features that are of particular benefit apart from their low cost are as follows:

- Once the oxidative halogen inactivates the microorganisms and is exhausted, N-halamines can be easily recharged, for example, by a dilute solution of NaOCl and can then continue to be effective in inactivating pathogens.
- They can be used for the production of textiles which will be able to kill pathogenic microorganisms with high resistance to many antibacterial agents.
- Skin irritation is low, so N-halamines can be used in wound dressings to prevent infection (Demir et al. 2017).
- N-halamines can be combined with other agents to yield multifunctional finishes, although there may be some reduction in oxidative chlorine-retention properties (Ma et al. 2019b).

Given their expected effectiveness against a wide range of pathogens, it is about time that the application of improved test methods on the antiviral effectiveness of N-halamine-treated fabrics to confirm their broad-spectrum effectiveness became the accepted routine in research reports.

Polyhexamethylene biguanides (PHMB) are polycationic amines wherein the cationic biguanide repeat units are separated by hydrocarbon chains and the most common is polyhexamethylene biguanide, $(C_8H_{17}N_5)_n$ where n, the degree of polymerisation, is typically selected to be between 11 and 16. The amine groups in PHMB are spaced out between sections of hydrocarbon chain six carbon atoms in length. The higher the degree of polymerisation, the stronger the attachment to the fibre surface and the more effective the antibacterial action. Their development and application for use in healthcare workers' uniforms was reported (Chen-Yu, Eberhardt, & Kincade 2007) and their application has been reviewed (Zhao & Chen 2016). Effective PHMB-based finishing agents are reported to be commercially available (Morais Guedes & Lopes 2016). Research into guanidine-based antibacterial treatments continues, with the accent on their durability (Cao et al. 2020; Li et al. 2017).

Triclosan is a phenolic antibacterial compound with the chemical formula 5-chloro-2-(2,4-dichlorophenoxy)phenol. It has been widely used as an antimicrobial agent for around 20 years, not just for textiles but also for plastics, consumer care products such as toothpaste, antibacterial soaps, and body washes because in small quantities (0.1%) it will inhibit the growth of microorganisms while at higher concentrations (0.3%) it will destroy them. However, its popularity is now falling dramatically for several reasons:

- toxic waste: residues in wastewater prove difficult to break down, so they end up contaminating streams, lakes, agricultural soils, and the wildlife therein.
- cross-resistance: stimulation by triclosan of the development of resistant strains of microorganism, not only because of bacteria developing resistance to triclosan but also because it has been indicated that the agent may stimulate resistance to some antibiotics
- long-term health risk: concerns that triclosan may potentially pose a long-term public health risk on account of absorption into the blood stream in humans with the possibility of consequent hormonal effects, although it has not been shown as yet to be carcinogenic or to be detrimental to breast-fed children or to the human embryo.

It is on account of issues of this kind plus the fact that manufacturers could not demonstrate their safety that the FDA banned over-the-counter sale in the USA in 2017 of antibacterial wash products containing any of 19 ingredients; one of which was triclosan, unless subjected to a pre-market review regarding its safety and effectiveness. Japan followed suit but there was no ban in Australia, whereas in Europe triclosan is under assessment as being 'persistent, bio-accumulative and toxic' and products containing it must be labelled 'very toxic to aquatic life with long-lasting effects, causes serious eye irritation and causes skin irritation' (ECHA 2021).

5.2.3 Other Finishes

5.2.3.1 Fluid-Repellent Finishing

There is considerable interest in the development of fabrics which are able to easily shed fluids and other soils likely to contaminate surgical gowns and other personal protective equipment during use (Mitchell, Spencer, & Edmiston 2015) and which can also prevent strike-through when splashed with blood or other bodily fluids. It remains difficult to achieve both desired performance aspects without coating the fabric to prevent penetration (which can lead to discomfort during wear) or resorting to the use of laminates with a semi-permeable central layer such as biaxially extended PTFE film such as in Gore Tex fabrics (W. L. Gore & Associates (UK) Ltd. Livingston, Scotland) and as was the case for a barrier fabric intended to prevent penetration of viruses (Parthasarathi & Thilagavathi 2015). There are, however, a number of ways to achieve fluid repellency, not least by so-called super-hydrophobic finishing treatments. Super-hydrophobic fabrics are those which demonstrate a (static) contact angle with a water droplet of over 150°, contact angle hysteresis of less than 10°, and low sliding angle. That high level of water repellency, said to be inspired by the lotus leaf's microscopically rough surface coupled with its waxy coating, cannot be achieved by a water-repellent surface alone; PTFE, for example, has a static contact angle with a water droplet of 120°. In practice, super-hydrophobic performance is often achieved through the application of nanosilver, nano zinc oxide, or nano silicon dioxide particles to create surface texture together with a suitable silane to counteract the nanoparticles' hydrophilic nature. If the fibre surface already possesses significant texture, as is the case for cotton, treatment with a silane alone can be effective in achieving super-hydrophobic performance (Lin et al. 2020). Regarding resistance to strike-through and super-hydrophobicity, droplets of liquid projected at increasing rates at a super-hydrophobic cotton fabric either suspended or supported by a solid surface fabric were described as 'bouncing',' pinning,' then 'splashing' as the velocity was increased and it was helpful, together with the qualitative descriptions, to see an attempt to quantify the different categories of dynamic behaviour (Tudu, Sinhamahapatra, & Kumar 2020), an approach which might hopefully lead to the development of a standard test method for strike-through. However, as a first step, the range of fluid types would need to be extended beyond just water. There is good reason to believe that the super-hydrophobic fabrics based on the presence of nanoparticles would work well against blood, because the platelets which are most likely to result in its adhesion to the fibre surface are an order of magnitude larger than the nanoparticle coating and the spaces between the particles, so surface contact is minimised.

5.2.3.2 Plasma Treatment

Gas plasma treatment of textiles offers the opportunity to bring about surface modification to the component fibres of a material without the application of heat or chemical finishing agents. The electrical discharge through the gas generates a variety of charged entities within the gas and these are capable of bringing about a surface etching effect. Different choices of gas result in different surface effects as different charged or excited components become attached to the reactive sites on the fibres exposed by the etching or its components may become polymerised onto the fibre surface. Argon, for example, brings about surface roughness, and oxygen or nitrogen increase fibre hydrophilicity, whereas sulfur heaxafluoride yields increased lipophilicity because fluorine-containing groups become attached to the surface if it is used, and fluorocarbons create a lipophilic surface by generating fluoropolymer surface films (McCoustra & Mather 2018). The remaining gas can be reclaimed once the treatment cycle is ended, so gas plasma treatment represents an eco-friendly way of bringing about surface modification as there is no waste released into the environment. It is also a useful way to bring about surface changes to delicate textile objects intended to be used as implants such as grafts/stents and there have been some European Union projects focused on medical textiles which demonstrated success in enhancing tissue growth on fibrous scaffolds and stimuli-sensitive poly (N-isopropylacrylamide)-grafted surfaces for wound dressings (CORDIS 2017). In an attempt to further stimulate interest in installing such equipment by textile companies in the EU, atmospheric plasma treatments were developed so as to keep the plasma treatment simple to apply industrially. However, despite its advantageous effects, the relatively gentle way in which surface modification can be achieved, and its environmental benevolence, plasma modification of textiles is not widely implemented.

5.2.3.3 Chitosan

Chitosan applied at low concentrations is often used to modify the surface properties of cellulose fibres and confer some antibacterial action (Mondal & Ahmed 2020). It is antimicrobial and non-toxic, and the antimicrobial action is attributed to the free amino groups on the chitosan; binding of the chitosan to the fibres by covalent linkages to permanently attach it is a compromise: it is necessary to carefully judge the extent of binding so as not to reduce the number of amino groups too much and affect the antimicrobial action. However, the chitosan will need to be cross-linked to the cellulose to improve its durability to laundering processes if it is intended to be used for bed linen or protective clothing. In other applications, it can be useful that its attachment to the surface is reversible, for example, if it is required that the antimicrobial chitosan is intended to be released from the textile beside a wound or from a textile implant (Strnad, Sauperl, & Zemljic 2010). Chitosan may be applied alone or used in conjunction with other agents such as silver nanoparticles (Xu et al. 2018, 2019) or zinc oxide (Ma et al. 2020) to enhance its antibacterial action or to create additional functionality.

5.2.3.4 Cyclodextrins

Cyclodextrins are oligosaccharides in which glucose residues are linked together to form ring structures, most commonly consisting of 6 (α-cyclodextrin), 7 (β-cyclodextrin), or 8 (γ-cyclodextrin) glycopyranose units. They are derived from starch by enzymatic action, and it is β-cyclodextrin that is most used (95% of consumption) (Voncina & Vivod 2013). The ring structures of cyclodextrins have their hydroxyl groups arranged around the outer edges of the ring, which makes them

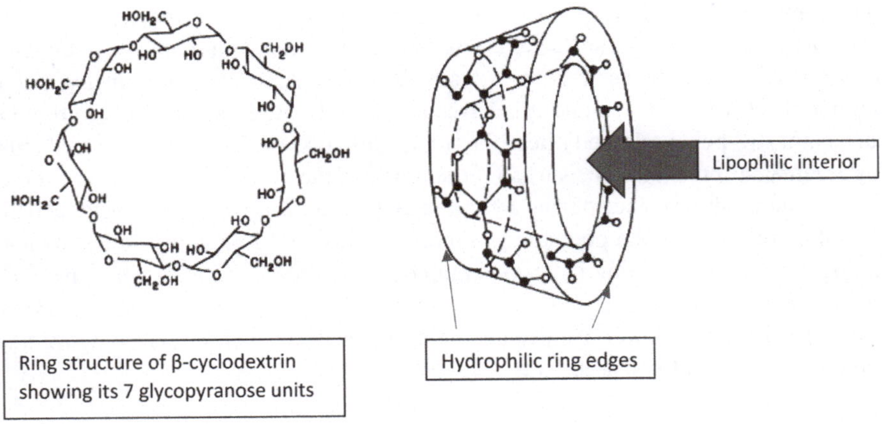

FIGURE 5.2 The chemical structure and the conical shape of the β-cyclodextrin molecule (adapted from Loftsson and Brewster, 1996; reproduced by permission of Elsevier Science and Technology Journals).

hydrophilic on the ring edges, but by contrast, the inside of the ring structure is lipophilic. Figure 5.2 illustrates how this feature originates in the case of β-cyclodextrin, the most-widely used type.

Because of this arrangement, cyclodextrins can form inclusion complexes with some drugs and with surfactants by entrapping lipophilic sections of the drug–surfactant molecules within the centre part of the ring structure (Dong et al. 2014). The host-guest entrapment is reversible and obeys Le Chatelier's principle (Mukhopadhyay et al. 2018), so it is possible for the entrapped species to be released at a predictable steady rate with no great initial surge, which is useful for drug release from a variety of medical textile materials such as sutures and scaffolds. Although cyclodextrins themselves may not be strongly attached to the fibre, modified forms such as the triazinyl complex become covalently attached to cellulose fibres in a manner similar to that of reactive dyes and are therefore firmly held and durable to repeated wet treatments (Ramanujam & Sundrarajan 2015). A treatment with the monochlorotriazinyl derivative of β-cylodextrin was intended to achieve four simultaneous effects: large wrinkle recovery angle (WRA), hydrophilicity, antibacterial capacity, and a good breaking resistance, so that the medical or sportswear garments made from such multifunctional cotton would be more comfortable and the results were that the finish did achieve its multifunctional purposes. It will be interesting to find out how the material performs in real-life setting given its strong performance when tested in the laboratory (Popescu, Petrea, & Popescu 2021).

Many surfactants show a considerable affinity for certain types of textile fibres and as is the case for drugs with a lipophilic section to the molecule, cyclodextrins can form inclusion complexes with surfactants where often a delicate balance exists between the lipophilic and hydrophilic segments of the molecule, particularly for non-ionic surfactants (Buschmann et al. 1998). Surfactant retained by fabrics can cause problems not only in dyeing processes conducted after scouring and bleaching operations but also following normal domestic laundering of clothing and bed linen. The characteristics of the surfactants (surface-active agents) in domestic detergents are not dissimilar to those of a direct dye with poor wash fastness. On rinsing, some but not all of it is removed and it behaves similarly if rinsed again and again, with surfactant still being released after 20 or more rinse cycles. This can cause problems for eczema sufferers as some surfactant retained in the fabric is released on contact with the moist skin surface during wear and may act as a skin irritant. Cyclodextrins should therefore have the potential to serve as a rinse-aid following domestic laundering, because by forming inclusion complexes with the adsorbed surfactants they can assist in their removal (Buschmann et al. 1998); the surfactant–cyclodextrin complex will have a lower affinity for the fibre because it is not surface active and should be more readily rinsed away.

5.2.4 Molecular Imprinting

Molecular imprinting of polymers involves casting the polymer to encapsulate a selected molecule, then removing that molecule so that a site is generated on the polymer surface which will accept further molecules of the same shape. Films of such imprinted polymers have proved successful in acting as detectors for specific molecules (Guan et al. 2008). It has taken longer to become able to prepare useful molecular imprinted electrospun nanofibres (Patel et al. 2020), but there are good reasons for doing so as shown by a recently successful example; the imprinted nanofibres held a greater drug load and released the drug at a steadier rate than 'naked' electrospun nanofibres, and based on the choice of polymer adjusting the nature and strength of drug–polymer interactions, the drug-release time could be greatly extended (Tamahkar, Bakhshpour, & Denizli 2019). The approach used here was based on soft molecular imprinting (Vozzi et al. 2010; Criscenti et al. 2018).

5.3 MULTIFUNCTIONAL FINISHING OF MEDICAL TEXTILES

A detailed review of the roles of apparel in the transfer of pathogens in healthcare settings drew attention to the greatly enhanced effectiveness of antibacterial finishing treatments when combined with fluid repellency (Mitchell, Spencer, & Edmiston 2015); finished fabrics fulfilling the preferred requirements of healthcare settings as expressed in the review, such as those possessed by Daltex® Smart Barrier, and products from Heathcoat Fabrics, are commercially available (Dalton & Low Medical 2020; Heathcoat Fabrics 2021). Such multifunctional finishing has drawn considerable attention as shown by reported research (Zhang et al. 2018, 2020; Lin et al. 2018; Song et al. 2019), with the purpose of capturing a series of beneficial improvements in fabric properties alongside antimicrobial action. One recent piece of research involved applying a thin, elastic xerogel coating as a finish by padding on woven 67% PET/33% cotton fabric by the sol-gel method to achieve antibacterial (vs both gram-positive and gram-negative bacteria) and antifungal effects, combined with photocatalytic cleaning, a high ultraviolet protection factor (over 50), and high abrasion resistance. The sol used was a hybrid Al_2O_3/SiO_2 sol modified with metallic nanoparticles of Ag/Cu powder and TiO_2 P25; this is a significant combination of nanoparticles, one set selected for its antimicrobial action (Ag/Cu) and the other for photocatalytic self-cleaning and UV-protection effectiveness (TiO_2 P25) (Kowalczyk, Brzeziński, & Kamińska 2018). Such multifunctional finishes may not always be achieved only with nanoparticles; in another case, it was with a quaternary ammonium salt plus a sulfopropylbetaine (Zhang et al. 2018, 2020).

5.4 ANTIMICROBIAL TESTING OF FINISHES

Antibacterial tests are carried out with what are considered to be representative and relatively safe examples from the two categories, namely gram-positive and gram-negative bacteria. Antiviral tests are done either with a surrogate for the virus or the virus itself. The surrogate may be used to indicate likely effectiveness but performance against each virus then needs to be tested individually to determine antiviral action of the textile against that specific pathogen.

5.4.1 Qualitative Antibacterial Tests

The Agar Diffusion Test is the basis for ISO 20645: 'Textile Fabrics Determination of Antibacterial Activity; Agar Diffusion Plate Test (01/12/2004)' and AATCC test method 147: 'Antibacterial Activity Assessment of Textile Materials: Parallel Streak Method.' Broadly speaking, the methods consists of placing the test specimen in intimate contact with nutrient agar, which has been previously streaked with an inoculum of a test bacterium (a standard strain of bacteria is used). After incubation, a clear area of interrupted growth underneath and along the sides of the test material provides a qualitative indication of antibacterial activity in the test specimen. The agar diffusion/qualitative methods are simple to perform, quick, and useful when a large number of samples have to be screened.

5.4.2 Quantitative Antibacterial Tests

Absorption or quantitative methods provide values of antimicrobial activity based on the reduction in bacterial growth brought about by the treated fabric but they are more time and material consuming than the qualitative methods, so more suited to detailed trials following initial screening by diffusion/qualitative methods.

The Suspension Challenge Test is the basis for AATCC test method 100: 'Antibacterial Finishes on Textile Materials.' This is the test intended to complement the qualitative AATCC test method 147, and in it swatches of test and control textile materials are tested quantitatively for antibacterial activity. Test and control fabrics are inoculated with test organisms. After incubation, the bacteria are eluted from the swatches by shaking in the known amount of neutralising solution. The number of bacteria present in this liquid is determined, and the percentage reduction in the treated specimen is calculated.

5.4.2.1 ISO 20743: Quantitative Test Methods to Determine the Antibacterial Activity of All Antibacterial Textile Products

The international standard originated as JIS L 1902, the Japanese Industrial Standard was established in 1990 as a test for antibacterial activity of photocatalytic products and efficacy under indoor lighting environment. It was adopted by the International Standards Organisation as the ISO 20743 test method in 2007 but with a wider brief, i.e., to specify quantitative test methods to determine the antibacterial activity of all antibacterial textile products including non-wovens. ISO 20743 is applicable to all textile products, including cloth, wadding, thread, and material for clothing, bedclothes, home furnishings, and miscellaneous goods, regardless of the type of antibacterial agent used (organic, inorganic, natural, or man-made) or the method of application (built in, after-treatment, or grafting). Based on the intended application and on the environment in which the textile product is to be used and also on the surface properties of the textile products, the user can select the most suitable of the following three inoculation methods on determination of antibacterial activity:

1. absorption method (an evaluation method in which the test bacterial suspension is inoculated directly onto specimens)
2. transfer method (an evaluation method in which test bacteria are placed on an agar plate and transferred onto specimens)
3. printing method (an evaluation method in which test bacteria are placed on a filter and printed onto specimens)

The colony plate count method and the ATP (ATP = adenosine triphosphate) luminescence method are also specified for enumerating bacteria (ISO 2021).

5.5 ANTIVIRAL TESTING OF FINISHES

Unlike antibacterial testing which can be carried out with what are considered to be representative examples of the two types, i.e., gram-positive and gram-negative bacteria, such an approach cannot be used with viruses. Useful initial information about the likelihood of a material being able to act as a barrier to the penetration of viruses can be determined from tests using a virus surrogate, as was the case in the assessment of the effectiveness of an antiviral surgical gown for liquid barrier protection (Parthasarathi & Thilagavathi 2015), but for greater information about performance against specific viruses, tests against each individual candidate virus must be carried out.

5.5.1 Test Methods Using a Surrogate

The ANSI/AAMI PB70 standard includes four standard tests to evaluate the barrier effectiveness of surgical gowns, isolation gowns, and surgical drapes. Based on the results of these standardised tests, four levels of barrier performance are defined, with Level 1 being the lowest and Level 4 being the highest level of protection. Only

Level 4 gowns are tested for viral penetration resistance and therefore only Level 4 garments are considered impermeable to viral penetration. ASTM F1671 is the test method used to measure the resistance of materials used in such protective clothing for penetration by blood-borne pathogens, using a bacteriophage under conditions of continuous liquid contact. As specified in ASTM F1671/1671M-13, antiviral performance can be measured using the bacteriophage X174 as a surrogate for Hepatitis B virus (HBV), Hepatitis C virus (HCV), and HIV. The ΦX174 bacteriophage is a non-enveloped 25–27 nm virus (similar to HCV, the smallest pathogen) with an icosahedral or nearly spherical morphology and excellent environmental stability. It is non-infectious to humans, has a limit of detection which approaches a single virus particle, grows rapidly, and can be cultivated to reach high titres similar to HBV (the most concentrated pathogen mentioned), and it is considered to be an excellent choice for the testing of barrier materials (Lytle et al. 1991). For protective clothing intended to provide protection against blood, body fluids, and other potentially infectious materials, it is also important to simulate the wetting characteristics of blood and body fluids; the surface tension range for blood and body fluids is approximately $42–60 \times 10^{-3}$ N/m, so the surface tension of the ΦX174 bacteriophage suspension needs to be adjusted to approximately the lower end of this surface tension range (42×10^{-3} N/m). Test samples were prepared by randomly cutting the protective clothing material into approximately 75 × 75 mm swatches. Test samples were exposed to approximately 60 ml of a ΦX174 bacteriophage suspension. At the conclusion of the test, the observed side of the test sample was rinsed with a sterile assay medium and then analysed for the presence of the ΦX174 bacteriophage. Surgical protective clothing 'pass/fail' determinations were based on the detection of penetration (Parthasarathi & Thilagavathi 2015).

5.5.2 Test Methods Requiring Tests with Each Individual Virus

It is necessary, if the efficacy of a fabric against particular types of virus is to be determined, to test each virus separately to determine the fabric's performance against that specific virus. The standard developed most recently to provide a test method of this type is BS ISO 18184:2019: 'Textiles: Determination of Antiviral Activity of Textile Products,' first published in June 2019. For this test method, a 20 mm × 20 mm sample of test material is cut (the overall mass should be 0.40 g and the weight can be made up with extra material if required). A total of nine control pieces and six test pieces are required for the test. Of these, three pieces of each material are used to test the effect of the fabric on cells without virus present (for cytotoxicity), three control pieces are used to recover the starting titre of virus, and the remaining pieces are inoculated with 200 µl of virus at a concentration of ~107 median tissue culture dose (TCID50 – giving a final concentration of 105) and left for the required contact time. When the required contact time has elapsed, the fabric is recovered in 20 ml of cell culture medium and enumerated onto an appropriate cell line. TCID50 is calculated following the appropriate incubation time. Antiviral activity is calculated by comparison of the antiviral test material to what was immediately recovered from the control fabric.

5.5.3 Suitability of Test Method to Intended Application

There are serious concerns that the test regimes applied to medical textiles to determine their bactericidal or virucidal effectiveness do not relate to what happens in practice. Under circumstances where the methods instituted by established standards organisations and used in their regulations by regulatory bodies fall short, it can be difficult to initiate and support change. It should be helpful when another respected organisation advises and intervenes, and this is what the Organization for Economic Cooperation and Development (OECD) has tried to do in relation to biocides. The OECD Environment Directorate in their 2008 *Guidance Document on the Evaluation of the Efficacy of Antimicrobial Treated Articles with Claims for External Effects* (OECD 2008), recommends a three-tiered approach to determining the efficacy of antibacterial-treated articles, namely:

Tier 1: *Proof of Principle* defines the basic industry standard tests that determine the efficacy of an antibacterial-treated article in a controlled laboratory environment.

Tier 2: *Simulated Use* defines the translational tests that mimic end-use scenarios, environments, and incubation times.

Tier 3: *In-Use Evaluation* substantiates direct health benefit claims or supports marketing initiatives by the development of clinical trials that take place in end-use environments under real-world conditions.

All of the qualitative and quantitative types of current standard test methods outlined earlier fit into the Tier 1 category, Tier 2 testing is still missing; however, for Tier 3, there are reports of a small number of clinical/on-site trials such as those applied to copper-treated textiles and surfaces (Marcus et al. 2017; Lazary et al. 2014; Sifri et al. 2016) which do fall into the Tier 3 testing category.

Work has been reported where it has been found that there can be discrepancies between the quantitative and qualitative test types and that the quantitative tests were the most reliable (Pinho et al. 2011). However, even a satisfactory quantitative test indication of antimicrobial action does not necessarily result in adequate performance in the practical setting (Rozman et al. 2017); the issue appears to be caused in part by higher loadings in the practical setting than in the laboratory-based test regime but could also be due to being exposed to very different environmental conditions in practice compared with those experienced by the pathogens during the test applied in the laboratory. A randomised controlled trial with 105 participants (hospital physicians, nurse practitioners, physician assistants, house staff, and nurses working in internal medicine units) was undertaken to compare the extent of bacterial contamination of uniforms and skin when healthcare workers wore one of two antimicrobial scrubs or standard scrubs. Bacterial colony counts were carried out on cultures taken from the healthcare workers' scrubs and wrists at the end of the working day. There was no evidence that either antimicrobial scrub product decreased bacterial contamination of healthcare workers' uniforms or skin after an 8-hour working day (Burden et al. 2013). Another case, where silver-treated uniforms were assessed against untreated items, found that prior to use the differences in antibacterial activity between control and silver-doped samples were highly significant, but evaluation of antibacterial activity performed on the experimental uniforms after they had been worn by healthcare workers provided results that were not always in agreement with the data obtained from fabric samples in vitro (Condò et al. 2015). Despite the fact that the effectiveness of an antimicrobial material was demonstrated in laboratory test, the effectiveness was not exhibited in the hospital environment. The bacterial load on medical workers' uniforms was much higher than the concentrations of microorganisms used in the laboratory test method, which could reduce antimicrobial efficiency because of the contamination remaining on the fabric and continued interaction between the antimicrobial agent and the heavy load of microbes that had already inactivated or that load physically inhibiting contact with the active agent. A recent review noted that in 2021 there is still a gap between scientific knowledge concerning the use of antimicrobial-impregnated fabrics in healthcare services, their potential or their ineffectiveness in bringing about a decrease in microbial contamination, and their applicability (Schneider et al. 2021).

It is at Tier 2 where current test methods fall seriously short. Realistic, reliable laboratory-based Tier-2 test methods need to be developed for medical textiles and validated for their alignment with practice (e.g., through their capacity to reliably predict outcomes from earlier clinical trials) before they could be considered for acceptance as standards The OECD gives guidance on their development in their 'Series on Testing and Assessment No. 287, series on Biocides No. 13: Guidance Document on Use and Development of Tier-2 Laboratory Based Test Used to Substantiate Claims for Efficacy of Biocide Treated Articles.' That document provides guidance on how the efficacy of treated articles can be assessed using Tier-2 laboratory-based protocols. In it, the OECD makes the point that:

> for any claim that a product inhibits growth, it is vital to demonstrate that growth on the material in question does occur under its normal conditions of use (not in some artificial laboratory test) and that many microorganisms demonstrate poor levels of survival when exposed to surfaces even when those surfaces do not contain a biocide. In both cases therefore, it will be necessary to have data that demonstrates that the target species (or at least representative surrogates) do indeed survive on the materials and under the conditions in which the articles are intended to be used. Having identified a situation in which microorganisms do grow, or survive and present a hazard, data which shows the beneficial effects of the treatment of a material or article needs to be generated.

The document includes a structure for possible claims for treated articles and treated materials, as well as guidance on different types of claims and how to support them by providing data that is relevant to the actual use. The guidance contains two example protocols to determine the efficacy of treated articles after contamination via the deposition of aerosols and splashes, or after deposition by hand contact (OECD 2019) and some organisations are now engaged in this type of development work and there is a claim that results are predictive of clinical trial performance, particularly in the case of their splatter assay (Hardwick 2019). Finally, the OECD sets down the basic requirements for a valid test as follows:

1. The test should be carried out on the final article.
2. An untreated variant of the test material must be included such that the impact of the treatment can be demonstrated.
3. Test conditions should reflect normal conditions of use in terms of humidity, temperature, contact frequency, durability, etc.
4. The test should employ organisms that are relevant to the end use of the article and the benefit being claimed.
5. Tests that employ a single species of organisms should be favoured over those that use consortia.
6. A minimum of three replicate test pieces of both treated and untreated materials should be employed.
7. The final data should include either some indication of the impact of service conditions on the performance of the treated material/article or data from an ageing study. The intention is to demonstrate how long the claimed benefit will be sustained.

5.6 DURABILITY TESTING OF FINISHES

It is encouraging to be able to report on thorough testing of the durability of the effects of antibacterial treatment with silver nanoparticles, not least because it demonstrated continued high levels of antibacterial effectiveness after 50 cycles of laundering (Xu et al. 2018, 2019; Wu et al. 2019), as did a guanidine-functionalised cotton fabric (Cao et al. 2020). Twenty years ago just 10 Launder-Ometer® (SDL Atlas, Rockville, S. Carolina, USA) washings used to be thought indicative of durability (Kim & Sun 2001) but while 20 laundry cycles may be a helpful indicator in the early stages of trials (Duan et al. 2020), 50 cycles is better for making a more realistic, final-performance claim. With 30–50 laundry cycles becoming more common in test reports, it is time for the higher number of treatments to be clearly specified and agreed upon as a minimum standard for durability claims, and where the treated fabrics are expected to be laundered in a hospital or commercial laundry, for the testing regime to match (or be shown to be comparable to) that type of laundry process.

5.7 SUITABILITY OF ANTIMICROBIAL TREATMENT TO INTENDED APPLICATION

It is not possible to be entirely certain which type of antimicrobial treatment on a textile might produce the desired effect in any particular application, which is why it is necessary to subject them to suitable tests at Levels 1, 2, and 3 of the OECD protocol. It may help to:

(i) examine the mechanisms of interaction between examples of antimicrobial agents
(ii) determine what has been found out about their effectiveness in different applications
(iii) see whether the mismatch between expectation and practice might have been able to be predicted or avoided using improved Level 1 test methods that were more reflective of the conditions experienced in practice

5.7.1 Mechanisms of Interaction between Antimicrobial Textiles and Pathogens

The antimicrobial agent in some cases is firmly bound to the fibres, for example, by covalent bonding between the agent and reactive groups on the polymer chains of which fibre is composed or by formation of active polymer on the fibre surface. Bound to the fibre, the agent is immobilised, so for agents such as these to be effective, the environmental conditions must be such that the microbes can arrive at the fibre surface and interact on their arrival as soon as they encounter the active agent bound there. The types of environments within which agents bound to the fibre might be expected to work most effectively are:

(a) those such as would exist within the body around an implant where microbes might arrive by diffusion through the surrounding liquid medium
(b) in a filter as contaminated air is drawn through the filter fabric thereby bringing the microbes into contact with the agent on the surfaces of the treated fibres within
(c) a reusable wipe, cloth, or fabric cleaning tool head intended to be used when wet

However, even in circumstances such as these, the agent might still not work sufficiently rapidly or well under typical conditions of use to have any practical value, or the achievable loading of agent on the fibre may be insufficient to bring about the desired effect, or the amount of contamination may overpower the agent's ability to exert its antibacterial effect.

For other agents, there is attachment of a weaker kind between the agent and the fibre (such as with nanoparticles deposited on, but not anchored to, the fibre surface, or with metal salts with affinity not only for the fibres within the textile but also with the surrounding aqueous medium); however, these attachments are not as effective or as durable as covalent bonding, and the active agent steadily leaches out of the fabric. Having said that, that is the way that these agents work, i.e., by leaking active agent out into any surrounding liquid where it can diffuse towards microbes, encounter them, and interact with them. If such an agent were to be found which worked by release of a volatile organic compound, the VOC's migration would not need to be surrounded by a liquid medium.

The differences in the ways that agents behave and interact with microorganisms mean that no single type can be expected to be suitable across all applications.

5.7.2 Tests for the Effectiveness of Antimicrobial Treatments in Different Applications

5.7.2.1 Implants

Experiments have been undertaken with silver treatments of various kinds on plastic biliary stents to determine whether the formation of biofilm can be prevented, or at least slowed down, so that the lifetime of the stent is lengthened by not becoming occluded so rapidly as an untreated device (Yamabe et al. 2021). The aim has been to try to establish whether a (cheaper) plastic tube stent treated with silver would last as long as the usual device, a self-expanding metal stent or SEMS, which also becomes occluded but over a longer period of time. Such a device is not a textile but it is informative to learn what facts have been assembled and what experiments were undertaken to try to determine whether the necessary effectiveness might be able to be achieved. Stent occlusion is brought about by the build-up of biliary sludge, the adhesion of which is assisted by formation of a biofilm on the surface of the stent. There are advantages from the very start gained from using silver in various forms as the antibacterial agent in antibacterial implants, not only because 60 ppm of silver ions are known to be effective in controlling the growth of most bacteria and fungi, but also because it has been employed for a long time in various medical treatments, mostly those involving topical application, where it is considered to be a valuable therapeutic agent. Silver-treated stents had also been trialled on patients where it was found that the antibacterial effect of stents with a silver content of 0.04 wt% was ineffective in many patients, whereas a silver content of 1.5 wt% was effective in several patients, and that antibacterial activity was improved by an increase in silver content. However, silver is toxic and there is a known limit to the amount of silver released internally which would be found acceptable (10 ppm) and a known level of silver required to control bacteria and fungi (0.1 ppm). Data on the release of silver ions indicated that following an initial surge (well inside the acceptable level), the Ag^+ release from a silver-nanoparticle-coated biliary stent was an effective, slow, and sustained process. Tests have been undertaken to determine the effectiveness of coating with silver particles, inclusion if silver particles within the plastic and by coating it with silver nanoparticles, in which the treated and untreated stents were immersed in infected bile for 4 weeks. Further in vitro experimentation is now necessary to determine how the lifetime of the plastic stent can be extended to match that of the SEMS (ca. 9 months).

5.7.2.2 External Applications

5.7.2.2.1 Wound Care

Work was undertaken in 2015 in an attempt to develop an improved way of testing the effectiveness of antibacterial treatments on textile materials intended to be used in wound care (Pinho et al. 2015), through adjustment of the approaches applied in AATCC 100: 'Assessment of Antibacterial Finishes on Textile Materials (2012)'; ISO 20743: 'Textiles—Determination of Antibacterial Activity of Textile Products (Adsorption Method) (2013)'; and JIS L 19002: 'Testing for Antibacterial Activity and Efficacy on Textile Products—Quantitative Method (Adsorption Test) (2008).' Searching for a more realistic test method, Pinho et al. (2015) found that moisture levels exerted the greatest effect on the activities of the antibacterial textiles used, that the test method for fabrics in contact with wound exudate should incorporate high moisture levels, and also that the medium within which the test was undertaken affected the efficacy of antibacterial action by the textile. They adopted synthetic sweat solution because it appeared to represent a viable option to predict the effect of the antibacterial textiles on an infected wound. Their method could be successfully applied to both leaching and non-leaching antimicrobial agents against gram-positive and gram-negative bacteria with the leaching types showing the best performance and they used a much higher loading of pathogen (300×) than the AATCC 100, ISO 20743, or JIS L 19002 methods. Comparison with those methods showed that by enabling a more realistic analysis of a treated fabric's performance under test conditions similar to those found on most types of wounds (exudate, infected skin, and sweat when in contact with infected wounds), the method developed by Pinho et al. (2015), 'Testing for Antibacterial Activity and Efficacy on Textile Products for Wound Dressing Application—Quantitative Method (2015),' was a better test than any of the other three for wound dressing applications of antibacterial textiles.

5.7.2.2.2 Fabrics in Contact with Patients, Healthcare Worker's Uniforms, and Workwear

It was found that newly laundered physicians' uniforms and infrequently washed coats show similar bacterial contamination after the working day (Burden et al. 2011). The presence of pathogens on the coats of healthcare workers is associated with the presence of pathogens on their hands, demonstrating the relevance of textile decontamination in patient care. Given that the transfer of gram-positive bacteria, particularly multi-resistant *Staphylococcus aureus* (MRSA) and vancomycin-resistant enterococci (VRE), within healthcare settings is of increasing concern, it was considered important to determine the persistence of a variety of such organisms and their non-resistant counterparts on medical textile materials. Five common materials were inoculated with microorganisms:100% cotton clothing fabric, 100% cotton terry towelling, 60/40 polyester/cotton blend as used in scrubs, 100% polyester as used in privacy drapes, and 100% polyethylene plastic splash aprons. The inoculated specimens were kept separate while left to dry under a safety hood with the fan running. All organisms were found to have survived for at least 1 day, and some of them survived for more than 90 days on the various materials underscoring the need for meticulous contact control procedures, careful disinfection, and the urgent need to develop effective antibacterial medical textiles for these types of application (and test methods which enable them to be more readily identified as such) to limit the spread of resistant bacteria. To begin with, given that the pathogens behave differently depending on the fabric that they are contaminating, it is not satisfactory to believe that there is a single representative type of fabric that should be used for treatment and testing, but instead, it should be what is used in the intended application (Neely & Maley 2000).

Other work involving the analysis of published data showed that at up to 206 days at room temperature survival of bacteria was the longest on polyester (PET) compared to 90 days for some species on cotton and blends; generally speaking, persistence was longer on synthetic polymer fibre types than on cotton (Kampf 2020). The greatest reliability in cleanliness would be shown if fabrics could be treated to have an antibacterial effect; otherwise they can be a source of pathogens and their transfer throughout the single period of wear, then, unless they are cleaned and sterilised after every use, contaminated textiles or fabrics may remain a source of transmission for days, weeks, or for some viruses, several years.

The ASCOT trial, part of the 'CDC Prevention Epicenters Program,' was undertaken to determine the effectiveness of antimicrobial-impregnated polyester/cotton scrubs treated with either silver alloy (within the fibres) or fabrics treated with a silane plus quaternary ammonium compound (such that the silane bound it durably to the fibre on the clothing worn by healthcare personnel) together with a fluid-repellent treatment, a hydrophobic fluoroacrylate copolymer emulsion. Neither of the antimicrobial-impregnated scrubs was effective at reducing contamination (Anderson et al. 2017).

Similarly treated fabrics of similar fibre composition may work better in some applications than others, so it is essential that the way the fabric is intended to be used is mimicked as closely as possible in any test for antimicrobial effectiveness. For example, silver nanoparticles and copper oxide are widely used antimicrobial substances for the impregnation of fabrics. The use of these treated fabrics with patients, such as in bed and bath linens and clothing, was more effective in reducing antimicrobial load than in health workers' uniforms (Schneider et al. 2021). It appears that for the treatment methods assessed here, the antimicrobial fabrics were more effective in applications where the individual was in more prolonged, repeated, or sustained contact with the material. Other cases, however, do show that some antibacterial treatments for fabrics indicated to be effective by traditional tests did demonstrate the hoped-for performance in the practical setting (Kampf 2020). Among chronic ventilator-dependent patients, a significant reduction of healthcare infections indicators, such as antibiotic treatment initiation events, fever days, and antibiotic usage, was described when healthcare workers wore copper-oxide-impregnated textiles instead of regular hospital textiles (Marcus et al. 2017) and copper-impregnated hospital linens were even described to reduce healthcare-associated *C. difficile* infections (Butler 2018). It is clear, however, that much work needs to be done to develop effective antimicrobial treatments for healthcare workers' scrubs, gowns, and uniforms, so it was surprising that a review published very recently suggested that despite some encouraging results, however, control to prevent too widespread use and regular checks on effectiveness become necessary to prevent over-exposure of nosocomial pathogens to any particular biocidal agent; to understand whether it still works becomes necessary because overuse is likely to enhance tolerance to any agent (Kampf 2018). Domestic applications of items with permanent biocidal impregnation should therefore be restricted if possible (Kampf 2018).

5.7.2.3 Furnishings, Fixtures, and Fittings

5.7.2.3.1 Drapes, Seating

The hazards presented by everyday objects can easily be ignored. Contamination with group A streptococci of a fabric-upholstered chair used by a healthcare worker in an office adjacent to a ward was suspected to have enhanced transmission to other healthcare personnel (Kampf 2020). Another example was an outbreak in Birmingham in the UK of meropenem-resistant *A. baumannii* in an intensive care unit where the major source appeared to be the curtains surrounding the patient' beds (Das et al. 2002). Outbreaks caused by bacterial spores on linen have also been reported (Cheng et al. 2017; Hosein et al. 2013).

5.7.2.3.2 Air Filters

N-halamines are one of the most effective antimicrobial agents against a broad spectrum of microorganisms and various studies have investigated the incorporation of antimicrobials into air filters to prevent viruses from entering the indoor environment. In one study, 1-chloro-2,2,5,5-tetramethyl-4-imidazolidinone (an N-halamine called MC) was coated on non-woven fabrics resulting in remarkably reduced avian influenza virus on the N-halamine-treated fabric in a short period of time. Aerosolised avian influenza (AI) viruses were completely inactivated when they passed through filters containing the coated fabric. The active chlorine in the N-halamine is stable, and the coating procedure is straightforward and inexpensive. At higher concentrations, the N-halamine completely inactivated AI viruses and disrupted their RNA, preventing them from being detected by real-time reverse transcriptase-polymerase chain reaction assay (Ren et al. 2018).

5.7.3 Predictability of Mismatch between Expectation and Practice

The antibacterial properties of five kinds of antimicrobial-finished textiles were examined against *Staphylococcus aureus*, including methicillin-resistant S. aureus (MRSA) strains, and *Pseudomonas aeruginosa*, under wet and dry conditions. Commercially available textile products containing silver, zinc, ammonium zeolite, and chitosan were found to be effective against methicillin-sensitive S. aureus (MSSA) for up to 6 hours' incubation under wet and dry conditions, and effective against MRSA for up to 24 hours' incubation, but only under wet conditions. Under dry conditions, all the antimicrobial textiles were ineffective against one strain of MRSA. When organic matter was added to the incubation mixture, the textile products containing silver, zinc, ammonium zeolite, and chitosan showed reduced antibacterial activity. The results suggested that there are differences in antibacterial properties among commercially available antimicrobial fabrics (Takai et al. 2002) and also that

(i) Determining effectiveness requires several hours of incubation,
(ii) Water content is an environmental factor that can affect effectiveness,
(iii) Some bacterial species and strains are not susceptible to antimicrobial fabrics, and

(iv) The antibacterial properties of fabrics shown in tests may be of limited value in the clinical setting.

Their conclusions suggest that some modifications of JIS L 19002 and ISO 20743, to include both dry conditions and resistant strains of bacteria, may make detecting effective antibacterial textile materials easier and help researchers to close in on possible Tier 2 laboratory-based assessment methods for antibacterial-treated textiles.

5.8 STERILISATION

Defining sterilisation as the complete absence of any viable microorganisms including spores makes it an absolute term; however, that absence cannot be proved by current microbiological techniques. Consequently, what the manufacturers of sterilising equipment do, having determined the effects of the variants such as treatment time, temperature, and concentration of sterilant on its lethality, is to build in large safety margins to ensure that any microorganisms present on the items being processed will not survive and then also to provide guidance on how and how frequently the proper performance of the steriliser must be checked (Wendt, Frei, & Widmer 2015).

Sterilisation is not necessary for all medical textiles as would be gathered from Spaulding's classification (Table 5.1). So while essential for implants and bandages/wound dressings, it is not required for bed linen, pyjamas or other patient coverings, pillowcases, bedcovers, uniforms, bed-screens, or furnishings, except in cases where resistant organisms are known to be present. However, it remains important to ensure that in all cases contamination is removed prior to reuse. Wipe-able pillows and mattress covers may appear to be an attractive option, but laundering (carried out commercially or within the hospital at temperatures > 60°C) has been found to be more controllable and more effective in achieving the required cleanliness (Hooker, Ulrich, & Brooks 2020). Laundering of used medical textiles is also essential in reducing the bioburden prior to any form of sterilisation. The laundering processes do need to be closely monitored, as there are a number of case studies that have linked small outbreaks of infection with inadequate laundering or infection control processes surrounding healthcare laundry and also studies demonstrating the survival of potential pathogens during laundering of healthcare textiles, which may increase the risk of infection (Owen & Laird 2020).

5.8.1 Physical Sterilisation Methods

5.8.1.1 Moist Heat Sterilisation

Steam sterilisation is the means by which moist heat in the form of saturated steam is applied under pressure, and the most widely used of all the methods available for sterilisation; nontoxic, inexpensive, rapidly microbiocidal, and able to rapidly heat up and penetrate fabrics, it is also the most dependable. The ideal steam for sterilisation is dry, saturated steam with a dryness fraction ≥97%. Pressurising the autoclave serves as a means of obtaining the high temperatures that need to be maintained for a given length of time to kill microorganisms. Two common steam-sterilising temperatures and times are 121°C for 30 minutes in a gravity-displacement steriliser (air flows out as the steam flows in at the beginning) and for wrapped healthcare supplies, 132°C for 4 minutes in a pre-vacuum steriliser (the air within the autoclave/cabinet is removed by vacuum before the steam is allowed to enter) (CDC 2019). It is recommended that steam sterilisation should be used whenever possible on all critical and semi-critical items that are heat and moisture resistant even when not essential to prevent pathogen transmission.

5.8.1.2 Low-Temperature Sterilisation

Low-temperature sterilisation can prove useful with items or devices which cannot withstand the high temperatures and/or moist conditions encountered in steam sterilisation. Single-use items such as N95 respirators, for example, cannot withstand steam sterilisation, so in cases of emergency and shortages such as those occurring during an epidemic, other treatments must be sought.

Radiation sterilisation can be carried out using electron beams, X-rays, gamma rays, or subatomic particles. Their attraction is that they do not consume expensive chemical agents or generate waste but they are all extremely dangerous and require shielding to protect their operators. X-rays and gamma rays have the advantage of being able to penetrate significant depths of materials needing to be sterilised but whereas continuous shielding is required for sources of gamma rays such as caesium-137, X-ray generators can be switched off at source when not in use.

For *ethylene oxide sterilisation*, the process begins by purging the sterilising cabinet with nitrogen gas to remove air or by evacuating the chamber, following which, items are exposed to ethylene oxide at 55°C. Ethylene oxide has several disadvantages. Unlike in the case of heat, sterilisation by ethylene oxide depends on contact by the gas so it does not sterilise where it cannot penetrate. Also, it is highly toxic, and where it has penetrated, all residual ethylene oxide must be removed, a time-consuming step which can take up to 12 hours to achieve, meaning that the whole sterilisation process can take over 16 hours to complete.

For *low-temperature hydrogen peroxide plasma sterilisation*, the low-temperature plasma is produced in a closed chamber with deep vacuum, an electromagnetic field, and a chemical precursor (hydrogen peroxide – H_2O_2 – or a mixture of H_2O_2 and peracetic acid). The H_2O_2 or its mixture together with the ultraviolet radiation and free radicals generated by the plasma are thought to be what rapidly destroy vegetative microorganisms including spores. Cellulose and certain nylons absorb H_2O_2 and interfere with the sterilisation process while some metal items corrode.

With *ozone sterilisation*, sterilisation takes place at a temperature between 25 and 35°C and unlike in the case of ethylene oxide, aeration following sterilisation is not required so the whole process can be completed in around 4 hours. Furthermore, no toxic chemicals or wastes are involved. Ozone can also be used in low-temperature laundry treatments for the decontamination and disinfection of garments or cleaning cloths (JLA 2021).

Liquid chemical sterilisation with 35% peracetic acid is approved in the USA but not in the EU or the UK. Intended for the treatment of surgical instruments, its advantage is that it is very rapid and treated goods do not require aeration, so the whole process takes only 30 minutes at 50°C but monitoring of the peracetic acid concentration is unreliable as is the monitoring of sterilising performance plus it is expensive to buy and operate (Wendt, Frei, & Widmer 2015).

5.9 SUMMARY

Textile finishing is the final stage in textile manufacture during which the characteristics of the textile item are able to be adjusted or determined. Apart from bleaching and sterilising, and mechanical consolidation, for medical textiles finishing may mean conferring to the textile surface hydrophilicity, or so-called super-hydrophobicity, depending on whether moisture absorption or fluid repellency is required. In some cases, it may be preferable to have the two sides of the fabric behave differently, particularly in the case of wound dressings. Finishing may also involve the process of impregnating or coating the textile with an agent or agents intended to confer specific properties in their own right or to assist in the uptake or retention properties of the active agent. How the agent is applied is capable of being very precisely controlled during finishing so that exactly the right amount of the agent needed to achieve the necessary performance is taken up by the fabric.

Antimicrobial treatments for medical textiles applied by finishing have received a great deal of exploration recently, particularly nanofinishes based on nanosilver, nanozinc oxide, or nanotitanium oxide, alongside durable organic antimicrobial agents, but much more attention needs to be paid to the appropriateness of the test methods supposed to demonstrate their effectiveness. For medical textiles intended for external use or those employed in reusable wipes or the cleaning devices used to maintain acceptable hygiene, the application of an approved test procedure to ensure that the finished medical textile demonstrates the promised antimicrobial performance and that such performance is durable to hospital/commercial laundering, particularly in the case of medical textiles used in high volumes, is of great importance. Test methods for the detection of pathogens, those used to establish the effectiveness of implanted devices treated with antibacterial agents, and those used to determine the effectiveness of barrier materials to pathogens including viruses appear to be effective. However, in the case of textiles treated with antimicrobial agents intended to act against the contaminants on PPE and workwear, the ability of current test procedures to predict how well the textile will perform in practice is very poor. Properly designed trials undertaken in realistic situations are few and far between and the trials which *have* been carried out show that existing antimicrobial treatments are ineffective in the practical setting.

There will always be a need for fabrics able not only to act as barriers but also to deactivate pathogens and therefore to keep staff and patients safe despite contamination during their treatment. The best hope for an effective treatment to date lies with a light-activated treatment (Parthasarathi & Thilagavathi 2015).

What is needed from other researchers in place of papers involving the continued use of test regimes unsuited to the intended application and reporting high levels of effectiveness not verified in the practical setting, is for them to take the lead in a concerted effort to overcome these deficiencies. Good researchers should recognise that for fabrics and garments to be able to demonstrate the antimicrobial action necessary to prevent cross-contamination under conditions which adequately represent those experienced by surgeons and healthcare professionals during their work, a new start needs to be made. The groundwork was prepared some years ago and set down in the 'three-tier' protocol published by the OECD in 2008 in their *Guidance Document on the Evaluation of the Efficacy of Antimicrobial Treated Articles with Claims for External Effects* (OECD 2008). For the protective garments and uniform wear intended for healthcare professionals, that protocol now needs to be properly addressed.

REFERENCES

Anderson, Deverick J., Rachel Addison, Yuliya Lokhnygina, Bobby Warren, Batu Sharma-Kuinkel, Laura J. Rojas, Susan D. Rudin et al. "The antimicrobial scrub contamination and transmission (ASCOT) trial: A three-arm, blinded, randomized controlled trial with crossover design to determine the efficacy of antimicrobial-impregnated scrubs in preventing healthcare provider contamination." *Infection Control & Hospital Epidemiology* 38, no. 10 (2017): 1147–1154.

Bae, Geun Yeol, Byung Gil Min, Young Gyu Jeong, Sang Cheol Lee, Jin Ho Jang, and Gwang Hoe Koo. "Superhydrophobicity of cotton fabrics treated with silica nanoparticles and water-repellent agent." *Journal of Colloid and Interface Science* 337, no. 1 (2009): 170–175.

Beringer, Jan. "Nanotechnology in textile finishing-state of the art and future prospects." *VDI BERICHTE* 1940 (2007): 35.

Boillot, C., C. Bazin, F. Tissot-Guerraz, J. Droguet, M. Perraud, J. C. Cetre, D. Trepo, and Y. Perrodin. "Daily physicochemical, microbiological and ecotoxicological fluctuations of a hospital effluent according to technical and care activities." *Science of the Total Environment* 403, no. 1–3 (2008): 113–129.

Burden, Marisha, Lilia Cervantes, Diane Weed, Angela Keniston, Connie S. Price, and Richard K. Albert. "Newly cleaned physician uniforms and infrequently washed white coats have similar rates of bacterial contamination after an 8-hour workday: A randomized controlled trial." *Journal of Hospital Medicine* 6, no. 4 (2011): 177–182.

Burden, Marisha, Angela Keniston, Maria G. Frank, Carrie A. Brown, Jeff Zoucha, Lilia Cervantes, Diane Weed, Kathy Boyle, Connie Price, and Richard K. Albert. "Bacterial contamination of healthcare workers' uniforms: A randomized controlled trial of antimicrobial scrubs." *Journal of Hospital Medicine* 8, no. 7 (2013): 380–385.

Buschmann, H.-J., U. Denter, D. Knittel, and E. Schollmeyer. "The use of cyclodextrins in textile processes—An overview." *Journal of the Textile Institute* 89, no. 3 (1998): 554–561.

Cao, Yihong, Jingwei Gu, Shu Wang, Zhuocheng Zhang, Huali Yu, Jianna Li, and Shiguo Chen. "Guanidine-functionalized cotton fabrics for achieving permanent antibacterial activity without compromising their physicochemical properties and cytocompatibility." *Cellulose* 27, no. 10 (2020): 6027–6036.

CDC 2019. "Guideline for Disinfection and Sterilization in Healthcare Facilities (2008) Last update: May 2019." Accessed June 4th, 2021. https://www.cdc.gov/infectioncontrol/pdf/guidelines/disinfection-guidelines-H.pdf.

Cerkez, Idris, Hasan B. Kocer, S. D. Worley, R. M. Broughton, and T. S. Huang. "Epoxide tethering of polymeric N-halamine moieties." *Cellulose* 19, no. 3 (2012): 959–966.

Chen-Yu, Jessie H., Darlene M. Eberhardt, and Doris H. Kincade. "Antibacterial and laundering properties of AMS and PHMB as finishing agents on fabric for health care workers' uniforms." *Clothing and Textiles Research Journal* 25, no. 3 (2007): 258–272.

Cheng, Vincent C. C, Jonathan H. K. Chen, Sally S. M. Leung, Simon Y. C. So, Shuk-Ching Wong, Sally C. Y. Wong, Herman Tse, and Kwok-Yung Yuen. "Seasonal outbreak of Bacillus bacteremia associated with contaminated linen in Hong Kong." *Clinical Infectious Diseases* 64, no. suppl_2 (2017): S91–S97.

Chin, Alex W. H., and Leo L. M. Poon. "Stability of SARS-CoV-2 in different environmental conditions–Authors' reply." *The Lancet Microbe* 1, no. 4 (2020): e146.

CORDIS. "Final Report Summary - PLASMAPOR (Plasma penetration into porous materials for biomedical, textile and filtration applications)" In Plasma Penetration into Porous Materials for Biomedical, Textile and Filtration Applications". 2017. Last updated 16 November 2017. https://cordis.europa.eu/project/id/279022/reporting.

Condò, Carla, Patrizia Messi, Immacolata Anacarso, Carla Sabia, Ramona Iseppi, Moreno Bondi, and Simona De Niederhausern. "Antimicrobial activity of silver doped fabrics for the production of hospital uniforms." *New Microbiologica*. (2015): 551–558.

Criscenti, Giuseppe, Carmelo De Maria, Alessia Longoni, Clemens A. Van Blitterswijk, Hugo AM Fernandes, Giovanni Vozzi, and Lorenzo Moroni. "Soft-molecular imprinted electrospun scaffolds to mimic specific biological tissues." *Biofabrication* 10, no. 4 (2018): 045005.

Dalton and Low Medical. "Surgical & Disposable Technical Data Sheet". 2020. Accessed June 4th, 2021. https://www.donlow.co.uk/media/uploads_file/2020/07/14/p1ed65tieliool3tt152pfb81jn54.pdf.

Das, Ira, P. Lambert, D. Hill, M. Noy, J. Bion, and T. Elliott. "Carbapenem-resistant Acinetobacter and role of curtains in an outbreak in intensive care units." *Journal of Hospital Infection* 50, no. 2 (2002): 110–114.

Debbabi, Faten, Sondes Gargoubi, Mohamed Adnene Hadj Ayed, and Saber Ben Abdessalem. "Development and characterization of antibacterial braided polyamide suture coated with chitosan-citric acid biopolymer." *Journal of Biomaterials Applications* 32, no. 3 (2017): 384–398.

Demir, Buket, Roy M. Broughton, Mingyu Qiao, Tung-Shi Huang, and S. D. Worley. "N-halamine biocidal materials with superior antimicrobial efficacies for wound dressings." *Molecules* 22, no. 10 (2017): 1582.

Dong, Chao, Ying Ye, Liying Qian, Guanglei Zhao, Beihai He, and Huining Xiao. "Antibacterial modification of cellulose fibers by grafting β-cyclodextrin and inclusion with ciprofloxacin." *Cellulose* 21, no. 3 (2014): 1921–1932.

Duan, Panpan, Qingbo Xu, Xujun Zhang, Jianing Chen, Weishi Zheng, Lin Li, Jing Yang, Feiya Fu, Hongyan Diao, and Xiangdong Liu. "Naturally occurring betaine grafted on cotton fabric for achieving antibacterial and anti-protein adsorption functions." *Cellulose* 27 (2020): 6603–6615.

ECHA. "Substance Infocard Triclosan." 2021. Accessed June 4th, 2021. https://echa.europa.eu/substance-information/-/substanceinfo/100.020.167.

Feng, Jicheng, Esther Hontañón, Maria Blanes, Jörg Meyer, Xiaoai Guo, Laura Santos, Laura Paltrinieri et al. "Scalable and environmentally benign process for smart textile nanofinishing." *ACS Applied Materials & Interfaces* 8, no. 23 (2016): 14756–14765.

Goldman, Emanuel. "Exaggerated risk of transmission of COVID-19 by fomites." *The Lancet Infectious Diseases* 20, no. 8 (2020): 892–893.

Gu, Jingwei, Lingjun Yuan, Ze Zhang, Xinhui Yang, Junxuan Luo, Zifan Gui, and Shiguo Chen. "Non-leaching bactericidal cotton fabrics with well-preserved physical properties, no skin irritation and no toxicity." *Cellulose* 25, no. 9 (2018): 5415–5426.

Guan, Guijian, Bianhua Liu, Zhenyang Wang, and Zhongping Zhang. "Imprinting of molecular recognition sites on nanostructures and its applications in chemosensors." *Sensors* 8, no. 12 (2008): 8291–8320.

Hardwick, M. "New Test Methods are needed for medical textiles." 2019. Accessed June 4th, 2021. https://specialtyfabricsreview.com/2019/12/01/new-test-methods-are-needed-for-medical-textiles/.

Heathcoat Fabrics. "Capabilities". 2021. Accessed June 4th, 2021. https://www.heathcoat.co.uk/capabilities/.

Holt, Brandon Alexander, Shawn Alan Gregory, Todd Sulchek, Shannon Yee, and Mark D. Losego. "Aqueous zinc compounds as residual antimicrobial agents for textiles." *ACS Applied Materials & Interfaces* 10, no. 9 (2018): 7709–7716.

Hooker, Edmond Anderson, David Ulrich, and Dane Brooks. "Successful removal of clostridioides difficile spores and pathogenic bacteria from a launderable barrier using a commercial laundry process." *Infectious Diseases: Research and Treatment* 13 (2020): 1178633720923657.

Hosein, I. K., P. N. Hoffman, S. Ellam, T-M. Asseez, A. Fakokunde, J. Silles, E. Devereux, D. Kaur, and J. Bosanquet. "Summertime Bacillus cereus colonization of hospital newborns traced to contaminated, laundered linen." *Journal of Hospital Infection* 85, no. 2 (2013): 149–154.

Irfan, Muhammad, Oleksandr Polonskyi, Alexander Hinz, Chiara Mollea, Francesca Bosco, Thomas Strunskus, Cristina Balagna, Sergio Perero, Franz Faupel, and Monica Ferraris. "Antibacterial, highly hydrophobic and semi transparent Ag/plasma polymer nanocomposite coating on cotton fabric obtained by plasma based co-deposition." *Cellulose* 26, no. 16 (2019): 8877–8894.

ISO. "(ISO 20743:2021(en), Textiles–Determination of Antibacterial Activity of Textile Products." 2021. Accessed October 1st, 2021. https://www.iso.org/standard/79819.htm.

JLA. "Ozone laundry disinfection." 2021. Accessed June 4th, 2021. https://jla.com/otex/laundry.

Kampf, Günter, Daniel Todt, Stephanie Pfaender, and Eike Steinmann. "Persistence of coronaviruses on inanimate surfaces and their inactivation with biocidal agents." *Journal of Hospital Infection* 104, no. 3 (2020): 246–251.

Kampf, Günter. "How long can nosocomial pathogens survive on textiles? A systematic review." *GMS Hygiene and Infection Control* 15 (2020).

Kampf, G. "Antiseptic stewardship: Biocide resistance and clinical implications. Antiseptic Stewardship: Biocide Resistance and Clinical Implications." (2018).

Karim, Nazmul, Shaila Afroj, Kate Lloyd, Laura Clarke Oaten, Daria V. Andreeva, Chris Carr, Andrew D. Farmery, Il-Doo Kim, and Kostya S. Novoselov. "Sustainable personal protective clothing for healthcare applications: A review." *ACS Nano* 14, no. 10 (2020): 12313–12340.

Kim, Hyung Woo, Bo Ra Kim, and Young Ha Rhee. Imparting durable antimicrobial properties to cotton fabrics using alginate–quaternary ammonium complex nanoparticles." *Carbohydrate Polymers* 79, no. 4 (2010): 1057–1062.

Kim, Young Hee, and Gang Sun. "Durable antimicrobial finishing of nylon fabrics with acid dyes and a quaternary ammonium salt." *Textile Research Journal* 71, no. 4 (2001): 318–323.

Kocer, Hasan B., Idris Cerkez, S. D. Worley, R. M. Broughton, and T. S. Huang. "Polymeric antimicrobial N-halamine epoxides." *ACS Applied Materials & Interfaces* 3, no. 8 (2011): 2845–2850.

Kowalczyk, Dorota, Stefan Brzeziński, and Irena Kamińska. "Multifunctional nanocoating finishing of polyester/cotton woven fabric by the sol-gel method." *Textile Research Journal* 88, no. 8 (2018): 946–956.

Lazary, A., I. Weinberg, J-J. Vatine, A. Jefidoff, R. Bardenstein, G. Borkow, and N. Ohana. "Reduction of healthcare-associated infections in a long-term care brain injury ward by replacing regular linens with biocidal copper oxide impregnated linens." *International Journal of Infectious Diseases* 24 (2014): 23–29.

Li, Shuhui, Jiangying Huang, Mingzheng Ge, Chunyan Cao, Shu Deng, Songnan Zhang, Guoqiang Chen, Keqin Zhang, Salem S. Al-Deyab, and Yuekun Lai. "Robust flower-like TiO_2@ cotton fabrics with special wettability for effective self-cleaning and versatile oil/water separation." *Advanced Materials Interfaces* 2, no. 14 (2015): 1500220.

Li, Yang, Pingxiong Cai, Zhang-fa Tong, Huining Xiao, and Yuanfeng Pan. "Preparation of copolymer-based nanoparticles with broad-spectrum antimicrobial activity." *Polymers* 9, no. 12 (2017): 717.

Liang, J., Y. Chen, K. Barnes, R. Wu, S. D. Worley, and T-S. Huang. "N-halamine/quat siloxane copolymers for use in biocidal coatings." *Biomaterials* 27, no. 11 (2006): 2495–2501.

Liang, Jie, Yongjun Chen, Xuehong Ren, Rong Wu, Kevin Barnes, S. D. Worley, R. M. Broughton, Unchin Cho, Hasan Kocer, and T. S. Huang. "Fabric treated with antimicrobial N-halamine epoxides." *Industrial & Engineering Chemistry Research* 46, no. 20 (2007): 6425–6429.

Lin, Huiping, Qingjian Hu, Tianyu Liao, Xinxiang Zhang, Wenbin Yang, and Shuang Cai. "Highly Hydrophobic cotton fabrics modified by poly (methylhydrogen) siloxane and fluorinated olefin: Characterization and applications." *Polymers* 12, no. 4 (2020): 833.

Lin, Jing, XiaoYu Chen, ChunYan Chen, JieTao Hu, CaiLong Zhou, XianFang Cai, Wei Wang et al. "Durably antibacterial and bacterially antiadhesive cotton fabrics coated by cationic fluorinated polymers." *ACS Applied Materials & Interfaces* 10, no. 7 (2018): 6124–6136.

Liu, Yuyang, John Haozhong Xin, and Chang-Hwan Choi. "Cotton fabrics with single-faced superhydrophobicity." *Langmuir* 28, no. 50 (2012): 17426–17434.

Loftsson, Thorsteinn, and Marcus E. Brewster. "Pharmaceutical applications of cyclodextrins. 1. Drug solubilization and stabilization." *Journal of Pharmaceutical Sciences* 85, no. 10 (1996): 1017–1025.

Lytle, C. D., W. Truscott, A. P. Budacz, L. Venegas, L. B. Routson, and W. H. Cyr. "Important factors for testing barrier materials with surrogate viruses." *Applied and Environmental Microbiology* 57, no. 9 (1991): 2549.

Ma, Wei, Lin Li, Xintong Xiao, Haishun Du, Xuehong Ren, Xinyu Zhang, and Tung-Shi Huang. "Construction of chlorine labeled ZnO–chitosan loaded cellulose nanofibrils film with quick antibacterial performance and prominent UV stability." *Macromolecular Materials and Engineering* 305, no. 8 (2020): 2000228.

Ma, Wei, Lin Li, Xuehong Ren, and Tung-Shi Huang. "Rational design of cotton substrates with enhanced UV–blocking, high antibacterial efficiency and prominent hydrophobicity." *Cellulose* 26, no. 9 (2019a): 5757–5768.

Ma, Zhipeng, Maoli Yin, Mengshuang Zhang, Zhenming Qi, Xuehong Ren, and Tung-Shi Huang. "Durable N-halamine antibacterial cellulose based on thiol-ene click chemistry." *Fibers and Polymers* 20, no. 2 (2019b): 244–249.

Marcus, Esther-Lee, Hana Yosef, Gadi Borkow, Yehezkel Caine, Ady Sasson, and Allon E. Moses. "Reduction of health care–associated infection indicators by copper oxide–impregnated textiles: Crossover, double-blind controlled study in chronic ventilator-dependent patients." *American Journal of Infection Control* 45, no. 4 (2017): 401–403.

McCoustra, Martin R. S., and Robert Rhodes Mather. "Plasma modification of textiles: Understanding the mechanisms involved." *Textile Progress* 50, no. 4 (2018): 185–229.

McDonnell, G., and P. Burke. "Disinfection: Is it time to reconsider Spaulding?". *Journal of Hospital Infection* 78, no. 3 (2011): 163–170.

Microban®. "Microban Zinc Additives." 2021. Accessed June 4th, 2021. https://www.microban.com/antimicrobial-solutions/technologies/zinc-additives.

Mishra, Rajesh, J. Militky, Vijaykumar Baheti, Juan Huang, B. Kale, Mohanapriya Venkataraman, V. Bele, V. Arumugam, Guocheng Zhu, and Yan Wang. "The production, characterization and applications of nanoparticles in the textile industry." *Textile Progress* 46, no. 2 (2014): 133–226.

Mitchell, A., M. Spencer, and C. Edmiston Jr. "Role of healthcare apparel and other healthcare textiles in the transmission of pathogens: A review of the literature." *Journal of Hospital Infection* 90, no. 4 (2015): 285–292.

Mohamed, Amina L., Mehrez E. El-Naggar, Th I. Shaheen, and Ahmed G. Hassabo. "Laminating of chemically modified silan based nanosols for advanced functionalization of cotton textiles." *International Journal of Biological Macromolecules* 95 (2017): 429–437.

Mokhtari, F., M. Salehi, F. Zamani, F. Hajiani, F. Zeighami, and M. Latifi. "Advances in electrospinning: The production and application of nanofibres and nanofibrous structures." *Textile Progress* 48, no. 3 (2016): 119–219.

Mondal, Md Ibrahim H., and Firoz Ahmed. "Cellulosic fibres modified by chitosan and synthesized ecofriendly carboxymethyl chitosan from prawn shell waste." *The Journal of The Textile Institute* 111, no. 1 (2020): 49–59.

Mondelli, Mario U., Marta Colaneri, Elena M. Seminari, Fausto Baldanti, and Raffaele Bruno. "Low risk of SARS-CoV-2 transmission by fomites in real-life conditions." *The Lancet Infectious Diseases* 21, no. 5 (2021): e112.

Morais, Diana Santos, Rui Miranda Guedes, and Maria Ascensão Lopes. "Antimicrobial approaches for textiles: From research to market." *Materials* 9, no. 6 (2016): 498.

Mukhopadhyay, Rahul Dev, Gourab Das, and Ayyappanpillai Ajayaghosh. "Stepwise control of host–guest interaction using a coordination polymer gel." *Nature Communications* 9, no. 1 (2018): 1–9.

Murugesh Babu, K., and K. B. Ravindra. "Bioactive antimicrobial agents for finishing of textiles for health care products." *The Journal of The Textile Institute* 106, no. 7 (2015): 706–717.

Neely, Alice N., and Matthew P. Maley. "Survival of enterococci and staphylococci on hospital fabrics and plastic." *Journal of Clinical Microbiology* 38, no. 2 (2000): 724–726.

OECD. "Guidance Document on the Evaluation of the Efficacy of Antimicrobial Treated Articles with Claims for External Effects; ENV/JM/MONO(2008)27, 18th November 2008." 2008. Accessed June 4th, 2021. https://www.oecd.org/env/ehs/pesticides-biocides/41692131.pdf.

OECD. "Environment, Health and Safety Publications Series on Testing and Assessment No. 287 Guidance Document on Use and Development of Tier-2 Laboratory-based Tests Used to Substantiate Claims for Efficacy of Biocide-treated Articles. Inter-Organisation Programme for the Sound Management of Chemicals, Environment Directorate, OECD, 1st March 2019". 2019. Accessed June 4th, 2021. https://www.oecd.org/officialdocuments/publicdisplaydocumentpdf/?cote=env/jm/mono(2018)20&doclanguage=en.

Owen, Lucy, and Katie Laird. "The role of textiles as fomites in the healthcare environment: A review of the infection control risk." *PeerJ* 8 (2020): e9790.

Pal, Anita, Y. C. Tripathi, Rakesh Kumar, and Lokesh Upadhyay. "Antibacterial efficacy of natural dye from Melia composita leaves and its application in sanitized and protective textiles." *Journal of Pharmacy Research* 10, no. 4 (2016): 154–159.

Parthasarathi, V., and G. Thilagavathi. "Development of tri-laminate antiviral surgical gown for liquid barrier protection." *The Journal of the Textile Institute* 106, no. 10 (2015): 1095–1105.

Patel, Kapil D., Hae-Won Kim, Jonathan C. Knowles, and Alessandro Poma. "Molecularly imprinted polymers and electrospinning: Manufacturing convergence for next-level applications." *Advanced Functional Materials* 30, no. 32 (2020): 2001955.

Petkova, Petya, Antonio Francesko, Ilana Perelshtein, Aharon Gedanken, and Tzanko Tzanov. "Simultaneous sonochemical-enzymatic coating of medical textiles with antibacterial ZnO nanoparticles." *Ultrasonics Sonochemistry* 29 (2016): 244–250.

Pinho, Eva, Graça Soares, Mariana Henriques, and Martin Grootveld. "Antibacterial activity of textiles for wound treatment." *AATCC Journal of Research* 2, no. 5 (2015): 1–7.

Pinho, Eva, Lúcia Magalhães, Mariana Henriques, and Rosário Oliveira. "Antimicrobial activity assessment of textiles: Standard methods comparison." *Annals of Microbiology* 61, no. 3 (2011): 493–498.

Popescu, Vasilica, Marioara Petrea, and Andrei Popescu. "Multifunctional finishing of cotton with compounds derived from MCT-β-CD and quantification of effects using MLR statistical analysis." *Polymers* 13, no. 3 (2021): 410.

Ramanujam, K., and M. Sundrarajan. "Biocidal activities of monochlorotriazine-β-cyclodextrine with MgO modified cellulosic fabrics." *The Journal of the Textile Institute* 106, no. 11 (2015): 1147–1153.

Ravindra, S., Y. Murali Mohan, N. Narayana Reddy, and K. Mohana Raju. "Fabrication of antibacterial cotton fibres loaded with silver nanoparticles via "Green Approach"." *Colloids and Surfaces A: Physicochemical and Engineering Aspects* 367, no. 1–3 (2010): 31–40.

Ren, Xuehong, Lei Kou, Hasan B. Kocer, Changyun Zhu, S. D. Worley, R. M. Broughton, and T. S. Huang. "Antimicrobial coating of an N-halamine biocidal monomer on cotton fibers via admicellar polymerization." *Colloids and Surfaces A: Physicochemical and Engineering Aspects* 317, no. 1–3 (2008): 711–716.

Ren, Tian, Teresa V. Dormitorio, Mingyu Qiao, Tung-Shi Huang, and Jean Weese. "N-halamine incorporated antimicrobial nonwoven fabrics for use against avian influenza virus." *Veterinary Microbiology* 218 (2018): 78–83.

Rezaie, Ali Bashiri, Majid Montazer, and Mahnaz Mahmoudi Rad. "Low toxic antibacterial application with hydrophobic properties on polyester through facile and clean fabrication of nano copper with fatty acid." *Materials Science and Engineering: C* 97 (2019): 177–187.

Rosenberg, Merilin, Krunoslav Ilić, Katre Juganson, Angela Ivask, Merja Ahonen, Ivana Vinković Vrček, and Anne Kahru. "Potential ecotoxicological effects of antimicrobial surface coatings: A literature survey backed up by analysis of market reports." *PeerJ* 7 (2019): e6315.

Rozman, Urška, Daniela Zavec Pavlinić, Emil Pal, Vida Gönc, and Sonja Šostar Turk. "Efficiency of medical workers' uniforms with antimicrobial activity." *Textiles for Advanced Applications* 255 (2017).

Rutala, William A. "APIC guideline for selection and use of disinfectants." *American Journal of Infection Control* 24, no. 4 (1996): 313–342.

Rutala, William A. "Disinfection, sterilization and waste disposal." In *Prevention and Control of Nosocomial Infections*. Baltimore: Williams and Wilkins, 1997, pp. 539–593.

Rutala, W. A. 1999 "Selection and use of disinfectants in healthcare." In *Infection Control and Hospital Epidemiology*, edited by Mayhall, C. G. Philadelphia: Lippincott Williams & Wilkins, 1999, pp. 1161–1187.

Salat, Marc, Petya Petkova, Javier Hoyo, Ilana Perelshtein, Aharon Gedanken, and Tzanko Tzanov. "Durable antimicrobial cotton textiles coated sonochemically with ZnO nanoparticles embedded in an in-situ enzymatically generated bioadhesive." *Carbohydrate Polymers* 189 (2018): 198–203.

Schneider, Guilherme, Felipe Lazarini Bim, Álvaro Francisco Lopes de Sousa, Evandro Watanabe, Denise de Andrade, and Inês Fronteira. "The use of antimicrobial-impregnated fabrics in health services: An integrative review." *Revista Latino-Americana de Enfermagem* 29 (2021).

Shaban, Mohamed, Fatma Mohamed, and Semsem Abdallah. "Production and characterization of superhydrophobic and antibacterial coated fabrics utilizing ZnO nanocatalyst." *Scientific Reports* 8, no. 1 (2018): 1–15.

Shahidi, Sheila, Necdet Aslan, Mahmood Ghoranneviss, and May Korachi. "Effect of thymol on the antibacterial efficiency of plasma-treated cotton fabric." *Cellulose* 21, no. 3 (2014): 1933–1943.

Sifri, Costi D., Gene H. Burke, and Kyle B. Enfield. "Reduced health care-associated infections in an acute care community hospital using a combination of self-disinfecting copper-impregnated composite hard surfaces and linens." *American Journal of Infection Control* 44, no. 12 (2016): 1565–1571.

Simmons, Bryan P. "CDC guidelines for the prevention and control of nosocomial infections. Guideline for hospital environmental control." *American Journal of Infection Control* 11, no. 3 (1983): 97–120.

Song, Lingjie, Liwei Sun, Jie Zhao, Xianghong Wang, Jinghua Yin, Shifang Luan, and Weihua Ming. "Synergistic superhydrophobic and photodynamic cotton textiles with remarkable antibacterial activities." *ACS Applied Bio Materials* 2, no. 7 (2019): 2756–2765.

Spaulding, Earle H. "Chemical disinfection and antisepsis in the hospital." *Journal of Hospital Research* 9, no. 1 (1957): 5–31.

Spaulding, E. H 1971 "The role of chemical disinfection in the prevention of nosocomial infections." In: *Proceedings of the International Conference on Nosocomial Infections*. Chicago, IL: American Hospital Association, 1970, pp. 247–254.

Strnad, Simona, Olivera Šauperl, and Lidija Fras-Zemljič. "Cellulose fibres functionalised by chitosan: Characterization and application." *Biopolymers* (2010): 181–200.

Takai, Kenichi, Tokuko Ohtsuka, Yoshiko Senda, Miyuki Nakao, Kouichiro Yamamoto, Junji Matsuoka, and Yoshikazu Hirai. "Antibacterial properties of antimicrobial-finished textile products." *Microbiology and Immunology* 46, no. 2 (2002): 75–81.

Tamahkar, Emel, Monireh Bakhshpour, and Adil Denizli. "Molecularly imprinted composite bacterial cellulose nanofibers for antibiotic release." *Journal of Biomaterials Science, Polymer Edition* 30, no. 6 (2019): 450–461.

The Textile Institute. "Textile Terms and Definitions". 2021. https://www.ttandd.org/content/textile-terms-and-definitions and 11th Edn; edited by Denton, M.J. and Daniels, P.N. The Textile Institute (2002).

Tian, Hongru, Yongshai Zhai, Cheng Xu, and Jie Liang. "Durable antibacterial cotton fabrics containing stable acyclic N-halamine groups." *Industrial & Engineering Chemistry Research* 56, no. 28 (2017): 7902–7909.

Tudu, Balraj Krishnan, Apurba Sinhamahapatra, and Aditya Kumar. "Surface modification of cotton fabric using TiO_2 nanoparticles for self-cleaning, oil–water separation, anti-stain, anti-water absorption, and antibacterial properties." *ACS Omega* 5, no. 14 (2020): 7850–7860.

Turalija, M., P. Merschak, B. Redl, U. Griesser, H. Duelli, and T. Bechtold. "Copper (i) oxide microparticles–synthesis and antimicrobial finishing of textiles." *Journal of Materials Chemistry B* 3, no. 28 (2015): 5886–5892.

Voncina, B., and Vivod, V. "Cyclodextrins in Textile Finishing. Published: January 6th 2013." 2013. Accessed June 4th, 2021. https://www.intechopen.com/books/eco-friendly-textile-dyeing-and-finishing/cyclodextrins-in-textile-finishing.

Vozzi, Giovanni, Ilaria Morelli, Federico Vozzi, Chiara Andreoni, Elisabetta Salsedo, Annagiulia Morachioli, Paolo Giusti, and Gianluca Ciardelli. "SOFT-MI: A novel microfabrication technique integrating soft-lithography and molecular imprinting for tissue engineering applications." *Biotechnology and Bioengineering* 106, no. 5 (2010): 804–817.

Wen, Wen, Zaixing Zhang, Lingxiao Jing, and Tonghua Zhang. "Synthesis of a Hein–Schiff base compound and its antibacterial activity on cotton fabrics." *Cellulose* 27 (2020): 7243–7254.

Wendt, C., Frei, R., and Widmer, A. Decontamination, disinfection, and sterilisation." In Volume 1, *Manual of Clinical Microbiology* (11th Edition), edited by J. Jorgensen, M. Pfaller, K. Carroll, G. Funke, M. Landry, S. Richter, D. Warnock. Washington, DC: ASM Press, 2015, pp. 183–216.

Wu, Yunping, Yan Yang, Zhijie Zhang, Zhihua Wang, Yanbao Zhao, and Lei Sun. "Fabrication of cotton fabrics with durable antibacterial activities finishing by Ag nanoparticles." *Textile Research Journal* 89, no. 5 (2019): 867–880.

Xu, Bi, and Zaisheng Cai. "Fabrication of a superhydrophobic ZnO nanorod array film on cotton fabrics via a wet chemical route and hydrophobic modification." *Applied Surface Science* 254, no. 18 (2008): 5899–5904.

Xu, QingBo, XiaTing Ke, LiWen Shen, NaiQin Ge, YanYan Zhang, FeiYa Fu, and XiangDong Liu. "Surface modification by carboxymethy chitosan via pad-dry-cure method for binding Ag NPs onto cotton fabric." *International Journal of Biological Macromolecules* 111 (2018): 796–803.

Xu, QingBo, WeiShi Zheng, PanPan Duan, JiaNing Chen, YanYan Zhang, FeiYa Fu, HongYan Diao, and XiangDong Liu. "One-pot fabrication of durable antibacterial cotton fabric coated with silver nanoparticles via carboxymethyl chitosan as a binder and stabilizer." *Carbohydrate Polymers* 204 (2019): 42–49.

Xue, Chaohua, Chen, Jia, Yin, Wei, Jia, Shun-Tian, and Ma, Jianzhong. "Superhydrophobic conductive textiles with antibacterial property by coating fibers with silver nanoparticles." *Applied Surface Science* 258 (2012): 2468–2472. DOI: 10.1016/j.apsusc.2011.10.074.

Yamabe, Akane, Atsushi Irisawa, Yasuhito Kunogi, Ken Kashima, Takahito Minaguchi, Akira Yamamiya, Naoya Izawa et al. "Development of biliary stent applying the antibacterial activity of silver: A literature review." *Bio-Medical Materials and Engineering Preprint* (2021): 1–9.

Zhang, Shaobo, Xinghui Yang, Bin Tang, Lingjun Yuan, Kui Wang, Xiangyu Liu, Xingli Zhu, Jianna Li, Zaochuan Ge, and Shiguo Chen. "New insights into synergistic antimicrobial and antifouling cotton fabrics via dually finished with quaternary ammonium salt and zwitterionic sulfobetaine." *Chemical Engineering Journal* 336 (2018): 123–132.

Zhang, Desuo, Ling Chen, Chuanfeng Zang, Yuyue Chen, and Hong Lin. "Antibacterial cotton fabric grafted with silver nanoparticles and its excellent laundering durability." *Carbohydrate Polymers* 92, no. 2 (2013): 2088–2094.

Zhang, Teng, Jingwei Gu, Xiangyu Liu, Dengshuai Wei, Huiling Zhou, Haihua Xiao, Zhuocheng Zhang, Huali Yu, and Shiguo Chen. "Bactericidal and antifouling electrospun PVA nanofibers modified with a quaternary ammonium salt and zwitterionic sulfopropylbetaine." *Materials Science and Engineering: C* 111 (2020): 110855.

Zhao, T., and Q. Chen. "Halogenated phenols and polybiguanides as antimicrobial textile finishes." In *Antimicrobial Textiles*. Woodhead Publishing, 2016, pp. 141–153.

Zhou, Chang-E., and Chi-wai Kan. "Plasma-assisted regenerable chitosan antimicrobial finishing for cotton." *Cellulose* 21, no. 4 (2014): 2951–2962.

Zhu, Tang, Junrong Wu, Ning Zhao, Chao Cai, Zhenchao Qian, Fangfang Si, Heng Luo et al. "Superhydrophobic/superhydrophilic janus fabrics reducing blood loss." *Advanced Healthcare Materials* 7, no. 7 (2018): 1701086.

6 Ensuring Regulatory Compliance

Peter J. Ogrodnik

6.1 INTRODUCTION

Chapter 6 provides an overview of the world of medical device regulations required for taking a design concept through to a marketable product. A brief glimpse of historical guidelines demonstrates how advancing technology has shaped new guidance such that the safety of users and those in the surrounding environment is maintained. This is a fast-changing area which, in the UK, will be affected by Brexit, though quite to what extent remains uncertain.

It is worth noting that over the past few years, the medical devices world has changed. Some of these changes are definite, for example, ISO 13485; some changes were enacted recently, for example, the EU Medical Devices Regulations; and other changes will have (as yet) an unknown impact, for example, the new UKCA system.

6.2 CHANGES TO LEGISLATION

The first is the new ISO 14971 (the risk management standard for medical devices) which was published in 2019. This is the version everyone should be using now.

In 2016, the new ISO 13485 (the quality-management standard for medical devices) was published; transition needed to be accomplished by Spring 2018. This is a change which is positive as it harmonises across boundaries; the FDA accepts ISO 13485:2016 as does the EU.

Finally, the European Union's new MDR (Medical Devices Regulations 2017/245) has been published and everyone must have transferred over by 26 May 2020 from the old Medical Devices Directive to remain compliant. However, due to the COVID outbreak this has been delayed and a staggered approach has been adopted. All new devices have to be compliant which depends on classification: all Class I, for example, must now be MDR compliant.

Equally the FDA has been tweaking rules and regulations too, but nothing as major as a brand-new set of rules, and unlike the EU, its rules are updated at least on an annual basis (and often sooner). Keeping up to date has never been so important.

One major important imminent change is Brexit. No one really knows what the implications were for the medical devices industry in the UK or even the marketplace.

DOI: 10.1201/9781003170570-6

However, we do know that if we are to sell devices into the EU and the USA, we must still follow EU and FDA rules. What happens in the UK will, hopefully, become clearer soon, but the importance of design control will, inevitably, remain the same because ISO 14971 and ISO 13485 are international standards. What will change imminently, however, is the UKCA replacement of CE and the likely effects of that are not known, so device developers and suppliers will need to remain alert.

6.3 THE MEDICAL DEVICES BODIES

The regulatory bodies concerned with medical devices exert considerable authority. Within Europe, each country has its own government body called the Competent Authority. Even though they are separate bodies they act in concert so that an application for a CE mark (the license to sell within the European Union) in one country counts in all the other member states. At the next level down is the Notified Body, the legal entity licensed by the Competent Authority to do the CE marking process. An applicant would work with and be audited by the Notified Body. The process is completely different in the USA; here the body is the U.S. Food & Drug Administration (FDA) and the relevant subset is the Center for Devices and Radiological Health (CDRH). The applicant talks direct to the FDA (via CDRH) and obtains a Clearance to Market.

It is important to know that the applicant/holder of the CE mark or FDA Clearance to Market is universally known as the Manufacturer and they are at the top of the regulatory chain for the device and ultimately responsible for the safety of that device (the designer, the subcontractor, the packager, etc. are subservient to them, but all are involved in the regulatory process). With manufacturer status comes further levels of responsibility, not only insurance, but reporting, vigilance, post-market surveillance, gathering clinical evidence, and much more. Canada has its own level of complexity (with CAMDCAS), and Japan's is even more complex, but the main thing to keep in mind is that the application processes are very different. Even so, the application is about how to present the design to the authorities, but how designing is done is always the same.

The manufacturer has the ultimate responsibility for liability. However, as with any other discipline, their insurers will try and pass liability down to sub-contractors. Hence it is important for sub-contractors to have relevant insurance in place – and that sub-contractors never exceed their particular level of experience. Nevertheless, the designer is at the hub of the activity. Without the designer nothing happens, no device exists, and there is nothing to present for sale; hence the product lives and dies at the designer's hand, so knowledge of the medical devices regime is fundamental, adherence to the structured design processes is essential, and communication with others involved is of paramount importance.

6.4 ESSENTIAL DEFINITIONS AND CHANGES TO THESE

It is important to be embedded in the discipline in which you practise design. Hence a car designer is embedded within the automotive industry, probably plays with their own car at night and weekends; almost certainly watches or takes part in motorsport; and will read every car magazine under the sun. So, it is with the medical device designer: we must tinker, read, observe, and play, but unlikely that we will ever be able to use our designs. Hence we operate remotely, but we also know that one day our design may just come and save us too. The lesson here is that we need to know as much about the end use as the end user. In fact, we need to know more than the individual end user, we need to consider all end users. I can promise you that if you understand your discipline well, your designs will be excellent and you will get great satisfaction in knowing that you have saved someone's leg, eye, or life.

The corollary is that you can also contribute to the loss of someone's leg, eye, or life. To this end, medical devices is one of the most highly regulated arenas to work in. The first staging post is to fully understand what a medical device is. Believe me, that this is one of the hardest battles you will have with your end users. Each one will think they are a special case and are, somehow, excluded – they are not, and neither are you. More importantly, you are the one who will end up in court.

The European Union and FDA have tidy definitions of a medical device. Within Europe this was laid down in law under the Medical Devices Directive 93/42/EEC as amended (most recently) by 2007/47/EC (European Commission 2016). The definition that was in force until Spring 2020 is as shown below:

> a) 'medical device' means any instrument, apparatus, appliance, material or other article, whether used alone or in combination, including the software necessary for its proper application intended by the manufacturer to be used for human beings for the purpose of:
>
> - diagnosis, prevention, monitoring, treatment or alleviation of disease,
> - diagnosis, monitoring, treatment, alleviation of or compensation for an injury or handicap,
> - investigation, replacement or modification of the anatomy or of a physiological process,
> - control of conception,
>
> and which does not achieve its principal intended action in or on the human body by pharmacological, immunological or metabolic means, but which may be assisted in its function by such means (EC 1993).

The definition is clear: if the device is to be used in any clinical environment, on humans, then it is a medical device. Note that the definition does not say that the device has to be used in a hospital or by a clinician – it is defined by its intended use, not by the user. The designer must state the intended use in their wording and it is important to get it right.

The new Medical Devices Regulations 2017/745 came into force in May 2020 and the new definition is:

> 'medical device' means any instrument, apparatus, appliance, software, implant, reagent, material or other article intended by the manufacturer to be used, alone or in combination, for human beings for one or more of the following specific medical purposes:

- diagnosis, prevention, monitoring, prediction, prognosis, treatment or alleviation of disease,
- diagnosis, monitoring, treatment, alleviation of, or compensation for, an injury or disability,
- investigation, replacement or modification of the anatomy or of a physiological or pathological process or state,
- providing information by means of in vitro examination of specimens derived from the human body, including organ, blood and tissue donations, and which does not achieve its principal intended action by pharmacological, immunological or metabolic means, in or on the human body, but which may be assisted in its function by such means.

The following products shall also be deemed to be medical devices:

- devices for the control or support of conception;
- products specifically intended for the cleaning, disinfection or sterilisation of devices as referred to in Article 1(4) and of those referred to in the first paragraph of this point. (EU 2017)*

As you can see, the definition has grown somewhat! But it is essentially the same, just more explicit so that some 'grey area' devices do not fall through the net – e.g., software. Compare this with the equivalent definition from the USA (taken from the Federal Food, Drug, and Cosmetic Act [FD&C Act]):

⃠ The term 'device' (except when used in paragraph (n) of this section and in sections 301(i), 403(f), 502(c), and 602(c)) means an instrument, apparatus, implement, machine, contrivance, implant, in vitro reagent, or other similar or related article, including any component, part, or accessory, which is –

(1) recognized in the official National Formulary, or the United States Pharmacopeia, or any supplement to them,
(2) intended for use in the diagnosis of disease or other conditions, or in the cure, mitigation, treatment, or prevention of disease, in man or other animals, or
(3) intended to affect the structure or any function of the body of man or other animals, and which does not achieve its primary intended purposes through chemical action within or on the body of man or other animals and which is not dependent upon being metabolized for the achievement of its primary intended purposes. (FDA 2004)

As with the EU, the FDA has updated their definition of a medical device; note the last paragraph:

an instrument, apparatus, implement, machine, contrivance, implant, in vitro reagent, or other similar or related article, including a component part, or accessory which is:

* To make things as clear as possible, all new definitions and guidelines will be made clear. Old ones will have an hour-glass symbol ⌛ indicating they have a limited shelf life. If they are now so old that they no longer exist, they will have a stop sign ⃠ indicating do not use any more: they are only there for comparison purposes.

1. recognized in the official National Formulary, or the United States Pharmacopoeia, or any supplement to them,
2. intended for use in the diagnosis of disease or other conditions, or in the cure, mitigation, treatment, or prevention of disease, in man or other animals, or
3. intended to affect the structure or any function of the body of man or other animals, and which does not achieve its primary intended purposes through chemical action within or on the body of man or other animals and

> which does not achieve its primary intended purposes through chemical action within or on the body of man or other animals and which is not dependent upon being metabolized for the achievement of its primary intended purposes. The term 'device' does not include software functions excluded pursuant to section 520(o).

Note that both EU and FDA clearly distinguish between a device and a pharmacological agent. Also note that the FDA has a much more detailed analysis of the role of software in medical devices (FDA 2019). It is important, therefore, to download a copy of 520(o) and to make full use of it if there is any software associated with the device.

Often devices need accessories or additional items for particular functions, these are covered too:

> (b) 'accessory' means an article which whilst not being a device is intended specifically by its manufacturer to be used together with a device to enable it to be used in accordance with the use of the device intended by the manufacturer of the device. (EC 1993)

And the MDR definition:

> 'accessory for a medical device' means an article which, whilst not being itself a medical device, is intended by its manufacturer to be used together with one or several particular medical device(s) to specifically enable the medical device(s) to be used in accordance with its/their intended purpose(s) or to specifically and directly assist the medical functionality of the medical device(s) in terms of its/their intended purpose(s). (EU 2017)

The importance of accessories will become more pronounced as we go further into the design process. Some people saw accessories as being devoid of regulatory control, as some form of 'get out clause.' The new MDR has tightened this up. If design is to be used with something from definition (a), then isn't this also a medical device, as are items used in the laboratory for assessment of things taken from the human body, and not necessarily in contact with that body?

> (c) 'device used for in vitro diagnosis' means any device which is a reagent, reagent product, kit, instrument, equipment or system, whether used alone or in combination, intended by the manufacturer to be used in vitro for the examination of samples derived from the human body with a view to providing information on the physiological state, state of health or disease, or congenital abnormality thereof (EC 1993)

But in the new regulations 'in-vitro diagnostic devices' have their own special regulation EU 2017/746, and in that regulation the definition is:

> 'in vitro diagnostic medical device' means any medical device which is a reagent, reagent product, calibrator, control material, kit, instrument, apparatus, piece of equipment, software or system, whether used alone or in combination, intended by the manufacturer to be used in vitro for the examination of specimens, including blood and tissue donations, derived from the human body, solely or principally for the purpose of providing information on one or more of the following:
>
> (a) concerning a physiological or pathological process or state;
> (b) concerning congenital physical or mental impairments;
> (c) concerning the predisposition to a medical condition or a disease;
> (d) to determine the safety and compatibility with potential recipients;
> (e) to predict treatment response or reactions;
> (f) to define or monitoring therapeutic measures.
>
> Specimen receptacles shall also be deemed to be in vitro diagnostic medical devices. (EU 2017)

The perennial question comes from the large 'made for the patient' market. Some people may hope that this offers an escape clause or a loophole, but it does not.

> (d) 'custom-made device' means any device specifically made in accordance with a duly qualified medical practitioner's written prescription which gives, under his responsibility, specific design characteristics and is intended for the sole use of a particular patient. (EC 1993)

What it does do is to allow for custom-made devices to exist but without the pre-market assessments required for mainstream devices. Because of over-exploitation of this type of categorisation, as such the EU has tightened the definition:

> 'custom-made device' means any device specifically made in accordance with a written prescription of any person authorised by national law by virtue of that person's professional qualifications which gives, under that person's responsibility, specific design characteristics, and is intended for the sole use of a particular patient exclusively to meet their individual conditions and needs.
>
> However, mass-produced devices which need to be adapted to meet the specific requirements of any professional user and devices which are mass-produced by means of industrial manufacturing processes in accordance with the written prescriptions of any authorised person shall not be considered to be custom-made devices. (EU 2017)

If this definition were not there, custom devices could not exist; it does not mean that the design rigour is any less stringent. It does not mean the medical practitioner takes the blame for any problems – they are not designers or engineers; designers and engineers still bear the responsibility and consequences for any design issues.

The next definitions are to do with power source, or to do with higher risk functions:

- 'active medical device' means any medical device relying for its functioning on a source of electrical energy or any source of power other than that directly generated by the human body or gravity. (EC 1990)
- 'active implantable medical device' means any active medical device which is intended to be totally or partially introduced, surgically or medically, into the human body or by medical intervention into a natural orifice, and which is intended to remain after the procedure. (EC 1990)

Once again, the new regulations have made changes. Most significantly, active devices are now a part of the new MDR:

> 'active device' means any device, the operation of which depends on a source of energy other than that generated by the human body for that purpose, or by gravity, and which acts by changing the density of or converting that energy. Devices intended to transmit energy, substances or other elements between an active device and the patient, without any significant change, shall not be deemed to be active devices.
>
> Software shall also be deemed to be an active device. (EU 2017)

Note the significance of 'software.' The last piece of the jigsaw is the new definition of an 'implanted' device:

> 'implantable device' means any device, including those that are partially or wholly absorbed, which is intended:
>
> - to be totally introduced into the human body, or
> - to replace an epithelial surface or the surface of the eye,
>
> by clinical intervention and which is intended to remain in place after the procedure.
>
> Any device intended to be partially introduced into the human body by clinical intervention and intended to remain in place after the procedure for at least 30 days shall also be deemed to be an implantable device. (EU 2017)

Once again these are very clear and it is the distilling of the legal wording into small chunks that has made these definitions understandable. Whichever of the above definitions the device being developed falls into, it is important to remember that it is a medical device governed by that definition. However, as technology advances, some products and processes become more dangerous than they were before, so there are two issues that designers have to consider:

1. keeping in constant touch with these important definitions
2. keeping up to date with advances in medicine and technology

There are several other requirements designers need to be aware of too. For medical devices there are sub-disciplines that need to be worked with. In the UK, the new system has all but copied the existing Active Implantable Devices (AID) (90/385/EC), and In-Vitro Diagnostics (IVD) (98/79/EC), but for the EU thinking needs to be in Medical Device Regulations terms (European Community 1990, 1993, 1998). However, at the time of this writing, there were only a handful of notified bodies with the capacity to assess new MDR applications – so designers must expect a long wait. Hence, a quick rule of thumb, until otherwise notified, in the UK the old MDD and its associated IVD and AID directives will be adequate – but with a long waiting list. For the EU, designers will be expected to be working to the new MDR.

The product may also fall within the jurisdiction of other directives, such as Electro-Magnetic Compatibility (EMC) or Powered Tools or other standards, that the device might have to adhere to. It is essential to have a copy of any legislative document that may be needed to hand; they are free to download.

6.5 CLASSIFICATION OF MEDICAL DEVICES

There are several reasons why classification is important.

- The first concerns the patient. The higher the level of risk a device poses to the patient, then the greater the reassurance that needs to be provided. Not all devices pose the same risk; consider, for example, a pacemaker compared to a support bandage. It is quite clear that the pacemaker poses the greater risk and, thus, should have more stringent controls attached to its design, manufacture, and eventual sales.
- The second reason concerns the manufacturer. Why should the registration process be as stringent for the support bandage as compared to the pacemaker?
- The third reason concerns the regulatory bodies as the classification indicates to them the level of risk to the patient and the nature of the beast they are dealing with, and hence the amount of effort they need to put in to the control. After all, governments have limited budgets too and they need to target their resources at the devices that pose the greater risk.

Although patient safety is a priority, one must not forget the users and their safety is just as important. All devices must obey the prime criteria 'do no harm.' However, for some devices to achieve a clinical goal, some harm is inevitable. This poses the question: 'Is the risk acceptable?'

The new Medical Devices Regulations and the new ISO 13485 – 2016 are both 'risk dominated': everything done in the design chain (and every other decision in fact) needs to be risk managed and failure to comply will cause the designer to fail in the creation of a medical device by being stopped by the regulatory bodies. Classification allows all participants in the regulatory process to understand the risk the device poses. In general, the higher the classification the more chance that the device could do some harm. Hence it should come as no surprise that devices such as replacement heart valves are high classification and inserts for shoes are low. However, that does not mean that lower-classification devices do not demand design rigour; the level of rigour is the same at all levels, and Table 6.1 illustrates how risk and classification are interlinked. Both the USA and EU classifications are given here for the purpose of illustration (but not for cross-referencing). Table 6.1 demonstrates that low-risk devices are Class I, and high-risk Class III (note in Canada there is also Class IV).

TABLE 6.1
Classifications in the USA and Europe

Risk	Low risk			High Risk
In Europe, the classifications are				
EU	I	IIa	IIb	III
In the USA, the classifications are				
USA	I / 510(k) exempt	II		III

6.5.1 Classification Rules

Each regulatory authority has its own set of classification rules. In the USA, these are stipulated within CFR21 Part 860 – Medical Device Classification Procedures (FDA 2010). Within the EU, they are currently stipulated within 93/42/EC Annex IX (EC 1993), but will soon be superseded by the new Medical Devices Regulations 2017/745, but is now to be found in Annexe VIII.* All documents are freely available on the World Wide Web, as are those for any other country. As a medical device designer, you must have an up-to-date copy of the classification rules to hand at all times.

There is a fundamental difference between the two systems. In the USA, classification is by precedent and is undertaken by the FDA; that is, you have a classification by comparison with decisions already made by a panel. In Europe, there is a long list of questions to answer, and you decide on your classification. However, attempts to cheat the system by 'under-classifying' will lead to failure.

The classifications are based on risk to the patient (as illustrated by Table 6.2). Risk is a very important aspect of design control; understanding risk to the patent (and to the clinical team/operator) is fundamental. The FDA process is not a good vehicle in helping to understand patient risk and classification, so the EU model is used here to help gain a picture of how classifications are made, and a copy of 93/42/EC Annex IX and the new MDR Annex VIII need to be to hand to assist.

Table 6.2 illustrates how the EC medical devices rules define the classification of a device. The symbols indicate that this rule defines this particular class of device. The new MDR has four new rules, but those new rules are spread throughout the

* At the time of writing this, the UK has left the EU and the medical devices framework. The new UKCA medical devices framework 'mirrors' the old MDD.

TABLE 6.2
EC Classification Rules in Comparison with the Classes They Define
☒ EU MDD & UK MDR : ☼ EU MDR

Rule \ Class in rule	Class I	Class IIa	Class IIb	Class III
# 1	☒ ☼			
# 2	☒ ☼	☒ ☼		
# 3		☒ ☼	☒ ☼	☼
# 4	☒ ☼	☒ ☼	☒ ☼	
# 5	☒ ☼	☒ ☼	☼	
# 6	☒ ☼	☒ ☼	☒ ☼	☒ ☼
# 7		☒ ☼	☒ ☼	☒ ☼
# 8		☒ ☼	☒ ☼	☒ ☼
# 9			☒ ☼	☼
# 10	☼	☒ ☼	☒ ☼	
# 11		☒ ☼	☒ ☼	☼
# 12	☒	☼	☼	
# 13	☼			☒
# 14			☒	☒ ☼
# 15		☒	☒ ☼	☼
# 16		☒ ☼	☼	
# 17		☼		☒
# 18			☒	☼
# 19		☼	☼	☼
# 20		☼	☼	
# 21			☼	☼
# 22				☼
Hip, knee, and shoulder replacements				☒

MDR; so, unfortunately, what was Rule 9 (for example) in the MDD may not be the same rule in the new MDR.

However, the same methodology applies: if you think your device is likely to be Class III, it will fall into the definitions described by one of Rules 6, 7, 8, 13, 14, and 17. It is best not to assume that these are the only rules that need to be considered; all rules need to be examined to make sure that classification is correct, so it is best to start at Rule 1 and go through to the end – crossing out the ones that do not apply; the one that is left at the end of the procedure is the one for the device.

The following definitions are close to becoming universal.

- *Invasive device*: a device that penetrates inside the body either through an orifice or through the surface of the body
- *Surgically invasive device*: Any device that enters the body other than through an established body orifice
- *Transient duration*: continuous use of less than 60 minutes
- *Short-term duration*: continuous use of not more than 30 days
- *Long-term duration*: continuous use of greater than 30 days (EC 1993 and MDR 2018)

The USA and Europe have their own particular wordings.

6.5.2 Custom-Made Devices

There are new rules around custom-made devices. Under the old MDD there was a 'loophole' that 'allowed' mass-produced items to fall under the definition of a custom-made device if it were 'prescribed' by a clinician for a given patient. Under the new MDR (and virtually everyone else's definition of a custom-made device), this is no longer the case.

⌛ MDD definition:

> 'custom-made device' means any device specifically made in accordance with a duly qualified medical practitioner's written prescription which gives, under his responsibility, specific design characteristics and is intended for the sole use of a particular patient.
>
> The abovementioned prescription may also be made out by any other person authorized by virtue of his professional qualifications to do so.
>
> Mass-produced devices which need to be adapted to meet the specific requirements of the medical practitioner or any other professional user are not considered to be custom-made devices.

MDR definition:

> 'custom-made device' means any device specifically made in accordance with a written prescription of any person authorised by national law by virtue of that person's professional qualifications which gives, under that person's responsibility, specific design characteristics, and is intended for the sole use of a particular patient exclusively to meet their individual conditions and needs.
>
> However, mass-produced devices which need to be adapted to meet the specific requirements of any professional user and devices which are mass-produced by means of industrial manufacturing processes in accordance with written prescriptions of any authorised person *shall not be considered* to be custom-made devices.

Although they are close, the fact that the words 'shall not be considered' suggest the new emphasis, despite the fact that this was already tightened in the modification to the original 93/42/EC in 2007. This new definition has major impacts on device manufacturers from orthotics and limb prostheses.

The FDA also tightened its definition in 2016:

Custom devices

(1) In general The requirements of sections 360d and 360e of this title shall not apply to a device that-

- (A) is created or modified in order to comply with the order of an individual physician or dentist (or any other specially qualified person designated under regulations promulgated by the Secretary after an opportunity for an oral hearing);
- (B) in order to comply with an order described in subparagraph (A), necessarily deviates from an otherwise applicable performance standard under section 360d of this title or requirement under section 360e of this title;
- (C) is not generally available in the United States in finished form through labeling or advertising by the manufacturer, importer, or distributor for commercial distribution;
- (D) is designed to treat a unique pathology or physiological condition that no other device is domestically available to treat;
- (E) (i) is intended to meet the special needs of such physician or dentist (or other specially qualified person so designated) in the course of the professional practice of such physician or dentist (or other specially qualified person so designated); or (ii) is intended for use by an individual patient named in such order of such physician or dentist (or other specially qualified person so designated);
- (F) is assembled from components or manufactured and finished on a case-by-case basis to accommodate the unique needs of individuals described in clause (i) or (ii) of subparagraph (E); and
- (G) may have common, standardized design characteristics, chemical and material compositions, and manufacturing processes as commercially distributed devices.

(2) Limitations

Paragraph (1) shall apply to a device only if-

- (A) such device is for the purpose of treating a sufficiently rare condition, such that conducting clinical investigations on such device would be impractical;
- (B) production of such device under paragraph (1) is limited to no more than *5 units per year* of a particular device type, provided that such replication otherwise complies with this section; and
- (C) the manufacturer of such device notifies the Secretary on an annual basis, in a manner prescribed by the Secretary, of the manufacture of such device.

It is worth noting the limit of 5 units per year, and 'custom-made device' is an area that has required even greater regulatory effort, and to the designer it means that a custom-made device requires more design and analytical input than a mass-produced one. The reason why this is the case is because the designer needs to prove it will not fail under normal use and thereby avoid a massive insurance claim. The type of defence based on the evidence that '4 million have worked just fine' is not available for an item which is a one-off.

6.5.3 Exemption?

The first question is whether the items are medical devices. Given the definition of a medical device, it could prove hard to justify a null response. But even so, it is worth taking the time to look at exemptions. It is common for people to think of calling their product a 'medical device' as a badge of honour or marketing tool, but that will lead to added costs. In virtually all markets, there are some things that one would think are medical devices, but under the current rules they have been granted an exemption and the list changes from day to day. For the UK, the list of exemptions is maintained by the MHRA; however, whichever country it was intended to operate in, such a list of exemptions (or in some cases, inclusions, as the list of medical devices is so small!) would be easily found on the Web, or by contact with the regulatory body concerned.

6.5.4 European Union Classification

The EU process is a step-by-step, rule-based process, hence it is always necessary to refer to the correct regulation and the correct annex. Under the MDR, it is Annex VIII. We start at Rule 1 and work our way upward.

> Rule 1: All non-invasive devices are in class I unless one of the rules set out hereafter applies. (same in both MDD and MDR)

Basically, the rule asks us the question: 'Is it invasive?' Clearly, being invasive is risky, so one would expect invasive devices to be high risk, and a non-invasive device must be less risky or so it should be. The first part of this rule says, 'all non-invasive devices can be assumed to be non-risky'; however, the second part says 'but if we have evidence that its particular use is risky then we have the right to make the classification higher.' It is therefore best to assume that all the rules need to be tested against the design idea to ensure further rules do not apply that may alter the classification category.

6.5.5 FDA Classification

Under the FDA process, the idea is to find a *precedent*, or something like the new device that has gone before. The first place to check is the database section of the FDA website (http://www.fda.gov/MedicalDevices/default.htm). The FDA hosts a classification database where a search can be carried out for precedents, namely the *product classification* database (Figure 6.1).

Using this search engine and the search text 'knee brace,' what is found is shown in Figure 6.2. As can be seen, it is not only Class I, but also 510(k) exempt. However, this is for the knee brace alone and not for any variations.

If nothing can be found on the FDA database, it will be necessary to apply to the FDA for a ruling on the classification, a step that can take a very long time.

6.6 RISK MANAGEMENT AND RISK ANALYSIS

Only one standard applies, namely ISO 14971: 2019.

6.6.1 Risk Management Process (ISO 14971)

To undertake this, one needs to adopt ISO 14971, and its latest version, with immediate effect. If software is being produced, it is necessary to refer to any software-specific guidance given in PD IEC – TR 8002. Figure 6.3 is extracted directly from the standard and illustrates a basic risk management process.

When designing a device, at every opportunity, potential hazards should be assessed, together with the risk of the hazard and whether this risk is acceptable. If the risk level is not acceptable, controls need to be placed (i.e., by design work) and then a hazard reassessment undertaken. If it is now acceptable, the work is done, otherwise more design work is required.

If Figure 6.3 appears daunting then there is an alternative, such as that of Figure 6.4.

Now this is where previous risk management texts tend to cause problems because, historically, there was a tendency to only undertake this exercise once a device was ready to progress for either CE mark or FDA application. If risk management is correctly conducted, then at this stage, all the individual risk assessments are assembled

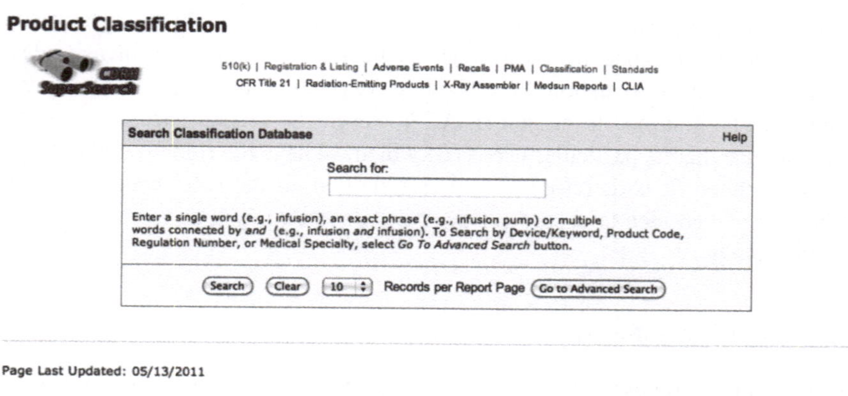

FIGURE 6.1 FDA product classification database window.

New Search | Back To Search Results

Device	Joint, Knee, External Brace
Regulation Description	Limb orthosis.
Regulation Medical Specialty	Physical Medicine
Review Panel	Physical Medicine
Product Code	ITQ
Premarket Review	Office of Device Evaluation (ODE) Division of Neurological and Physical Medicine Devices (DNPMD) Physical Medicine and Rehabilitation Devices Branch (PMDB)
Submission Type	510(K) Exempt
Regulation Number	890.3475
Device Class	1
Total Product Life Cycle (TPLC)	TPLC Product Code Report
GMP Exempt?	Yes

Note: This device is also exempted from the GMP regulation, except for general requirements concerning records (820.180) and complaint files (820.198), *as long as the device is not labeled or otherwise represented as sterile.*

Note: FDA has exempted almost all class I devices (with the exception of reserved devices) from the premarket notification requirement, including those devices that were exempted by final regulation published in the *Federal Registers* of December 7, 1994, and January 16, 1996. It is important to confirm the exempt status and any limitations that apply with 21 CFR Parts 862-892. Limitations of device exemptions are covered under 21 CFR XXX.9, where XXX refers to Parts 862-892.

If a manufacturer's device falls into a generic category of exempted class I devices as defined in 21 CFR Parts 862-892, a premarket notification application and fda clearance is not required before marketing the device in the U.S. however, these manufacturers are required to register their establishment. Please see the Device Registration and Listing website for additional information.

Implanted Device?	No
Life-Sustain/Support Device?	No
Third Party Review	Not Third Party Eligible

FIGURE 6.2 FDA result of 'knee brace' classification.

into one document. After all, if all assessments state that there is little risk (there can never be no risk), then the culmination should be the simple conclusion: '*risk is outweighed by the clinical benefit.*'

It is quite common to see, in a Technical File, a risk analysis that is some years old. This is not acceptable because the process is a loop that allows for events such as design changes, changes in staff, changes in material properties, changes in suppliers, new knowledge from the post-market surveillance, customer complaints, and non-conforming products. It is cyclic and is not static. Risk analysis for a given device should be reviewed at least annually, and at every_design change (no matter how small). The first step on the path, however, is to be able to perform a risk analysis.

6.6.2 Risk Analysis

This is the precursor to all that follows. In essence, a clinical evaluation follows an overall risk analysis – however, in practical terms they are so interlinked that it is impossible to separate them. Hence, risk analysis as a tool is introduced for use in the overall evaluation of the device. An overall risk analysis is essential for

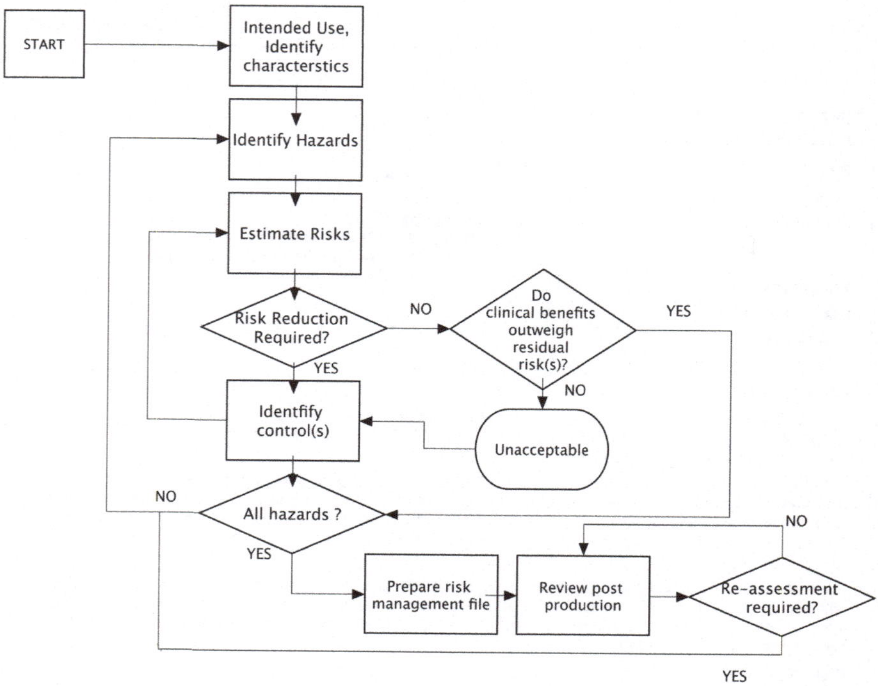

FIGURE 6.3 Risk management example flow chart.

all medical devices, be that in the USA or in the EC, and unlike many other disciplines the ISO standard '*Medical Devices – Application of Risk Management to Medical Devices – ISO 14971 2019* must be used. The first, and largest portion of the document, concerns risk management. Every design must have a risk management procedure, and this standard actually provides it– so there should be no mistake. A sub-section concerns risk assessment, which is prescriptive within the guideline. The way findings are presented is not prescribed but the remainder of it is legislated. Using this standard is essential in both the EU and the USA. ISO 14971 is so embedded in medical devices that purchasers, such as the NHS, will ask if you are using it. As an ISO standard it is international; so EC, FDA, and just about every other regulatory body accept it.

The important thing to consider with risk analysis is the simple principle of cause and effect. Risk analysis begins with the effect(s) and then determination of the root causes(s). In essence, it involves imagining what could 'happen' and then determining what could lead to that 'happening' and then seeing what can be done to 'control it' to 'stop it happening.' The essence of ISO 14971 is that there must be a risk management procedure in place and it helps by providing both the procedure (so there is no need to develop your own, all you need do is make it work for your company) and sample risk analysis forms.

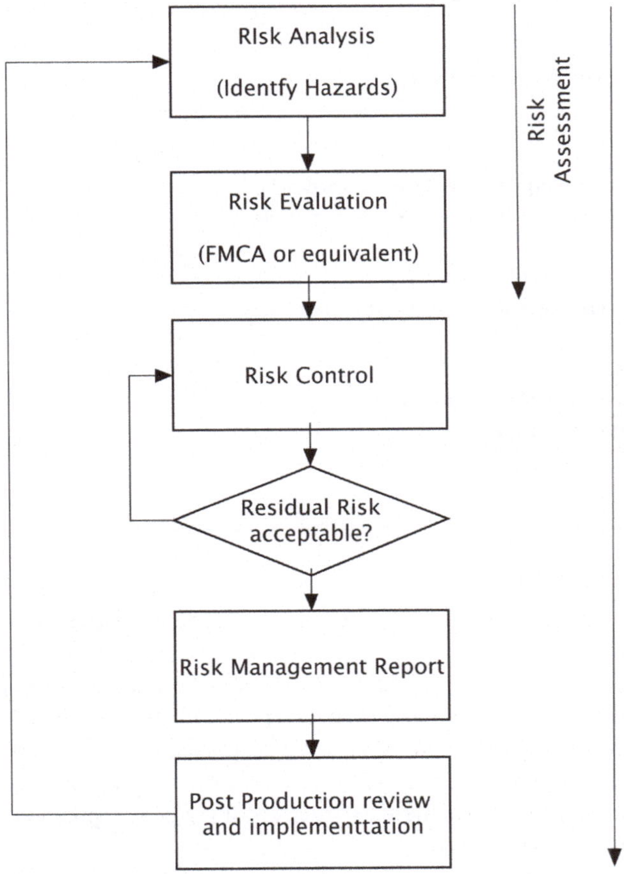

FIGURE 6.4 An alternative risk management depiction.

6.6.3 Identifying Hazards

This aspect of the clinical evaluation process is to ascertain risks and hazards. The first port of call is Annex C of ISO 14971. Table 6.3 illustrates one small sub-section of Annex C. The whole table, if worked through, helps identify risks pertaining to the device being developed.

Please note this is only an extract from ISO 14971, and if the intention is to create software then PD IEC- TR 8002 '*Medical Device Software, Part 1: Guidance on the Application of ISO 14971 to Medical Device Software*' needs to be consulted as well.

The whole aim of Annex C of the regulations is to get the designer thinking about risks when the device is in the real world, as opposed to the design office. It is essential to consider all aspects related to the device and its place of use, which may mean gaining some experience of the place of use or consulting someone who has that experience. In considering a single-use device that is supplied non-sterile

TABLE 6.3
Sub-section of Annex C ISO 14971

Sub-section	Applicable/Not Applicable	Comment
c.2.8 Is the medical device supplied sterile or intended to be sterilised by the user, or are other microbiological controls applicable?		
Factors that should be considered include		
2.8.1. Whether the medical device is intended for single use or reuse packaging		
2.8.2. Shelf-life issues		
2.8.3. Limitation on the number of reuse cycles		
2.8.5. Method of product sterilisation		
2.8.6. The impact of other sterilisation methods not intended by the manufacturer		

and that relies on the end user using steam sterilisation process before use, some of the comments that may be used are illustrated in Table 6.4. It is not a complete table.

Some of the questions posed by Annex C will not be related to the particular device under development. If so, what is necessary is to simply state N/A and then state in the comments why that is so. Also, some sections are repetitive. When completing this table, it is essential to consider issues at the hospital, at the suppliers, and in the warehouses and to use these questions to think of *any* potential risk – no matter how negligible it may seem.

Once related areas have been identified (using Annex C); it is also necessary to think of the appropriate hazards to be inserted in the comments column. Annex E to ISO 14971 helps to imagine such issues and it can be helpful to use the following 'W' questions. Table 6.5 gives provides examples of common hazards.

Who: Hazardous to whom? The patient? The end user? Other devices!
What: What makes this a hazard?
Why: Why is it hazardous?
Where: Does the local environment cause an issue? (If not obvious, you may have to describe in more detail. Things like electric shock, scalding need no expansion – apart from potential degree.)
When: When is this likely to occur (not just in time but procedurally)?

It is expected that that this will be a lengthy, time consuming process. However, at the end of the process, it should be possible to have thought of any potential hazard for every possible end user.

Risk analysis is a mandatory exercise and should be done correctly. If there is a good product design specification (PDS) in the first instance, then these risks will have, already, been mitigated.

TABLE 6.4
An Example of a Completed Annex C

Sub-section	Applicable/Not Applicable	Comment
c.2.8 Is the medical device supplied sterile or intended to be sterilised by the user, or are other microbiological controls applicable?	YES	Single use device to be steam sterilised before use.
Factors that should be considered include		
2.8.1. Whether the medical device is intended for single use or reuse packaging	YES	Can it be, mistakenly, used non-sterile? Can it be mistakenly reused? Does the packaging make its sterility status obvious?
2.8.2. Shelf-life issues	YES	Will the device deteriorate over time on stock shelf, in transit, or in hospital? Once sterile how long will the device remain sterile and in what conditions?
2.8.3. Limitation on the number of reuse cycles	YES	Will re-sterilisation (due to not being used) cause issues? How many times can it be re-sterilised without having detrimental effects?
2.8.5. Method of product sterilisation	YES	Can the device be washed/cleaned in normal clinical machines? Do we have a certificate stating it is sterilisable? Have we checked that it can be sterilised using normal clinical methods? Have we checked that the sterility conforms to standard procedures in all states it is being sold? Will the device store heat and hence can burn/scald patient end users?
2.8.6. The impact of other sterilisation methods not intended by the manufacturer	YES	What happens if the device is ETO sterilised? What happens if it is irradiated? Do either have detrimental effects? Do either cause any issues related to usability?

6.6.4 Assessing Level of Risk

If the device was designed using a well-constructed PDS, then this analysis should return a 'safe to use' result meaning that any risk of use is outweighed by the clinical benefits. For example, X-rays are an ionising radiation and hence dangerous. However, modern medicine and dentistry find the X-ray machine essential in diagnosis. Whilst it is impossible to remove all the risks, they can be reduced to levels where the benefits outweigh the risk, and as a consequence, all hospitals, dentists, and veterinary practices have an X-ray machine. The same arguments must be applied to other medical devices by being able to prove, using the risk analysis, that 'the medical benefits outweigh the risk' and in order to make this statement, the risks/hazards must be considered and then for each one, the root cause or (if applicable, the root causes) identified. As an illustration, Table 6.6 is a typical FMCA pro forma that has been modified from the ISO 14971 to coincide with terms already encountered.

Use of Annex C will identify potential failures/hazards. The relevant section number of ISO 14971 Annex C is entered into Box 1. There may be a number of different failure modes for a particular hazard; a single failure mode is entered into Box 2. Each failure mode hazard will have a particular effect (note this is related to the patient, the end user, or the surrounding environment – Box 5); this is explained in Box 3. Now the root cause, or the root causes, must be identified (Box 4); it is very likely that each hazard/failure will have several potential root causes.

Table 6.7 is a summary of the potential root causes as stated in ISO 14971. It is by no means comprehensive but provides a starting block to develop from. As stated earlier, a comprehensive PDS and design procedure will have anticipated all of these root causes and designed them out!

For each cause we now assess the risk (Box 6). A level of severity (S) and a likelihood of occurrence (L) are determined. Our assessment of RISK level (RPN) is

$$RPN = S \times L$$

Guidelines are required to set values of L and S. ISO 14971 suggests values but also lets the company to allocate their own appropriate levels; those given in Table 6.8 are commonplace.

Note that severity is based on potential for injury; company embarrassment is not a consideration. Table 6.9 illustrates a 'severity and likelihood table' for hazards unrelated to injury; here company embarrassment *is* a consideration. To ensure there is not a variety of forms dependent on the application it is worth considering use of the terms 'bystander' and 'environment' in relation to Table 6.5. Clearly the company's hazards can influence the patient or the end user (for example, using the wrong material!); what is needed, however, is a definition where 'the company' can sit, and a suitable position is the 'bystander' column.

Once the FMCA table is complete to the first RPN column, we assess if the risk is acceptable or not. Table 6.10 illustrates a typical risk evaluation table. ISO 14971 allows the designer to devise their own threshold values, but it is very common to have the following three zones:

1. a low-risk zone (no controls required)
2. a medium-risk zone (controls should be examined)
3. a high-risk zone (controls need to be implemented to reduce risk)

TABLE 6.5
Some Examples of Hazards (Modified from ISO 14971:2019)

Examples of Energy Hazards	Examples of Biological and Chemical Hazards	Examples of Operational Hazards	Examples of Information Hazards
Electromagnetic energy	**Biological**	**Function**	**Labelling**
Electricity	Bio-burden?	Effects due to:	Instructions for use adequate?
Line voltage	Bacteria?	Incorrect or inappropriate use?	Are the indications clear?
Is it connected to mains supply?	Viruses?	Incorrect measurement?	Contraindications clear?
Leakage current	Other agents (e.g. prions)	Erroneous data transfer?	**Operating instructions**
Electric fields	**Chemical**	**User error**	Written with the end user in mind?
Will it produce a magnetic field?	Any acids or alkalis?	Effects of:	Inadequate specification of pre-use checks?
EMC compatibility?	Any processing residues?	Lack of attention?	
Light	Any contaminates	Forgetfulness?	**Warnings**
Does it emit light?	Any additives or	Lack of training?	Any side effects?
Will it cause temporary blindness (flash)?	processing aids?	Ignoring the rules?	Any hazards likely with reuse?
Is it a laser?	Any cleaning, disinfecting, or testing agents?		**Specification of service**
			and maintenance
Radiation energy	**Biocompatibility**		Any special service instructions before reuse?
Ionising radiation	Toxicity of chemical		
Non-ionising radiation	constituents		
UV sunburn?			
Thermal energy			
Ductile-brittle transition?			
Burning/scalding?			

(*Continued*)

TABLE 6.5 (CONTINUED)
Some Examples of Hazards (Modified from ISO 14971:2019)

Examples of Energy Hazards	Examples of Biological and Chemical Hazards	Examples of Operational Hazards	Examples of Information Hazards
Mechanical energy			
Gravity			
– Can it fall?			
Vibration			
– Can it affect the user?			
Stored energy			
Moving parts			
Moving and positioning of patient			
– infrasound energy			
– sound			
High pressure fluid injection			
– Will it 'inject'?			

TABLE 6.6
Example Risk Analysis Pro forma

RISK ANALYSIS

Characteristic	1				Life cycle Phase			Design, Manufacture and supply	Comment					
Failure/ Hazard	2													
Effect	3													
Root Cause(s)	Hazard Relevance ✓ = relevant				Estimation of Risk: Likehood × Severity at start of lifecycle phase L × S = RPN			Risk reduction activities (Gray Black Zones) (if practical): Comment if required (white only)	Estimation of residual risk at the end of this lifecycle phase			Can the risk be reduced further? (Gray)	Action proposed to protect frok residual risk, . implementation and verification of efficacy?	Additional hazard introduced by risk control measures? If so, what action taken?
	Patient	User	Bystander	Environment	L	S	RPN		L	S	RPN			
4	5				6			7	8			9	10	11

TABLE 6.7
Example of Root Causes (Source: ISO 14971)

General Category	Examples of Causes
Incomplete requirements	Inadequate specification of: – design parameters – operating parameters – performance requirements – in-service requirements (e.g., maintenance, reprocessing) – end of life
Manufacturing processes	– Insufficient control of changes to manufacturing processes – Insufficient control of materials/materials compatibility information – Insufficient control of manufacturing processes – Insufficient control of subcontractors
Transport and storage	– Inadequate packaging – Contamination or deterioration – Inappropriate environmental conditions
Environmental factors	– Physical (e.g., heat, pressure, time) – Chemical (e.g., corrosions, degradation, contamination) – Electromagnetic fields (e.g., susceptibility to electromagnetic disturbance) – Inadequate supply of power – Inadequate supply of coolant
Cleaning, disinfection, and sterilisation	– Lack of, or inadequate specification for, validated procedures for cleaning, disinfection, and sterilisation – Inadequate conduct of cleaning, disinfection, and sterilisation
Disposal and scrapping	– No or inadequate information provided – Use error
Formulation	– Biodegradation – Biocompatibility – No information or inadequate specification provided – Inadequate warning of hazards associated with incorrect formulations – Use error
Human factors	Potential for use errors triggered by design flaws, such as – confusing or missing instructions for use – complex or confusing control system – ambiguous or unclear device state

(*Continued*)

TABLE 6.7 (CONTINUED)
Example of Root Causes (Source: ISO 14971)

General Category	Examples of Causes
	– ambiguous or unclear presentation of settings, measurements, or other information – misrepresentation of results – insufficient visibility, audibility, or tactility – poor mapping of controls to actions, or of displayed information to actual state – controversial modes or mapping as compared to existing equipment – use by unskilled/untrained personnel – insufficient warning of side effects – inadequate warning of hazards associated with reuse of single-use medical devices – incorrect measurement and other metrological aspects – incompatibility with consumables/accessories/other medical devices – slips, laps, and mistakes
Failure modes	– Unexpected loss of electrical/mechanical integrity – Deterioration in function (e.g., gradual occlusion of fluid/gas path, or change in resistance to flow, electrical conductivity) as a result of ageing, wear, and repeated use – Fatigue failure

TABLE 6.8
Example Table of Severity Levels

	L		S
5	<u>frequent</u> 1/100 uses or once per day	5	<u>catastrophic</u> Death
4	<u>probable</u> 1/1000 uses or once per week	4	<u>critical</u> Major injury (loss of limb, etc.): life-threatening injury
3	<u>occasionally</u> 1/10,000 uses or once per quarter	3	<u>serious</u> Minor injury requiring treatment
2	<u>remote</u> 1/1,100,000 uses or once per year	2	<u>minor</u> Minor injury NOT requiring treatment
1	<u>improbable</u> 1/1,000,0000 uses or once every 3–5 years	1	<u>negligible</u> Minor irritance to patient or end user

TABLE 6.9
Example Table of Severity Levels Related to Non-personal Injury Hazards

L		S	
5	frequent 1/100 uses or once per day	5	catastrophic Litigation
4	probable 1/1000 uses or once per week	4	critical Loss of CE mark/FDA clearance to market/recall of device
3	occasionally 1/10,000 uses or once per quarter	3	serious Receipt of formal complaint
2	remote 1/1,100,000 uses or once per year	2	minor Non-conforming product/failure to meet order/item lost in post
1	improbable 1/1,000,0000 uses or once every 3–5 years	1	negligible e.g., typing errors on delivery note

If the value of RPN falls into any of the white areas, then risk is adequately controlled. In the following comments section (Box 7), all that is necessary is to add a statement stating what the control method is/methods are.

However, it is very likely that at the first round there will be a value that is in the grey or black sections of Table 6.10, hence Box 7 is reserved for any description of remedial action you have undertaken to control the risk. A new level of RPN should be determined and entered into Box 8 (note that S will not change, only L does). It is not worth completing this section unless the controls take the value of RPN to a value recognised as being acceptable –As Far as Possible (or As Far As Practicable). Hence Box 7 should contain a complete description of the control measures in place. In some cases, a simple statement that an international standard is being used is enough; in others, it may be necessary to put in some more text.

If all is fine, then in Box 9, the acronym 'AFLAP' is entered. That does not mean that it is not worthwhile to reduce the risk anymore because it would cost too much; it literally means it *cannot* be reduced any further with current knowledge. Somewhere in these boxes it is necessary to make the statement that the risk is outweighed by the clinical benefit, which can be written in Box 9 using the phrase 'AFAP: residual risk is outweighed by the clinical benefit.'

If the residual risk is unacceptable, it is necessary to go back to the drawing board – but with a good PDS this eventuality should not happen. If the risk is significant, it is necessary to assess if the residual risk is outweighed by clinical benefit, and it may be necessary to instigate further controls.

Box 10 is simple, if there is any residual risk can anything further be done? Sometimes there are little things that are not directly under the designer's control but

TABLE 6.10
A Typical Risk-Evaluation Table

S / **L**	**Negligible:** **1**	**Minor:** **2**	**Serious:** **3**	**Critical:** **4**	**Catastrophic:** **5**
Frequent: 5	5	10	15	20	25
Probable: 4	4	8	12	16	20
Occasional: 3	3	6	9	12	15
Remote: 2	2	4	6	8	10
Improbable:1	1	2	3	4	5

Key:
Dark : Unacceptable (>10) – Risk *must* be controlled and RPN reduced.
Grey: Significant (>4 and <11) – Risk controls to be investigated to reduce RPN.
White: Insignificant (<5) – RPN need not be investigated further.

which can be used to increase safety. For example, consider the window-cleaner on a ladder. The window-cleaner can tie himself to the ladder to avoid falling off, and this will reduce the risk of falling off. However, it does not stop someone walking into the ladder and causing the window-cleaner to become unsteady and fall. The chances of this happening can be reduced by putting up warning signs around the ladder; this has not changed the design of the ladder, nor of the safety harness – but it has, potentially, reduced the risk of a fall a bit further.

Box 11 is less simple as changes needed to be made to reduce risk may have a knock-on effect; inadvertently, new risks may have been introduced trying to mitigate previous risks. This box forces the designer to look at that outcome. So, for example, using the ladder case above, a trip hazard has just been introduced for the pedestrian, hence another table.

Whilst at first sight this form and its associated processes look problematic, this is not the case. They have been established to make the designer think of the effects of their choices and to let others question those choices in a stable, coherent, and internationally accepted manner. However, a full and thorough examination of the simplest of devices can result in a folder containing at least 50 of these forms/tables with at least three root causes on each page!

6.6.5 Other Risk Assessment Methods

There are numerous forms one can adopt to assess risk rather than that presented above and there are software solutions (based on spreadsheets), but they all address same issues: identify the hazard, identify the severity, and identify the likelihood.

One simple version (not suitable above a Class I device) is presented in Table 6.11. In this case, no numbers are used, just degrees of hazard and degrees of likelihood.

To complete Table 6.11, one simply circles the relevant box. One cannot get away without using the 'AFLAP' statement in the assessment, nor the use of the statement

TABLE 6.11
Simple Risk analysis table

Hazard:

Control:

Severity \ Frequency	Rarely (possible, but unlikely)	Occasional	Frequent (likely to occur)
High (likely to cause death or severe injury)	MODERATE	MAJOR	CRITICAL
Medium (likely to lead to a complaint)	MINOR	MODERATE	MAJOR
Low (cosmetic defect)	NIL	MINOR	MODERATE

Assessment:

Residual Risk:

'risk is outweighed by clinical benefit.' Furthermore, one still needs to analyse any residual risk.

6.6.6 Risk Management Procedure Document

Once completed it is necessary to produce a risk analysis report, one that contains every completed risk analysis table/form. These individual forms are collated and together they define whether the device has any residual risk that is not acceptable. The front page of this report should summarise, and someone competent must sign it off confirming that the 'clinical benefits of the device outweigh any risks due to its use.'

It is essential to encapsulate the process within a single document, and since it is ISO 14971 the basic format is given.

Page 1: A copy of the ISO 14971 risk management process flow chart (as given in Figure 6.1)
Page 2: A statement on how hazards are ascertained (Annex C, PD IEC-TR8002, etc.)
Page 3: A copy of the form used
Page 4: A copy of the risk assessment chart being used
Page 5: A statement on:
 (a) 'risks whose probability cannot be estimated' and
 (b) 'post production' risk management

The answer to (a) is difficult, it is impossible to judge something if the data is not there. So a simple statement such as: *There are some occasions when quantitative estimates of probability cannot be accurately judged but changes in technology are reviewed periodically by [Company Name].* At least suggests the issue has been recognised. It does not, however, provide a license to ignore it; it just means some estimates of RPN may be incorrect and are liable to change. The standard states: 'In such cases, the risk estimate should be made on the basis of a reasonable worst-case estimate of probability' (ISO 2012).

The answer to (b) is a little easier as it requires it to be stated that the risk analysis will be periodically reviewed. A simple statement such as:

> Data is proactively sought from users regarding products in the post production stage as per the requirements of ISO 13485:2016. This information is fed into the 'Company's' monitoring and analysis process and the risk analysis is revised and reviewed according to the ISO 14971:2019 standard.

Page 6: This is blank pro forma for the risk management folder title page (Part 1 of the technical file's risk management file or the company's risk register as described in the next section). This pro forma is laid down by ISO 14971:2019.

The individual who signs the risk analysis *must be qualified to do so*, i.e., a member of staff with formal, professional qualifications such as a chartered engineer, licensed engineer, professional risk assessor, an individual with an ISO 14971 training certificate, or those with postgraduate qualifications in medical devices design. Thus, the individual signing it off cannot be the managing director or CEO just because of their position – they have to be qualified to do so. To avoid such issues arising another line can be added below the signature line: '*qualifications*.'

As a controlled document, it requires a title – such as 'Risk Management Procedure,' it needs approval, a version number, and a date of approval.

6.6.7 Risk Management Folder in the Technical File

An essential element of the Technical File (for CE marking) or the Design History File (DHF) (for FDA 510(k) and clinical assessment approval) is a risk-management folder/risk register. Before any application for a CE mark or for an FDA 510(k), this document must be in place. As virtually all regulatory bodies accept ISO 14971:2019 as the basis for risk management, then the file will always contain the following:

(a) statement of clinical benefit outweighing residual risk
(b) (optional) pre-assessment of hazards on which risk analysis is performed (e.g., Annex C as presented earlier)
(c) complete dossier of all individual risk assessments
(d) (optional) company risk management procedure

It is worth noting that if there is more than one technical file/DHF, then each time the risk management procedure is updated, it is necessary to update this section of *each* technical file. It can be more efficient to simply have a statement on the title page that states: 'this risk analysis was conducted using the risk management procedure XXX.'

6.6.8 Risk Management and Internal Procedures

As a part of compliance with ISO 13485, MDR, and the FDA CFR21, one needs to risk manage the whole of the process, not just the products themselves. Both are interlinked, of course, but it is much easier to claim in a product's risk analysis that it has been manufactured to minimise risk given that the procedures have already been analysed. The best way to evidence this is through a company *risk register.*

The best way to think about a risk register is a simple folder structure as illustrated in Figure 6.5.

The basic tenet of the risk register is that an analysis of hazards associated with each of the procedures is undertaken. Consider, for example, a situation where one of the procedures concerns ordering components from a supplier. Questions arise as to the hazards involved and who will they affect. Regarding the groups that may be affected: the patient, the company's reputation, the safety of the product itself. Further questions arise concerning the sort of hazards that could be associated with a supplier. They could make the component out of specification, that is, not to drawing. They could use the wrong materials. They could deliver the component late, and that could delay an operation. In the case of suppliers, there needs to be a supply agreement in place; that is, the risk control mechanism, but the designer should still assess the risk. The whole point of the process is to find out where processes have risk pinch-points and then to concentrate on those. Knowing where the risks are means something can be done about them.

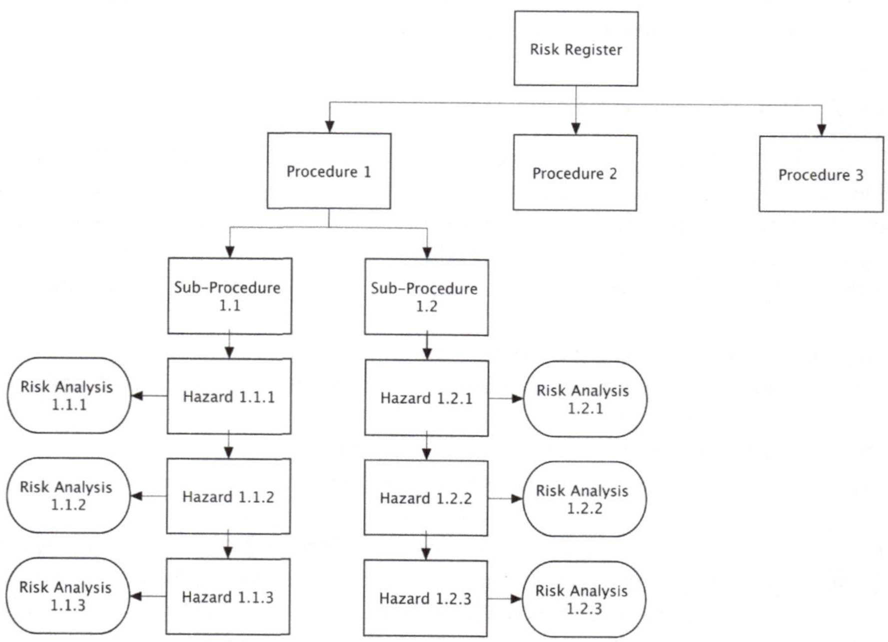

FIGURE 6.5 Example of a risk register structure.

Concerning what to look for, the main sub-groupings which need to be addressed in the investigations (lifecycle phase) are:

- design
- manufacture
- supply
- use

It is probably wise to divide the risk register into these sub-sections.

6.6.9 Software

The two standards that apply are BS EN 60601 Annex H and PD ISO/TR 80002-1 (ISO 2010 and British Standards 2015). In fact, it was deemed so important that elements of the PD ISO were brought into the new ISO 14971: 2019!

These documents help inform the process of hazard identification which developers can then answer and code appropriately for. SOUPs (Software of Unknown Provenance) are major headaches as coding libraries available for download are not always reliable. However, PD ISO/TR 80002 is detailed and in the appendices provides a useful plethora of hazards and typical solutions/control measures for those hazards. Table 6.12 is an extract which demonstrates this.

6.7 STANDARDS, COURSES, AND CERTIFICATION

It should come to little surprise that ISO 14971 is something that should be on the designer's bookshelf, but it must be remembered that standards bodies have strict

TABLE 6.12
An Extract from PD ISO/TR 80002 Illustrating Potential Hazards (BSI, 2009)

Software causes	Risk control measures	Verification types: Inspect ion	Test (unit, integration)	Analysis: static / dynamic / timing
Arithmetic				
Divide by zero	Run-time error traps, defensive coding	◆	◆	D
Numeric overflow/underflow	Range checks, Floating-point data representations	◆	◆	D
Floating point rounding	Robust algorithms	◆		
Improper rang e/bounds checking	Defensive coding	◆	◆	S
Off-by-one (OBO)	Defensive coding	◆	◆	

copyright laws – not surprisingly; so it is not acceptable to copy these documents and share them with friends, family, and casual acquaintances.

It is important not to forget that the risk analysis must tie in with the essential clinical evaluation (verification and validation in FDA speak) for the device, so these documents will need to be referred to too.

6.7.1 Courses and Certification

Attending an ISO 14971 course has two major benefits: first, for the training; and second, the ability to sign off risk-analysis front sheets.

6.8 BIOCOMPATIBILITY

It is important not to underestimate the importance placed on biocompatibility. Evidence must be provided that the materials used comply with the essential requirements for a medical device which is why the materials selection pro forma is so important to materials selection records. Even if the material is deemed 'safe' an '*eagle eye*' must be kept pointed at recall notices, the news channels and any other sources of 'product recall' information – just in case any material concerned is being used in the device. However, if the intention is to use a material that has not been used before, there are a new series of considerations. Biocompatibility comes into play when a device is communicating with tissue. It would be wrong to assume this is only by direct contact; it can also be indirect (it could be by emission or vapour). If the device communicates with tissue, then its biocompatibility must have been tested at some time, and biocompatibility testing is an expensive and time-consuming business. Initially it was thought that only inert materials were biocompatible; but the definition has changed due to the growth in using substances that can be implanted into the body that are not inert (e.g., re-sorbable implants). There has been much debate but the current definition of biocompatibility states:

> Biocompatibility is: 'The ability of a material to perform with an appropriate host response in a specific application' (Williams 1999).

Known as the Williams definition, this was adopted by the European Society of Biomaterials. It is brief and to the point. It states that if you have a material communicating with a host, it should do what it is supposed to do without harming the host – as in this further definition that expands on the former (and, not surprisingly, also written by Williams).

> Refers to the ability of a biomaterial to perform its desired function with respect to a medical therapy, without eliciting any undesirable local or systemic effects in the recipient or beneficiary of that therapy, but generating the most appropriate beneficial cellular or tissue response in that specific situation, and optimising the clinically relevant performance of that therapy. (Williams 2003)

Therefore, if the intention is to use a material that communicates with a body, then it has to be proven to behave in the way it is supposed to behave and not cause any

TABLE 6.13
A Selection of ISO Biocompatibility Standards and Their FDA Consensus Number

Standard	Title
BS EN ISO 10993 family	Biological evaluation of medical devices.
BS EN ISO 10993-1	Biological evaluation of medical devices. Evaluation and testing within a risk management process.
FDA consensus Recognition Number 2-156	Biological evaluation of medical devices. Evaluation and testing within a risk management process (biocompatibility).
BS EN ISO 7405	Evaluation of biocompatibility of medical devices used in dentistry.
FDA consensus Recognition Number 4-179	ISO 7405 - Evaluation of biocompatibility of medical devices used in dentistry.
BS EN ISO 11979-5	Opthalmic implants. Intraocular lenses. Biocompatibility.
FDA consensus Recognition Number 10-48	Opthalmic implants. Intraocular lenses. Biocompatibility.

deleterious effects. It is worth noting that these effects can be local or systemic and may not present until many years later. It should be no surprise that there are numerous guidelines and standards associated with this topic. A good rule of thumb is to use what has been used before unless there is a very good reason not to do so.

Table 6.13 is very brief but ISO 10993 has 16 parts; all having slightly different nuances on biocompatibility. They are revised frequently as new evidence emerges. There are specific tests for particular disciplines so if, for example, work was being carried out in dentistry it is necessary also to meet the relevant standards for that discipline. It is important that one makes sure that this search is done for one's own discipline and for the state in which it is the intention to sell, be that the USA or the EU; or elsewhere. It will prove essential to produce a biocompatibility report for all communicating devices – whether the material is in common use or not, and that report *must* meet the requirements of ISO 10993.

6.9 TECHNICAL FILES

It is very important to remember that all medical devices, whatever their classification, require a technical file or, as it is now known, Technical Documentation. It is beyond the scope of this text to describe the methodology or structure but there are a host of references to seek such details from (e.g., Ogrodnik 2019).

REFERENCES

British Standards. "BS EN 60601-1-2:2015+A1:2021. Medical electrical equipment. General requirements for basic safety and essential performance. Collateral standard: Electromagnetic disturbances. Requirements and tests." 2015. Accessed June 10, 2021. https://shop.bsigroup.com/ProductDetail/?pid=000000000030357107.

European Commission. “Meddev 2.7/1 (4) guidelines on medical devices.” 2016. Clinical evaluation: A guide for manufacturers and notified bodies under directives 93/42/EEC And 90/385/EEC.” 1–65.

European Community. “Medical devices directive. 93/42/EEC.” 1993. Accessed June 10, 2021. https://www.legislation.gov.uk/eudr/1993/42/contents.

European Community. “Active implantable devices directive. 90/385/EEC”. 1990. Accessed June 10, 2021. https://eur-lex.europa.eu/LexUriServ/LexUriServ.do?uri=CELEX:31990L0385:en:HTML.

European Community. “In-vitro diagnostics directive. 98/79/EEC”. 1998. Accessed June 10, 2021. https://eur-lex.europa.eu/legal-content/EN/TXT/?uri=CELEX:31998L0079.

European Union. “In-vitro diagnostic devices regulations. 2017/746”. 2017. Accessed June 10, 2021. https://eur-lex.europa.eu/legal-content/EN/TXT/PDF/?uri=CELEX:32017R0746.

European Union. “Medical devices regulations. 2017/745”. 2017. Accessed June 10, 2021. https://eur-lex.europa.eu/legal-content/EN/TXT/PDF/?uri=CELEX:32017R0745.

FDA. “Federal Food, Drug, and Cosmetic Act (FD&C Act) CFR21.” 2004 and ongoing. Accessed June 10, 2021. https://www.fda.gov/regulatory-information/laws-enforced-fda/federal-food-drug-and-cosmetic-act-fdc-act.

FDA. “Changes to existing medical software policies resulting from section 3060 of the 21st century cures act.” 2019. Accessed June 10, 2021. https://www.fda.gov/regulatory-information/search-fda-guidance-documents/changes-existing-medical-software-policies-resulting-section-3060-21st-century-cures-act

ISO. “ISO 14971:2019, medical devices - Application of risk management to medical devices.” 2019. Accessed June 10, 2021. https://www.iso.org/standard/72704.html.

ISO. “PD ISO/TR 80002-1:2009, medical device software. Guidance on the application of ISO 14971 to medical device software.” 2010. Accessed June 10, 2021. https://shop.bsigroup.com/ProductDetail?pid=000000000030164114.

Ogrodnik, Peter J. *Medical Device Design: Innovation from Concept to Market.* Academic Press, 2019.

Williams, David Franklyn. *The Williams Dictionary of Biomaterials.* Liverpool University Press, 1999.

7 Implantable Medical Textiles

7.1 INTRODUCTION

An implantable medical device means any active medical device which is intended to be totally or partially introduced, surgically or medically, into the human body or by medical intervention into a natural orifice, and which is intended to remain there after the procedure is completed (Medicines and Healthcare Products Regulatory Authority 2021). Such devices may be biologically active or biologically inert. Those that fall under the medical textile remit include sutures, vascular grafts, meshes, and resorbable polymer structures such as scaffolds for cell growth.

7.2 DESIRABLE PROPERTIES IN IMPLANTABLE MEDICAL TEXTILES

Implantable medical textiles can be used in almost every organ of the body. They ideally should have biomechanical properties that are comparable to the tissue in which they are implanted without causing any adverse effects. In addition, they need to be biocompatible, bio-adhesive, bifunctional, and resistant to corrosion from bodily fluids. The materials used should be non-irritant, non-toxic, and non-carcinogenic.

For biologically active implants, the active material may be required to be released at a particular rate over a given time frame and so the method of incorporation of the active molecule into the implant is critical to ensure these properties. Resorbable implants that gradually disappear with time need carefully selected/adjusted working profiles such that if structural support is required for a given period of time, the implant can indeed provide this adequately and does not lose critical mechanical properties too soon.

7.3 SUTURES

Sutures are used in surgery to oppose tissues to allow wound healing. The ideal suture should allow healing tissue to recover sufficiently to keep the wound closed together before the suture is either removed or absorbed. Suture materials must fulfil specific roles which are dictated by factors such as the location they are intended to be used in, the type of tissue being closed, and the type of surgery being undertaken.

DOI: 10.1201/9781003170570-7

Sutures need to demonstrate a number of characteristics which can be summarised as follows:

- Tensile strength – the ability of the suture to resist damage and deformation
- Shape memory – the ability of the material to return to or maintain its original shape
- Capillarity – the extent to which the suture material allows the passage of adsorbed fluid
- Pliability – the ease of handling of the suture material
- Knot security – sutures must be able to be tied effectively such that the knots do not slip
- Low coefficient of friction – the ease with which a suture passes through the skin

Some of the related properties need to have standard methods for their measurement as values can vary substantially, for example, rate of extension needs to be set at a practically suitable rate when testing knot strength (Carr et al. 2009, 51–56). In braided structures, it was found that the variation of braid angle had an important influence on breaking load and elongation of the suture and on the slippage ratio for knots. Tests have shown that the presence of a knot lowered the breaking load of the suture strand and that the rupture occurred consistently at the knot region (Ben Abdessalem et al. 2009, 247–252).

Both absorbable (usually synthetic absorbable or SA sutures) and non-absorbable sutures are used in surgery and may be manufactured from natural or synthetic polymer materials in monofilament or in a multifilament form (Barrows 1986, 233–257). Figure 7.1 shows a selection of current sutures within use.

Synthetic absorbable sutures are made from biodegradable copolymers which undergo degradation within the patient's body by enzymatic digestion or hydrolysis. Various different linear polyether/polyester materials, such as poliglecaprone 25 (a copolymer of polyglycolic acid and ε-caprolactone), polyglactin 910 (a polylactic acid–polyglycolic acid copolymer made from 90% polyglycolic acid and 10% polylactic acid), and poly(*p*-dioxanone) (a polyether-ester synthetic polymer) are used for their different absorption and tensile strength retention profiles (see Chapter 4). For example, poliglecaprone 25 degrades rapidly whereas polyglactin 910 degrades at a slower rate. Knowledge of this is critical in preventing wound dehiscence (wound opening owing to suture failure before healing). Poly(l-lactic acid) or PLLA is another biodegradable material that can be used. Used as a single polymer material, it is too stiff and inflexible itself for monofilament suture purposes due to its high glass transition temperature and crystallinity; however, it can be modified by combining it with another polymer. For example, the properties of PLLA are able to be adjusted by blending PLLA (90%) with poly (lactide-co-ϵ-caprolactone) or PLCL (10%), thereby lowering the Tg with consequent reduction in stiffness and improvement in flexibility in monofilament form (Viju, Thilagavathi, and Gupta 2010, 835–841), similar effects achieved in a simpler way to those which would result from copolymerisation of polylactic acid and polyglycolic acid. Poly(*p*-dioxanone) is also

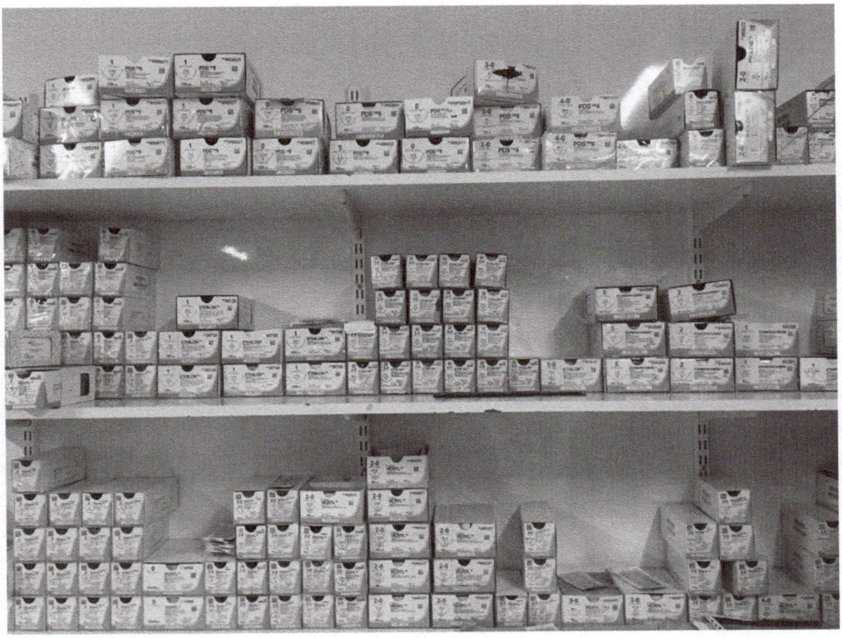

FIGURE 7.1 A range of sutures currently used in the operating theatre.

a stiff material, but not as stiff as PLLA or PGA, which has allowed it to be used as a monofilament suture rather than in braided form.

There are some roles where the function of the suture is more critical than in others; for example, the failure of a suture in the anastomosis (join) of a large vessel may be fatal whilst the dehiscence of a subcutaneous (inner part of the skin) fat plane or overlying skin may cause an unwelcome, unsightly scar but not a fatality. Traditionally, skin is often closed with a non-absorbable nylon or absorbable poliglecaprone 25. Non-absorbable sutures require removal which necessitates a healthcare attendance whilst the absorbable will gradually dissolve without the need for removal.

Absorbable suture materials are also used in novel and specialist applications such as the so-called ‘catgut embedding acupuncture’ where sutures are implanted into an acupoint based on the theory of acupuncture. The ideal embedding materials are required to have excellent swelling, mechanical, and antibacterial properties; two absorbable polymers have been assessed and regarded as suitable, namely polyglycolic acid and polylactic acid in the form of monofilaments. Various ways of optimising their performance have been explored:

- Chitosan coating: The treatment of polyglycolic acid with chitosan altered its rate of degradation offering the possibility of control over this feature (Fu and Zhang 2019, 270–280).
- Coating method: The method used to apply the chitosan coating was important and this consisted of pre-treatment, spray-coating, and rolling

and drying (Fu and Zhang 2019, 1557–1572). The application of a 3% chitosan coating proved most effective (Viju, Thilagavathi, and Gupta 2010, 835–841).

- Hydrophilicity and swelling behaviour: Surface modification of polygycolic acid monofilaments either by ultrasonic treatment in a 50/50 v/v solution of ethanol/H_2O_2 at 250 W ultrasonic power for 30 minutes or by cold oxygen plasma treatment, improved both key properties for acupoint embedding therapy (Fu and Zhang 2019, 3839–3849; Fu, Lu, and Zhang 2019, 4071–4082; Fu et al. 2019, 3556–3566).

Mostly, however, sutures are employed in the repair of wounds, and are largely successful in this respect, but problems do occur. Poor clinical outcomes in wound repair include surgical site infection, delayed or excessive wound healing, poor cosmetic outcome, incisional hernia formation, and perineal pain (Stadelmann, Digenis, and Tobin 1998, 26S–38S). It may be that development of new sutures and biomaterials should be directed towards these avenues.

7.3.1 Healing of Wounds

Different tissues within the body exhibit different mechanical and biological characteristics and, in general, for stronger tissues, a stronger suture is required. Fascial planes, for instance, are comparatively tough and aid in keeping structures in various compartments within the body. Condensations of fascia can form ligaments, for example, the palmar fascia in the hand condenses to form the carpal tunnel ligament. Pathology here can create carpal tunnel syndrome. In comparison, subcutaneous fat is a relatively soft tissue to close and the quantity that can be closed varies widely between individuals.

Different tissues heal at different rates; therefore, any successful suture must maintain a sufficient strength over the time taken for the wound to heal and not interfere with the native biology. The healing of stomach and colon tissue in dogs, for example, has been demonstrated to differ from that of their skin wounds. The gastrointestinal tissues are more metabolically active with a markedly elevated rate of both collagen and non-collagenous protein synthesis so that after 21 days, the breaking strength of the wound does not increase significantly (Hastings et al. 1975, 701–707).

Most surgical wounds heal by what is known as primary intention, where wound edges are re-approximated using sutures, staples, clips, or glue. Some wounds are left open to heal by secondary intention, where they heal from the 'bottom up.' This may be done because wound closure is not appropriate due to infection or because wound edges cannot be approximated. Some wounds break down following closure and may partially or completely reopen.

Acute wounds undergo faster healing than chronic wounds, and thus for the acute wound an absorbable polymer suture that loses its mechanical integrity at a fast rate may be appropriate. In the healing of an acute wound, there is an orderly progression through inflammation, fibroblast proliferation, and maturation.

(i) *Inflammation*
In the acute inflammatory phase, there is local vasodilatation of vessels allowing an influx of inflammatory cells and growth factors. These trigger a cascade of cytokines that ultimately tell platelets to clot to prevent blood loss, immune cells to upregulate and move from a dormant to an active phase to fight infection and finally to stimulate relevant cells to proliferate to aid in wound closure.
(ii) *Fibroblast proliferation*
Within 2–3 days, fibroblasts appear and relevant extracellular matrix. Collagen and glycosaminoglycans are produced to aid in wound healing. There is also angiogenesis to produce capillaries required for scar formation.
(iii) *Maturation*
By 3 weeks, wound remodelling begins. This can last up to 2 years in the healthy individual. During this phase, there is reorganisation of new cells into a more organised structure, determined by mechanical factors and an increase in tensile strength.

By contrast, chronic wounds are all unique and heal in a different manner from that of acute wounds. One of the unique features is that the wounds contract. This does serve a useful role in that it reduces the size of the wound but can cause disorganised structural integrity, loss of function, and cosmetic deformity. Chronic wounds also produce granulation tissue (which acute wounds do not) composed of numerous capillaries and a support matrix rich in fibroblasts, inflammatory cells, endothelial cells, pericytes, and myofibroblasts, each of which have their own function. The problem with granulation tissue is that it has been converted from a cell-rich, highly vascular medium to a relatively avascular and acellular matrix of collagen with slower cell turnover. Finally, in chronic wounds there is a dysregulation of growth factors in comparison to acute wounds (Stahelmann, Digenis, and Tobin 1998, 26S–38S).

Surgical site infection is a serious global health issue that can lead to significant morbidity, need for re-intervention and treatment, and, in very serious infections, the possibility of fatality (Awad 2012, 234–237; Brown, Tanner, and Padley 2014, 1171–1187; Liu et al. 2018). Different types of surgical wounds carry different risks for surgical site infection (SSI). Wound class is assessed using the classification system adopted by the Centres of Disease Control and Prevention (Centre of Disease Control and Prevention 2021). For example, dirty wounds such as a bowel perforation or a known infected wound carry an increased risk compared with wounds in clean surgery, such as a thyroid or arthroplasty operation. Whilst there is a view that the method of surgical wound closure may impact on SSI risk, there is limited background evidence on mechanisms for SSI prevention. It has been suggested that the better the seal the closure method obtains, the better the barrier to microbial contamination (Gurusamy et al. 2014).

In plastic surgery, the most common wound complications are tissue reactivity, infections, and wound dehiscence. It is well known that choice of suture material is imperative to appropriate wound closure. The 'perfect' suture material would be of uniform calibre (possess uniform linear density), be readily available, be reasonably inexpensive and easy to sterilise, elastic, supple, and have good tensile strength.

In one study, 1000 plastic surgical wounds were evaluated at days 3, 7, and 14 post operation for three outcomes of interest: tissue reactivity, wound dehiscence, and local infection. Monofilament non-absorbable sutures included in the study were composed of nylon whilst the multifilament absorbable sutures were of catgut, polyglycolic acid, and polyglactin. Multifilament non-absorbable synthetic sutures were of braided polyamide and polyester and there were natural sutures made of silk.

There was no significant difference between commonly used sutures in terms of tissue reactivity and wound site did not create a significant difference either. In two-layer wounds, silk demonstrated an increased risk of tissue reactivity when compared with the monofilament sutures. With regard to internal suture materials, polyglactin 910 showed a 66% increase in risk of tissue reactivity when compared with polyglycolic acid. Thinner sutures showed a statistically significant protective effect.

With regard to wound dehiscence, the type of suture material in one- and two-layer wounds did not make a significant difference. Nevertheless, patient characteristics, for example, the existence of comorbidities did play a role. Suture material did not appear to make a difference to the rate of infection, although the overall infection rate was only 1.7%, hence this was a small sample size (Gabrielli et al. 2001, 38–45).

In gastrointestinal surgery, a Cochrane review investigated the optimal method for laparotomy wound closure. The review asked the question: 'Does the type of suture material, or type of closure prevent complications?' With regard to sutures, there was no difference at 1 year or more of follow-up of the incidence of incisional hernia between absorbable and non-absorbable sutures. Nor was there any difference in risk of wound infection. However, absorbable sutures did reduce the risk of sinus or fistula tract formation when compared to non-absorbable sutures and the review suggested that absorbable sutures could be used to reduce the risk of chronic drainage from the wound and that monofilament sutures should be considered for abdominal closure to reduce the risk of incisional hernia (Patel et al. 2017).

A further Cochrane review in obstetrics assessed the role of absorbable sutures for repair of perineal damage at the time of childbirth. Women stitched with synthetic materials had less pain in the first 3 days after delivery and required fewer pain-relieving drugs in the 10 days after giving birth compared to those stitched with catgut. However, there was evidence that synthetic sutures were not always readily absorbed and some women required the sutures to be removed (Kettle, Dowswell, and Ismail 2010).

7.3.2 Advances in Suture Materials

More recently, there has been interest in developing bio-active and bio-inert polymers for closing surgical incisions and wounds. This has modified the function of the suture to an active medical device that biologically interacts with the host environment to prevent suture failure and to promote a positive healing response. Modifications to sutures that alter their overall function include coating the suture to achieve advantageous bioactivity, creating sutures with barbs to obviate the need for knots, or creating sutures where the knot may be adjusted to achieve different degrees of tightness of wound closure.

In 2003, antimicrobial-coated Vicryl® Plus (Ethicon) made from polyglactin 910 was introduced. The coating contains a broad-spectrum antimicrobial agent based upon triclosan and has been shown to reduce surgical site infection by up to 30% (Henriksen et al. 2017, 833–841; Wang et al. 2013, 465–473). Work into antimicrobial sutures continues (Chen et al. 2018) as well as into other biologically active modifications such as the addition of antimicrobial grapefruit seed extract (Lee et al. 2013, 40–43), growth factors such as BMP-12 (Chamberlain 2015, 916–927), and even stem cells (Hansen et al. 2016, 249–260).

Barbed sutures, such as those illustrated in Figure 7.2, are sutures that have barbs or projections on the surface which penetrate into the tissues and hold them without necessitating the need for knots. The knotless, barbed suture was first described in 1967 by McKenzie in tendon repair in the hand (McKenzie 1967, 440–447). In an orthopaedic study, it has been shown to lead to a shorter operation time and lower total cost when used instead of standard sutures and yielded similar post-operative function and a lower total complication risk (Zhang et al. 2016). Animal studies of

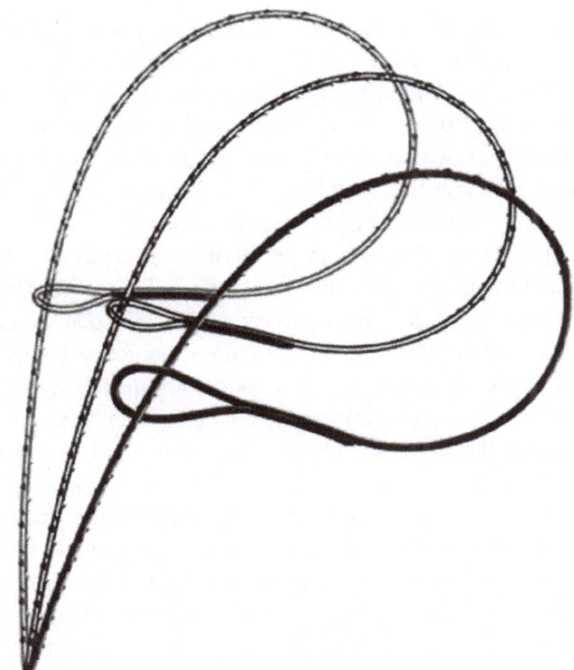

FIGURE 7.2 A example of a barbed suture. Reproduced with kind permission granted by Medtronic, Hertfordshire, UK, 2020.

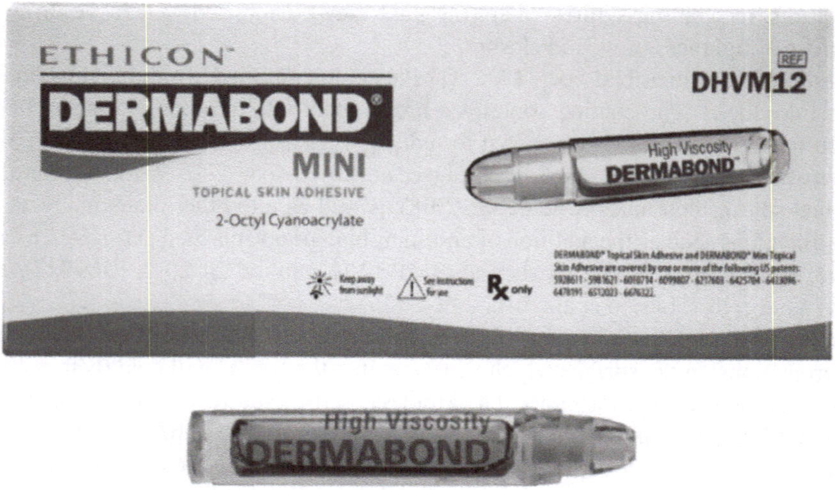

FIGURE 7.3 Dermabond. An example of an adhesive used to close wounds. Reproduced with kind permission granted by Ethicon, Johnson & Johnson, Belgium, 2021.

gastrointestinal closure confirm that the speed of closure was significantly faster than that achieved by traditional sutures with no significant increase in complication rate (Demyttenaere 2009, 237–242). Finally, a Cochrane review explored whether adjustable sutures may be of benefit in ophthalmological surgery for strabismus but could reach no reliable conclusion due to the lack of data in this area (Hassan, Haridas, and Sundaram 2018). There is still tremendous scope for innovation and design of sutures and further trials may elucidate the potential benefits.

As mentioned earlier in this section, in addition to sutures, wounds and lacerations may be treated with adhesive glue, as shown in Figure 7.3. One study on traumatic wounds demonstrated no difference at 1 year between wounds treated with octylcyanoacrylate (glue) and sutures. In a busy Emergency Department, adhesive glue is quicker to apply than suturing and does not require local anaesthetic, making it appealing for use on combative or paediatric patients, and with a premorbid patient, speed is vital; hence these may be influencing factors in this situation when clinicians have to decide what to use (Quinn et al. 1998, 645–649). One currently available product provides a microbial barrier with 99% protection in vitro for 72 hours against organisms commonly responsible for surgical site infections (Bhende et al. 2002, 251–257). A recent Cochrane review called for more comparative studies with large sample sizes to explore the relative frequency of incidence of wound complications between sutures, tissue adhesives, tapes, and zippers (Goto et al. 2020).

7.4 VASCULAR GRAFTS, STENTS, AND VALVES

The primary purpose of the vascular system is to serve as a non-thrombogenic conduit for blood flow. The structure and function of the vascular tree vary depending upon location. As well as providing the human body with 'plumbing,' the vessels are also biologically active and can regulate blood flow, blood pressure and focus the delivery of blood to tissues according to their metabolic requirements. Their metabolic needs are met by their own unique blood supply, the vasa vasorum. The body has an incredible ability to form new or accessory blood vessels called collaterals, around those native vessels with compromised flow. They are of course in no way as good as the originals and, over time, in the presence of disease may become inadequate with regard to maintaining appropriate perfusion.

There are three types of vessels: arteries, veins, and capillaries. Arteries generally deliver oxygenated blood to the tissues and veins take deoxygenated blood away from the tissues. Arteries and veins are composed of three distinct layers: tunica intima, tunica media, and tunica adventitia. In arteries, the intima is composed of a single layer of epithelial cells (endothelium) supported by a basement membrane and elastic lamina. The media contains circular smooth muscle cells and an elastin-rich cellular matrix, whereas the adventitia is composed of loose connective tissue, fibroblasts, nerve endings, and vasa vasorum (blood supply to the vessel) (Orlandi and Bennett 2010, 1706–1713). Arteries can be divided into large elastic arteries, medium muscular arteries, and small arteries. Veins are capacitance vessels that operate under low-pressure conditions and are larger and thinner walled than arteries. There are fewer smooth muscle cells in the tunica media. The basic structural components allow for the vasculature to regulate blood flow by changing luminal area and wall thickness. The differences in structural composition explain the higher pressure system in arteries or vessels leaving the pump, compared to the lower pressure in veins which fills the pump. As the vessels are living tissues, damage to them or the introduction of foreign material results in endothelial dysfunction leading to an inflammatory response, resulting in hardening and narrowing of the vasculature called atherosclerosis.

Grafts can be used to 'replumb' the whole or segments of diseased vessels. They can be used to bypass sites of severe narrowing or occlusion or to strengthen weakened vessels by re-establishing a channel of flow that excludes the compromised wall, for example, an aneurysm (enlargement of an artery due to weakness in the arterial wall). Arterial grafts may be constructed by weaving, knitting, or braiding; the first was commercially available in the USA in 1957 and the period between 1957 and the 1970s saw the commercial introduction of many more synthetic-fibre prostheses (Pourdeyhimi 1986, 1–30). However the graft is constructed, it must be able to withstand the pressures generated within the vessel that it is grafted to. The graft must also be incorporated into the vessel, and in the case of an aneurysm repair, anchored sufficiently from the inside to prevent pressured blood leaking between graft and vessel wall. It is believed that the success of a textile vascular graft, in the healing process after implantation, is due to the porous micro-structure of the wall. Indeed, it has been demonstrated that the type of fabric in textile vascular grafts and the degree of porosity and their permeability affect both the local fluid dynamics and the level of penetration of platelets through the wall, thus indicating their importance as design parameters (Valencia, Garcia, and Bustamante 2018, 858–870).

Grafts can be exceptionally sophisticated with regard to their design and performance with the ability to manufacture seamless grafts by knitting (Sing and

Wang 2016, 380–392), weaving (Moghe and Gupta 2008, 467–477; Li et al. 2013, 1017–1023), or braiding (Xing et al. 2020, 1537–1548; Freitas et al. 2010, 1027–1034) and including bifurcations or trifurcations (Li et al. 2013, 1017–1023), as illustrated in Figure 7.4. Following initial manufacture, treatments are applied to improve performance; compaction (to reduce permeability), crimping (to prevent kinking), and sterilisation are those to note (Pourdeyhimi 1986, 1–30). The performance of the graft can be modelled (not least to explore flow at bends in the stent) to enable informed choices to be made (Ben Abdessalem et al. 2005, 117–122). For example, in a comparative study between knitted and braid structures made from polypropylene, it was concluded that the braid structures performed better in that instance (Stoeckel, Bonsignore, and Duda 2002, 137–147).

In another example, to minimise radial compliance mismatch between native arteries and vascular prostheses over the entire blood pressure range, a biomimetic woven prosthesis sample with a bilayer wall was developed. In this design,

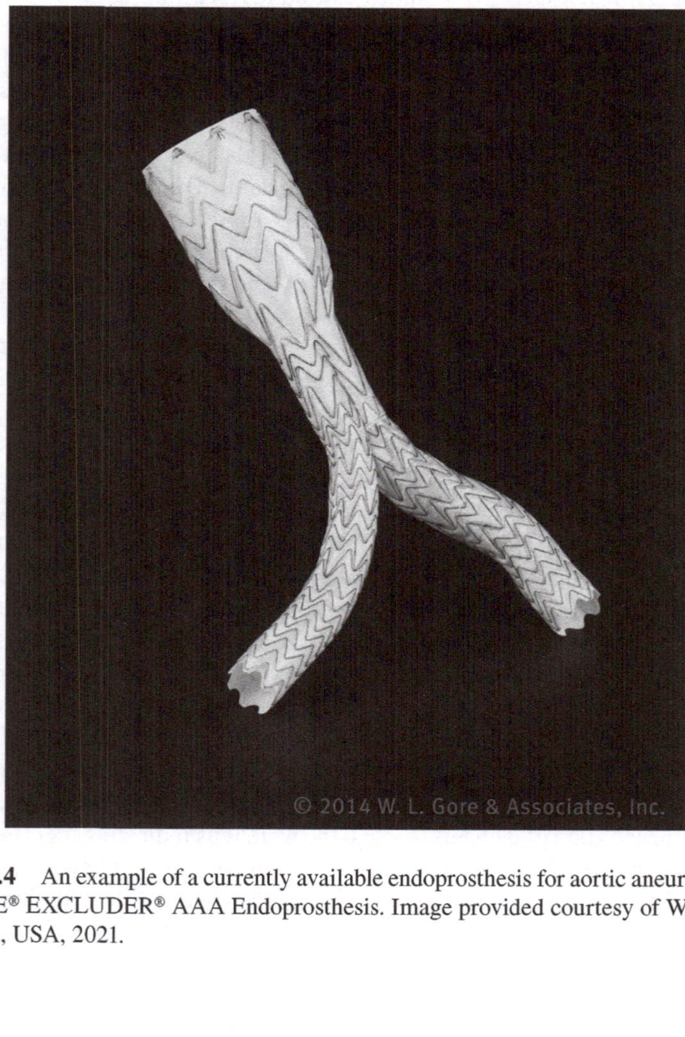

FIGURE 7.4 An example of a currently available endoprosthesis for aortic aneurysm repair. The GORE® EXCLUDER® AAA Endoprosthesis. Image provided courtesy of W.L. Gore & Associates, USA, 2021.

poly(trimethylene terephthalate) (PTT) filaments were utilised as the circumferential yarns in the inner layer to increase the radial compliance of the inner wall whilst poly(ethylene terephthalate) (PET) filaments formed the outer layer to provide a strong and more rigid external prosthesis wall. The two layers were joined together axially along the sample's length by a stitched weave. By means of its woven design, the cross section of the tubular sample consisted of a circumferentially crimped outer layer woven around the inner layer. The bilayer wall structure allowed only the inner layer of the sample to deform radially under small loads equivalent to low normal physiological (diastolic) blood pressures. As the load increased, the inner layer stretched until it came into contact with the outer layer. At higher (systolic) pressures, further loading caused both layers of the wall to deform together. As a result, the prosthesis showed a high degree of pressure-induced compliance when the load was within the normal diastolic pressure range and an appropriately lower compliance at higher systolic pressures (Chen et al. 2012, 106–111).

A stent is a tube that is inserted into the lumen of a vessel or duct to keep the passageway patent. It is used in narrowed and occluded arteries to enlarge, or re-establish, the arterial lumen and increase flow to the end organ. Vascular stents placed are generally left in situ; however, if migration, narrowing, or occlusion of the stent were to occur and result in further problems, this would necessitate the need for removal. This is in contrast to, for example, stents placed in the biliary system which normally are removed. Attention is being paid to the suitability of biodegradable materials for stents, to circumvent the need for removal. Particular attention is needed to ensure that a stent (knitted in this case) made from such a material (polylactic acid or PLA, in this instance) can withstand the radial forces likely to be exerted over the required length of time (Wang et al. 2019, 4230–4238).

Grafts and stents made from nanofibres of absorbable or non-absorbable polymers (Moktari et al. 2016, 119–219), also appear to offer many advantages over those made from conventional yarns, not least because of their high degree of porosity, which, in the case of a tubular woven nanofibre graft can be adjusted by controlling thread density (Joseph et al. 2018, 19449–19458). The yarns made from bundles of nanofibres are relatively fragile so great care had to be taken not to damage them during the (novel robotic) weaving process. Nevertheless, the resulting graft was robust, suturable, kink-proof, and non-thrombogenic. The woven nanofibre graft is claimed to possess significant advantages over nanofibrous nonwovens owing to its regular and controlled hierarchy of nanofibres which yields super-hydrophilicity from an otherwise lipophilic polymer material. It was considered that this characteristic contributed to the observed enhanced protein adsorption, cell attachment and spreading.

Grafts may be inserted by a traditional open method or by an endovascular approach. In an endovascular approach, the site of interest is approached via the vessels from a distant site, most commonly via the common femoral, radial, or brachial artery. The arterial system is then used as a transport route to reach the target site. This is all done with intra-operative image guidance. The graft is preoperatively sized and fenestrated to allow blood flow to branches from the main vessel. It is placed under radiological guidance. Pre-operative imaging (computed tomography or CT) can allow for precise measuring and planning prior to intervention. Some fenestrated stents require customised measurements based on the patient's specific anatomy. For the UK, NICE guidelines from 2018 do not advocate the use of endovascular repair due to long-term complications and higher costs to the National Health Service for unruptured aneurysms. The same guidelines support open surgery rather than endovascular techniques (NICE 2018).

The heart acts to pump blood around the circulatory system. It is divided into a right and left and each side contains two chambers: an atrium that receives blood and passes it to the ventricle which pumps blood to either the lung (right side of the heart) or body (left side of the heart). The connection between the atrium and ventricle is separated by a valve, the bicuspid (also called mitral valve) or tricuspid, and the outflow pipes from the ventricles also contain valves, the pulmonary valve or aortic valve. The valves act to control blood flow by allowing blood to flow only in one direction. If blood flows in the opposite direction, the shape of the valve is such that the leaflets close to prevent this from happening.

Valves may become diseased and become incompetent, similar to the atherosclerotic process leading to calcification of the leaflets. This creates turbulent blood flow, detectable to the clinician as an audible murmur, and may allow blood to flow in the incorrect direction. This has an effect upon the structure of the heart which has to work harder to pump blood effectively and over time can become enlarged, weaker, and less effective. Diseased valves may be replaced by artificial valves; typically, porcine, bovine, or metallic. Both tissue and metallic valves have their own set of drawbacks and, as such, there is scope for design of artificial fibre heart valves that may overcome some of the limitations of current techniques. Although still called 'metallic,' it is becoming more common for this type of valve to be manufactured from carbon.

Polyester textiles have been proposed as an alternative solution to replace heart valve leaflets as they are less fragile than biological tissue. Methodical shaping processes allow for precise dimension setting of the textile material to replicate the tissue being replaced and early in vivo tests in sheep models have confirmed efficacy of prototypes manufactured by this method (Heim, Durand, and Chakfe 2011, 1303–1309). One of the drawbacks of uncoated polyester in the sheep modelling is that there is limited tissue ingrowth onto the structure and the fabric has a tendency to stiffen due to calcium deposition (Heim, Durand, and Chafke 2013, 361–367). Even prior to this, how the fabric is constructed had already been identified as an important factor that would affect longevity of textile-based valves, due to changing flexural properties with time, before biology was accounted for (Heim and Gupta 2009, 1001–1013). Attention has also been turned towards using polyethylene terephthalate as a fibre to reduce fibrotic tissue ingrowth and increase longevity, though durability is currently limited under accelerated cyclic loading (Amri et al. 2018, 221–230).

One other method of incorporating textiles into artificial heart valves involves using textiles as a reinforcement to tissue-engineered valves. The BioTexValve incorporates multifilament fibres, arranged similarly to the collagen bundles in the native aortic leaflet, fixed by a thin electrospun layer that is directly deposited on the pattern. The textile-based leaflets are subsequently positioned in a 3D mould with components that form a fibrin gel containing human vascular smooth muscle cells and upon fibrin polymerisation, a complete valve is obtained. At 21 days, the valve demonstrated excellent functionality under aortic pressure and flow conditions in a mock circulation (Moreira 2016, 2113–2121).

7.4.1 Current Problems with Grafts, Stents, and Valves

Graft revision of vascular intervention is frequently required beyond the first six weeks with up to 40% of femorodistal bypass surgery grafts (a vessel that bypasses a blockage and connects the femoral artery with an artery below the knee) requiring re-intervention within 5 years. Intervention can range from angioplasty ('ballooning') the compromised segment via an endovascular approach, placing a stent within the graft, or revision surgery. Despite there having been considerable enthusiasm for endovascular aortic aneurysm reconstruction (EVAR) (Brewster et al. 2006, 426), the same issue arises for endovascular intervention where up to 30% of patients need a re-intervention within 5 years after EVAR (Karthikesalingam et al. 2010, 657–663). This may be due to a variety of problems. Graft-related problems include occlusion, migration, and infection. EVARs also suffer from ongoing aneurysm sac expansion due to filling despite the graft in place, a phenomenon called endoleak. There are five types of endoleak:

- Type I, where the landing zone does not seal sufficiently, resulting in blood filling the sac in between the graft and blood vessel wall.
- Type II, where filling from arteries feeding the sac takes place.
- Type III, where filling happens between individually placed graft components.
- Types IV and V are rare and are not discussed here.

Graft thrombosis is influenced by both general and local factors. These include cardiac function, haematological properties of blood, proximal and distal bypass targets, and bypass conduit. Infra-inguinal bypass patency of autologous vein is better than Dacron (PET) or PTFE (Pereira et al. 2006, 510–517). For femoropopliteal bypass grafts (a graft connecting the femoral artery to the popliteal artery in the above-knee segment), patency at 5 years is similar when Dacron or PTFE are used (Takagi et al. 2010, 232–236). A heparin-bonded PTFE graft significantly reduced the overall risk of primary graft failure by 37% in a one-year multicentre RCT (randomised controlled trial) in Scandinavia. The heparin-bonded graft was superior to PTFE and with no difference in primary graft patency at 5 years for above-knee bypass (Ambler and Twine 2018; Lindholt et al. 2011, 668–673). The risk for ischaemic complications due to thrombosis or embolism and the need for emergency limb revascularisation are greater with occlusion of prosthetic grafts compared to venous grafts as the thrombus in the prosthetic graft extends into the outflow artery and is at a higher risk of breaking off, embolising and resulting in distal infarction (Jackson et al. 2000, 498–505).

A Cochrane review in 2018 demonstrated a clear primary patency benefit for autologous vein when compared to synthetic materials for above-knee bypasses. In the long term (5 years), Dacron confers a small primary patency benefit over PTFE for above-knee bypass. More research is required to determine which graft is superior for a below-knee bypass (Ambler and Twine 2018).

Graft infection is relatively uncommon but has a high amputation and mortality risk (Yeager 1992, 485–491). Treatment is aimed at patient survival, eradication of infection where possible, and revascularisation by a method that is durable and does not itself become infected. Sometimes intervention will need to be in a staged approach, for example, in aorto-enteric fistula disease (communication between the aorta and small bowel). Infection of foreign material is notoriously difficult to completely eradicate. Grafts have been manufactured that incorporate antimicrobials. At present, Rifampicin bonding of Dacron grafts does not appear to reduce graft infection, nor does silver-coating of the graft (Gao et al. 2010, 472–477; Stewart, Eyers, and Earnshaw 2006). If explantation of grafts or redo-bypasses are not possible, then the patient may be committed to lifelong antibiotic therapy.

The development of aneurysms was frequent with early PTFE grafts. Manufacturing appears to have eliminated this. Dacron undergoes late degradation and dilatation, and this becomes clinically significant in 2–3% of cases. After 5–10 years, disruption can occur at points of stress, for example, under a ligament, and cause a false aneurysm (Damme et al. 2005, 249–255). Distraction of the graft may cause spontaneous rupture or anastomotic disruption of PTFE axillofemoral grafts (White et al. 1990, 625–627).

In a similar manner to grafts, one of the most common problems with stents is thrombosis within the stent itself. Whilst rare, it carries a high mortality of 45% and a recurrence rate of 20%. Risk factors are multifactorial including biology of the endothelium, blood flow, blood constituents and viscosity, and patients factors as a whole (Gori et al. 2019, 243–256). Reducing the risk of stent thrombosis has attracted much attention over the years and still continues to do so with large randomised, controlled trials aimed at modifying factors that are known to affect the risk (Lopes et al. 2020, 781–783). Most notably smoking cessation, anticoagulation for thrombotic blood disorders, and antiplatelet therapy can optimise risk reduction.

As discussed earlier within this section, manufacturing tissue valves with textiles is still in the rudimentary phase. Nevertheless, it is gaining more attention as it offers a potential solution to the issues encountered with biological and metallic heart valves. Current challenges which need to be addressed with textile valves include fibrous ingrowth, a lack of flexibility of valve leaflets and wear and fatigue profiles over time. Some of the issues, such as regurgitation of blood through the pores within the fabric can be overcome if rapid tissue ingrowth can be stimulated (Yousefi et al. 2017, 476–486).

7.4.2 Advances with Grafts, Stents, and Valves

In small-diameter vessels, synthetic grafts are of limited use due to poor patency rates (Pashneh-Tala 2016, 68–100). Whilst there has been some improvement in patency by seeding autologous endothelial cells onto the luminal surface of synthetic grafts, the grafts have been unable to exceed the performance of autologous vessels

(Deutsch et al. 2009, 352–262). Synthetic polymer scaffolds have been used to create vascular grafts. A porous scaffold produced from a biodegradable copolymer mesh of poly (l-lactide) and poly-caprolactone reinforced with polyglycolide has been seeded with cells prior to inflammation. The grafts were implanted into large vessels and results were somewhat promising though not without room for improvement (Hibino et al. 2010, 431–436; Mirensky et al. 2009, 1127–1133). A variety of other fibre types, both synthetic and natural, have been used to create scaffolds on which to seed cells. Current understanding of the underlying molecular process in replacing the engineered graft by host cells is limited. Better understanding of this process will enable the construction of grafts with the potential for long-term graft success.

There is a greater understanding of in-stent thrombosis; it is typically multifactorial and affected by patient factors, anticoagulation, and the device itself. Drug-eluting stents were bulky and cumbersome initially and required meticulous insertion. Issues involved chronic inflammation that caused impaired endothelialisation, slower strut healing, adverse vessel remodelling, and neoatherosclerosis. Following these initial findings, a number of modifications were undertaken to improve performance.

Biodegradable polymers were introduced to reduce long-term implications of a permanent polymer implant. The polymers can be modified such that they also elute drugs. Various polymers and coatings have been trialled including poly(l-lactic) polymer stents and silicon carbide stent coatings which have demonstrated various outcomes in trials. Fully bioresorbable stents were introduced in 2012. The most studied device was the polylactic acid Absorb, but despite initial encouraging results at short-term and mid-term follow-up, a two- to threefold increase in the rate of in-scaffold thrombosis was witnessed when compared to everolimus-eluting stents. The stent was eventually withdrawn from the market in September 2017 (Gori et al. 2019, 243–256).

With the advent of new material design and manufacture and the progress in the preparation of well-arranged nanofibre assemblies, the area of graft, stent, and valve design is likely to continue to expand as solutions to the problems witnessed in clinical practice are sought.

7.5 IMPLANTABLE MESH PRODUCTS

The development of mesh has been undertaken to address a variety of problems, from augmenting tendon and ligament repairs through to providing a mechanical barrier to prevent hernias or a mechanical support to manage pelvic floor dysfunction.

7.5.1 Tendons and Ligaments

Tendons connect muscle to bone and are made from fibrous connective tissue. Their main function is to transfer forces from muscles to bone to produce joint motion. Examples include the Achilles tendon at the ankle, patella tendon at the knee, and rotator cuff tendons in the shoulder. Tendons are subject to many types of stresses through their lifetime and overuse may lead to a tendinopathy and eventually tendon rupture. This results in loss of function of the affected joint. For example, the

Achilles tendon is the thickest and strongest tendon in the body and withholds stress approximately 12.5 times the individual's body weight when running. Repair of a defect can be undertaken as a primary procedure or augmented with autologous tendon, such as that of flexor hallucis longus, which increases load to failure. This remains a topic of interest in the foot and ankle community (De la Fuente et al. 2017, 78–83; Schmidtberg et al. 2019, 1505–1512).

Ligaments connect bone to bone and are also soft tissue structures made from fibrous connective tissue. They offer three main functions: to restrict motion, stabilise joints, and provide proprioception (awareness of the position and movement of the body) to a joint. Examples include the anterior cruciate ligament (ACL) within the knee and glenohumeral ligaments (GHL) of the shoulder. Ligament rupture can lead to joint instability which over time can cause wear to the cartilage within the joint and eventually lead to osteoarthritis.

Both tendons and ligaments have poor healing capacity and when ruptured must either be repaired or reconstructed. Prior to the implementation of artificial ligaments, autologous tendons and allografts were the most popular methods of managing these conditions; however, the risk of donor-site morbidity, weakening of adjacent anatomic tissues, and the transmission of diseases in an era stricken with the fear of hepatitis and HIV made the use of artificial grafts increasingly attractive. Artificial ligaments, therefore, began to be adopted in the 1980s and 1990s as advances in biomaterials allowed for them to be trialled. In particular, there was significant interest in ACL reconstructions. Early results were very encouraging which resulted in large numbers of different artificial ligaments being developed, though later results identified high complication and failure rates, resulting in many of these prostheses being discontinued.

When constructing the ideal artificial ligament some basic properties should always be present, including high tensile strength, abrasion resistance, and no immune reaction. In addition, the prosthesis should be capable of mimicking the native ligament/tendon and allow ingrowth of the surrounding tissue in a physiological manner. Although, the ideal artificial ligament remains elusive (Tsukazaki et al. 2003, 355–362), efforts have been made to develop systems to help with ligament repair. One example of a ligament reconstruction augment is the Ligament Advanced Reinforcement System, LARS. This is a synthetic ligament scaffold manufactured from polyethylene terephthalate. It is available in different forms for use in soft tissue applications such as those around the knee, shoulder, foot, and ankle. LARS ligaments have also been used in ACL repair and demonstrated positive results in short- and mid-term follow-up. In comparative trials, the LARS ligament has been demonstrated to be superior to other ligament equivalents manufactured from polyester (Iliadis et al. 2016). There have, however, been some reports of local soft tissue reactions. There were also reports of early increased laxity in the knee which was due to insufficient tissue ingrowth into the graft (Lavoie, Fletcher, and Duval 2000, 157–163). The Leeds–Keio ligament, invented in partnership between the University of Leeds in the UK and Keio University in Tokyo, Japan, is also manufactured from polyester fibres and was developed specifically for ACL reconstruction. It was made such that the mechanical structures mimicked those of the native ACL but its clinical efficacy was controversial with varying results from clinical trials. Complications such as synovitis from particle wear and poor functional recovery were frequently reported between 1991 and 2004. More recently, there has been some focus on creating artificial ligaments that mimic the normal anatomical ligament. Attention has therefore turned towards braided ligaments, where fibre choice, braid angle, and number of braids can be varied to alter mechanical properties. In addition, combining several braids mimics the normal structure of the anterior cruciate ligament bundles, as shown in Figure 7.5. Laboratory trials proved promising with artificial ligaments mimicking the normal loading cycles of a native ACL, as demonstrated in Figure 7.6 (Jedda et al. 2008, 273–280; Turki, Marzougui, and Ben Abdessalem 2015, 912–918).

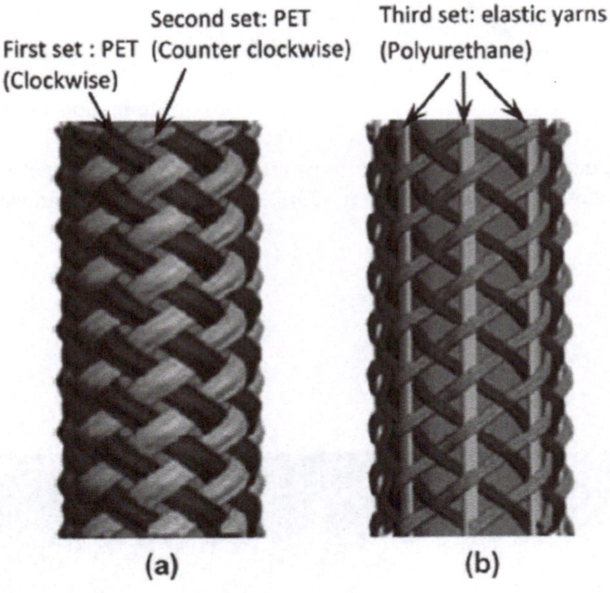

FIGURE 7.5 An example of braided ligaments; (a) biaxial braid, (b) triaxial braid. Picture reproduced from Turki et al. (2015). Permissions kindly granted by Taylor & Francis, 2021.

Artificial tendons are also available and are commonly used to augment primary and delayed primary repairs. Examples of these include repair of quadriceps or patella tendons where commercially available tapes are available, as shown in Figures 7.7 to 7.9. Other ways to augment a repair include using patches such as Pitch Patch™ (Neoligaments, Leeds, UK), a permanent implant constructed from a knitted polyester fabric that encourages tissue ingrowth and can be used to reinforce rotator cuff tendon repair, as shown in Figures 7.10–7.11. Artificial ligaments and tendons possess unique advantages to autologous repairs such as no donor-site morbidity, early recovery, and no risk of disease transmission; however, post-operative complications such as infection, local soft tissue reactions, and rupture of the graft have emerged.

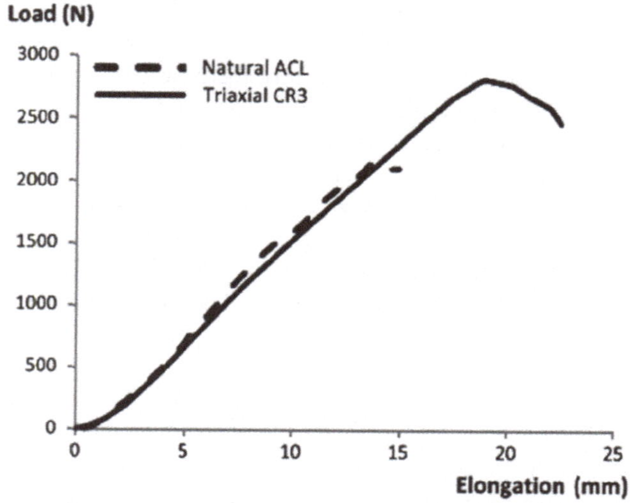

FIGURE 7.6 Load-elongation curves of the natural ACL and the preloaded artificial triaxial ACL. Picture reproduced from Turki et al. (2015). Permissions kindly granted by Taylor & Francis, 2021.

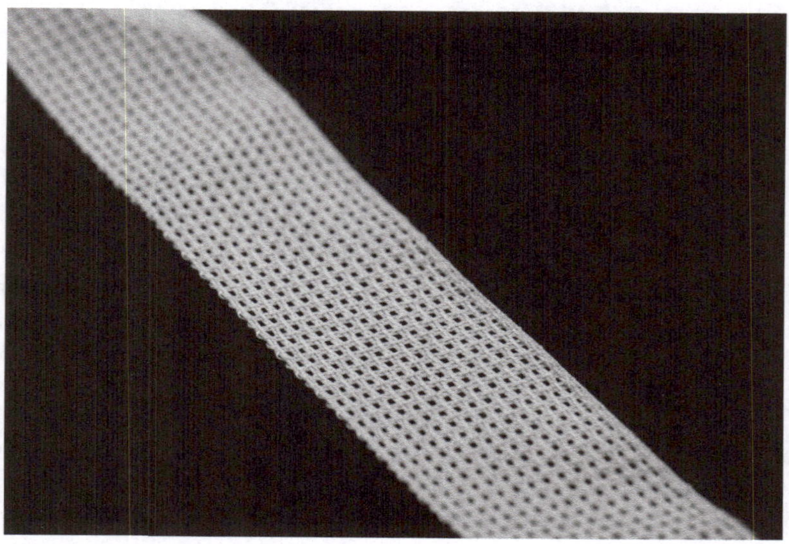

FIGURE 7.7 An example of a braided tape used in tendon reconstruction. The implant comprises a wide, open weave Poly-Tape. PatellaTape System™. Reproduced with kind permission granted by Neoligaments™, a division of Xiros, Leeds, UK, 2021.

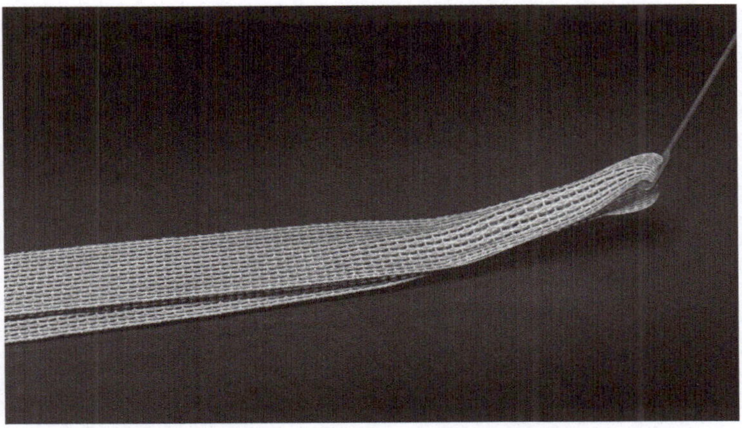

FIGURE 7.8 – An example of a braided tape used in tendon reconstruction. PatellaTape System™. Reproduced with kind permission granted by Neoligaments™, a division of Xiros, Leeds, UK, 2021.

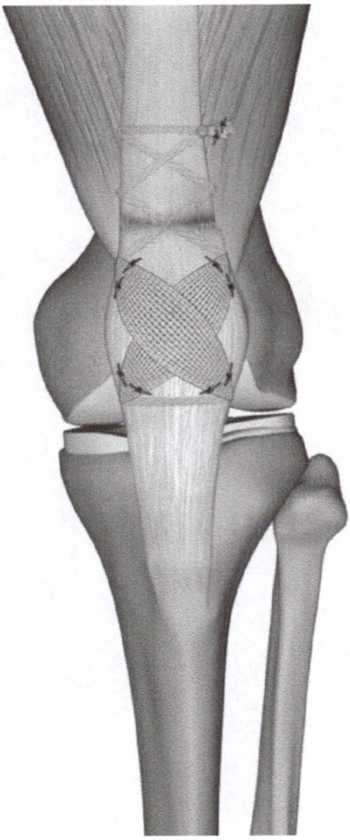

FIGURE 7.9 An example of a braided tape used to repair the quadriceps tendon. The implant comprises a wide, open weave Poly-Tape. QuadsTape System™. Reproduced with kind permission granted by Neoligaments™, a division of Xiros, Leeds, UK, 2021.

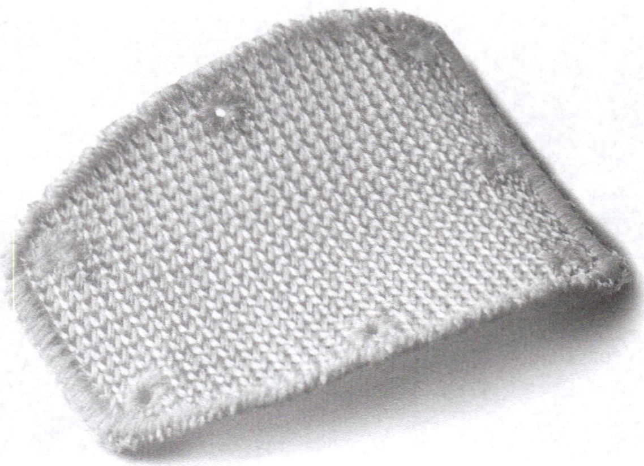

FIGURE 7.10 An example of a knitted augment used as a patch in a tendon repair for the rotator cuff tendons of the shoulder. This may be used when the tear cannot be completely repaired using normal methods or the quality of the soft tissue is poor. Pitch Patch™. Reproduced with kind permission granted by Neoligaments™, a division of Xiros, Leeds, UK, 2021.

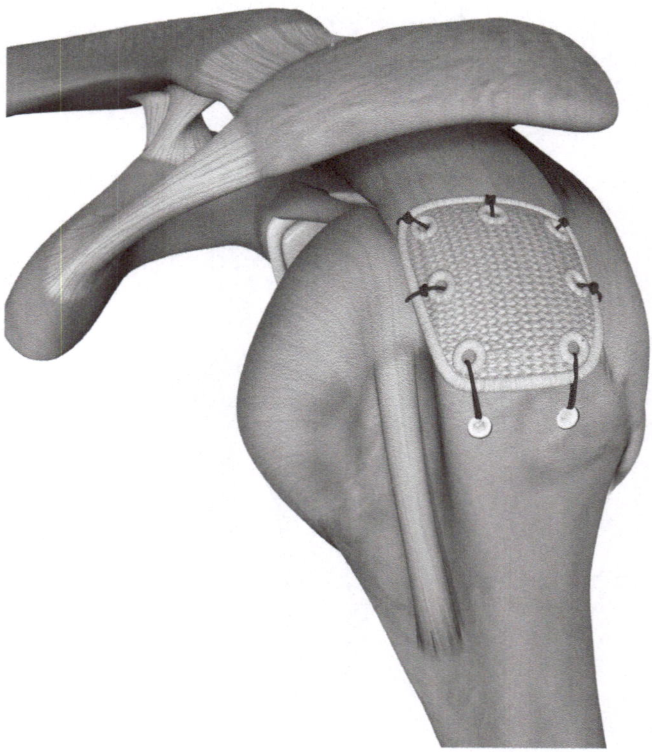

FIGURE 7.11 An example of a knitted augment in rotator cuff repair in the shoulder. Pitch Patch™. Reproduced with kind permission granted by Neoligaments™, a division of Xiros, Leeds, UK, 2021.

7.5.2 Hernial Repair

Implantable synthetic mesh is used to treat a hernia – a protrusion of an organ through the body wall of the cavity that normally contains it. Hernias are very common and their treatment is one of the most frequently performed surgical procedures worldwide, estimated at around 20 million cases per year (HerniaSurg Group 2018, 1–165; Kingsnorth and LeBlanc 2003, 1561–1571). The lifetime risk of groin hernia is between 27 and 43% for men and 3–6% for women (HerniaSurg Group 2018, 1–165; Kingsnorth and LeBlanc 2003, 1561–1571). The global incidence of hernia is also increasing due to escalating levels of obesity and global access to open surgical intervention (risking incisional herniae).

Hernias are predominantly described by their location. Abdominal wall hernias can occur primarily through acquired weaknesses in the groin, the abdominal wall, or by the side of stomas. They can occur post-operatively through a weakness in the repair of the fascia (a strong connective tissue layer in the abdominal wall). Congenital causes of hernias are common, but these are not repaired with synthetic mesh as it is not able to 'grow' with the patient.

The development of synthetic meshes has resulted in the advancement of surgical technique away from bolstering the tissue with sutures towards using a mesh to close a defect. In groin hernias, mesh repair reduces the risk of hernia recurrence compared to non-mesh repair (2 vs 5%) (EU Hernia Trialists Collaboration 2002, 322–332) and reduces post-operative pain, resulting in a shorter hospital stay and quicker return to normal activity (Lockhart et al. 2018). The risk of hernia recurrence is also reduced in mesh repair of parastomal hernias and laparoscopic repair of inguinal hernias (Jones et al. 2018). In 2002, the European Union Hernia Trialist Collaboration Group evaluated 58 randomised control trials to conclude, unanimously, that the use of mesh was superior to other techniques, especially highlighting reduced recurrence and post-operative pain (EU Hernia Trialists Collaboration 2002, 322–332). Today the use of mesh has virtually replaced sutured techniques in the developed world. Figure 7.12 shows an intra-operative example of mesh being placed.

7.5.2.1 Types of Mesh and Surgical Considerations

During a hernia operation, the hernia contents are dissected and 'reduced' into the cavity which would normally contain it. Mesh allows the surgeon to patch the 'defect' allowing ingress of new tissue into its knitted structure (incorporation), without the surgeon needing to pull tissues together, under tension, to do so. Viable tissues under tension are liable to 'pressure necrose' and fail, due to the same mechanics which caused the weakness in the first place. Without mesh, techniques to reduce (not eliminate) tension include extensive tissue dissection to allow the release of surrounding tissue; this is associated with more pain, bleeding, and risks of post-operative swelling due to fluid (seroma) or retained blood (haematoma) within the tissues.

To perform adequately, the mesh needs to be able to withstand the tensions and extensibility experienced within the abdominal wall; these can be calculated and

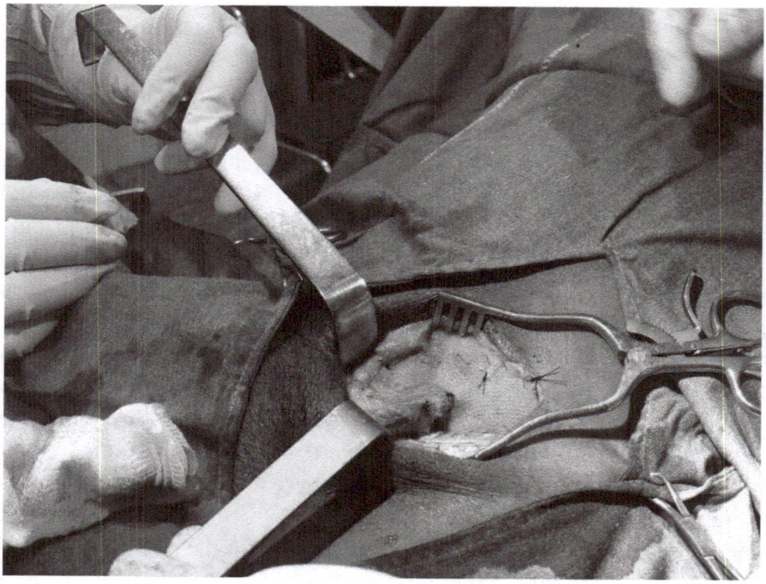

FIGURE 7.12 An example of a hernial mesh augment inserted into the abdomen. Image kindly provided by Mr Steve Lindley, General Surgeon, UK, 2021.

measured. The hernia-repair mesh needs to be able to withstand at least 180 mmHg (20 kPa) before failing, indicating a tensile strength requirement of 16 N/cm and extensibility in males of 23% ± 7% and 15% ± 5%, and 32% ± 17% and 17% ± 5% in females when tissue is stretched in the vertical and horizontal directions, respectively (Baylón et al. 2017, 47). As a result, 'mesh failure' is almost never encountered as the cause of hernia recurrence.

Since the advent of laparoscopic or 'keyhole surgery,' surgeons have been able to offer a minimally invasive technique to repairing hernias. This relies on the use of mesh. There are several techniques to treat groin hernias by the use of mesh, each of which is defined by the approach taken to undertake the repair. Transabdominal pre-peritoneal (TAPP) repair involves the surgeon entering the abdominal cavity and peeling the lining of the cavity (the peritoneum) down to access the plane to place the mesh. The totally extraperitoneal repair (TEP) technique does not involve penetration of the abdominal cavity, instead entering the abdominal wall itself, and, after dissecting out the hernia, placing the mesh in this plane. Both have their place in modern practice, depending on surgeon preference. The benefit over an open repair seems to be reduced post-operative pain and length of stay in hospital. There is some evidence suggesting less chronic pain in cases where sutures are not used to fixate the mesh (EU Hernia Trialists Collaboration 2002, 322–332). There is most evidence that laparoscopic techniques are superior for patients with bilateral hernias (avoiding debilitating bilateral open groin incisions) or those with hernia recurrence (as you are repairing the hernia via unadulterated tissues) (HerniaSurg Group 2018, 1–165).

Synthetic meshes have been made from a variety of materials that have evolved with experience and technology, an example is shown in Figure 7.13. Meshes may be manufactured from PTFE, polypropylene or polyester. Expanded PTFE, whereby a sheet of PTFE is created first and then stretched to create micropores, is an inert, microporous hydrophobic material that can be used intra-peritoneally due to the low risk of host inflammation reaction that is often associated with mesh. However, incorporation into the abdominal wall is limited. By contrast, polypropylene and polyester repair materials can be made in the form of porous meshes that allow a good integration in the abdominal wall by colonisation of the prosthesis with collagen fibres from the host. Polypropylene absorbs little if any moisture and in these applications is usually knitted or woven to the required design. Polyester is also woven into a variety of designs for similar purposes; it is slightly less lipophilic than polypropylene (Lacour et al. 2017, 517–528). Synthetic meshes are often characterised by 'weight' and porosity; varying between ultralightweight approximately <30 g/m^2 and heavyweight >90 g/m^2. Porosity is characterised by the size of the pore; microporous

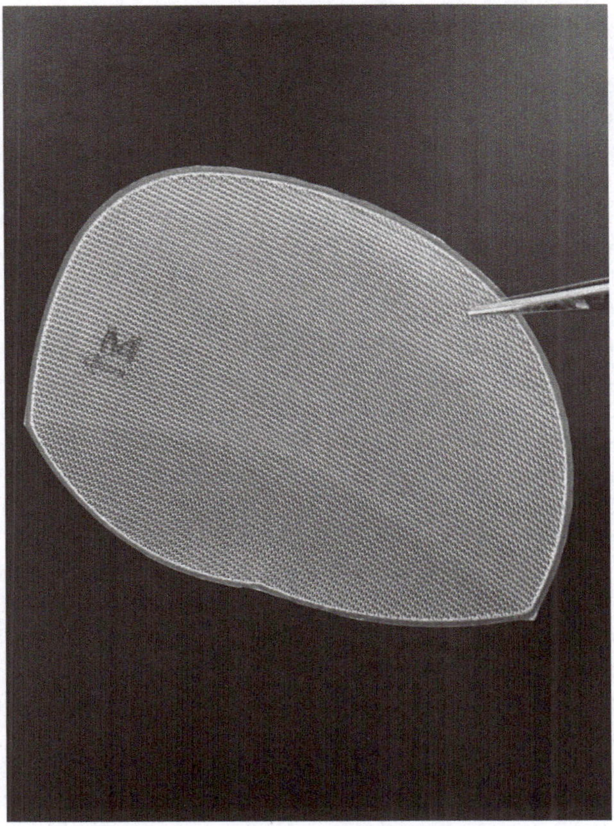

FIGURE 7.13 An example of a hernial mesh augment used in hernial repair. Image kindly provided by Mr Steve Lindley, General Surgeon, UK, 2021.

being <100 μm and large pores being 1000–2000 μm. Biocompatibility appears to be proportional to the pore size of the mesh (Novitsky and Martin-del-Campo 2018, 25–30). Initial thoughts that mesh for hernia repair needs to be high in tensile strength and be able to promote an aggressive fibrotic reaction to maximise incorporation into tissues have been refined. While incorporation is necessary, significant fibrosis is associated with more pain and movement restriction (Scheuerlein et al. 2013, 170–178). The maximum abdominal pressure required for meshes to withstand is about one-tenth of that of most meshes (Brown and Finch 2010, 272–278). Smaller surface areas lead to reduced fibrosis. These two realisations have led to the development of lightweight meshes. Pore sizes above 75 μm allow infiltration of macrophages and fibroblasts for collagenation. Microporous mesh replaces integration capability with the bridging of pores with granulomas. Granuloma bridging creates a firm inflexible capsule around the mesh which has more potential to shrink (Bilsel and Abci 2012, 317–321). Post-operative pain following Lichtenstein hernia repair with lightweight mesh is also less than with heavy mesh (Scheuerlein et al. 2013, 170–178). Shrinkage, adhesion formation, infection, and recurrence are all still possible with lightweight mesh, so the quest for the ideal mesh continues.

Covered or composite mesh has been developed to reduce the risk of adhesion formation, to satisfy concerns of bowel attachment, fistulation, and subsequent infection. Such meshes can be useful when considering repair of complex hernias which may require the placement of an intraperitoneal mesh (placed on the lining of the abdominal cavity – IPOM or intraperitoneal onlay mesh technique), rather than undertaking the risks of dissecting a large hernia defect. They require a specific orientation, so that the covered aspect does not attach to viscera, whereas the other surface can adhere to the peritoneum (Bilsel and Abci 2012, 317–321).

The most challenging hernia operations involve large defects which are contaminated with bowel content. These conditions make permanent prosthetic mesh unsuitable due to inevitable infection or high risk of intestinal fistulation. Developments in biologic meshes derived from porcine tissue (such as Permacol or Strattice) or bovine tissue employ acellular collagen matrices to provide a scaffold for native tissue penetration (Bilsel and Abci 2012, 317–321). These are expensive and so they are usually reserved for use in abdominal wall reconstruction. There are also absorbable meshes available, typically composed of copolymerised forms of polylactic acid, polyglycolic acid, polyglactin, and/or polycaprolactone; with these, one of the issues that needs to be taken into account is that the degradation rate needs to be slower than the native healing to ensure sufficient reinforcement of tissue walls while that healing takes place (Grant and Ramshaw 2018, 173–178). As a result, recurrence rates are very high, at >50% (Bilsel and Abci 2012, 317–321), and so planning of definitive hernia repair should be considered, or the cost of biologic meshes could be justified.

There is a massive unmet surgical need in less economically developed countries. Two of the barriers to satisfying this need are education and resources. The cost of imported commercial synthetic mesh is approximately $100 per treatment and, therefore, largely prohibitive (Freudenberg et al. 2006, 1785–1789). Tongaonkar

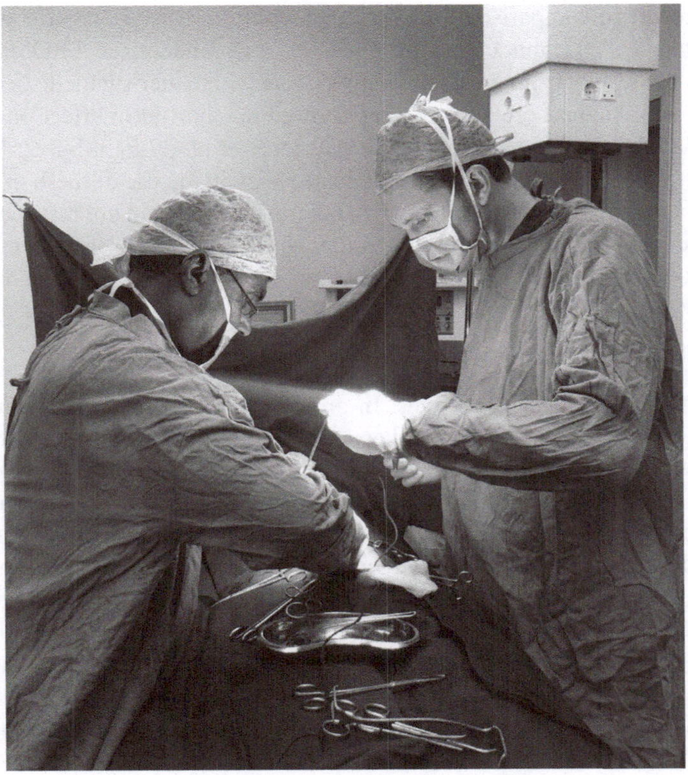

FIGURE 7.14 Hernial repair for a humanitarian organisation. Image kindly provided by Mr Steve Lindley, General Surgeon, UK, 2021.

demonstrated that ubiquitous cheap mosquito net could be sterilised and safely replace commercial mesh in the treatment of hernias in rural India. Mosquito net often includes a copolymer of polyethylene and polypropylene and is similar in properties to commercial hernia mesh. Subsequent studies have built on this discovery to prove its safety and efficacy (Ahmad et al. 2019, 429–435). International hernia charities such as Operation Hernia and Hernia International focus their work on promoting the adoption of the Lichtenstein tension-free repair in resource-challenged settings with impressive results. Figure 7.14 shows the author of the hernial section repairing a hernia whilst undertaking humanitarian work in Pakistan.

7.5.3 Urogynaecology

Prolapse of the bladder or rectum into the vagina, 'cystoceles' and 'rectoceles' respectively, are frequent conditions with significant morbidity. Mesh has a role in treatment options here too. Using mesh has been shown to provide a statistically significant advantage to anatomical outcome when used in anterior vaginal wall prolapse repair in comparison to native tissue with no deleterious effects on functional outcome. The multicentre, prospective, and randomised PROSPECT trial compared the results from the use of native tissue with either synthetic or biological mesh repair in vaginal prolapse surgery showed no short-term effect on outcomes such as effectiveness and quality of life (Glazener et al. 2017, 381–392; Vollebregt et al. 2011, 1518–1527). There is current controversy in the use of mesh in the repair of pelvic organ prolapse. Mesh erosion and chronic pelvic pain are material but relatively infrequent complications of this technique (Royal College of Obstetricians and Gynaecologists 2019).

7.5.4 Problems with Mesh

Mesh repair is not without problems. In groin hernias, a Cochrane review showed that wound infection and seroma (collection of fluid) were more common than in a hernia repair without mesh (Lockhart et al. 2018). Permanent mesh for vaginal prolapse was associated with a higher rate of de novo stress incontinence and bladder injury (Maher et al. 2016). In general, chronic pain following hernia repair cannot be avoided entirely. Mesh repair is associated with less pain than suture repair due to its tension free characteristics. Laparoscopic, non-sutured mesh could be associated with less chronic pain than in open inguinal hernia repairs with mesh (Eklund et al. 2010, 600–608) due to the avoidance of suturing which may trap and irritate peripheral nerves. Furthermore, there were reports of vaginal mesh erosion and chronic pain. In 2011, transvaginal permanent mesh was voluntarily withdrawn from the market, though lightweight transvaginal permanent mesh was still available until banned in 2018. Hitting the headlines of national newspapers in the UK in 2017, NICE in updated advice in December 2017 said that evidence on the safety of the procedure showed there were serious, but well-recognised safety concerns and recommended that the use of mesh in prolapse should be restricted to research only (NICE 2017). The latest update is that mesh can be implanted but that a register must be maintained to track patients and outcomes (Royal College of Obstetricians and Gynaecologists 2019). Mesh for these patients has currently been withheld until certain conditions can be met (Royal College of Obstetricians and Gynaecologists 2019).

7.5.5 Future Developments with Mesh

The search for the ideal mesh continues. Future efforts will likely focus on challenges associated with chronic pain, and materials resistant to chronic infection.

In an effort to decrease fibrotic response and to prevent adhesions that can occur with meshes, both polyester and polypropylene meshes have been coated with a range of anti-adhesive barriers including collagen, titanium, polyglactin, and omega-3 fatty acids (Novitsky and Martin-del-Campo 2018, 25–30). The use of coatings has been associated with less post-operative pain as shown by short- and long-term follow up but this may be attributed to the weight of the mesh rather than the coating (Novitsky and Martin-del-Campo 2018, 25–30). Polyester and polypropylene meshes have also been coated with polyethylenimine with promising results (Scheuerlein et al. 2013, 170–178).

There has also been work directed at the process of manufacture of the mesh. Most meshes are woven but one type is made from randomly orientated microfibres of polypropylene, which is expected to be more biocompatible. The integration of drugs and cells into meshes is also being trialled; for example, fibroblast cells and mesenchymal stem cells have been coated onto three commercial meshes and demonstrated a positive integration, but this research is still in its infancy (Brown and Finch 2010, 272–278).

7.6 OPHTHALMIC USES

The human eye is a highly specialised and complex organ which provides us with the gift of vision. It allows people to receive and process visual details by focusing light received from an object onto the light-sensitive nerve fibre layer called the retina. The retina converts this light energy into nerve impulses which are transmitted to the brain via the optic nerve. The brain processes these nerve impulses and creates an image that is consciously appreciated as vision (Kolb 1995).

Over the last few decades, significant research has been carried out on the use of biomaterials in ophthalmology to improve and help provide vision. There are various ocular conditions, such as astigmatism, keratoconus, cataract, advanced glaucoma, and ocular trauma, that have benefited from the use of ocular biomaterials. Biomaterials have been used extensively in the development of contact lenses, intraocular lenses, glaucoma filtration implants, keratoprostheses, intracorneal implants, orbital implants, and scleral buckles. There are also various viscoelastic agents that are used during intraocular surgeries (Giordano and Refojo 1996, 301–317).

For a better understanding of the eye and the use of biomaterials in the eye, a brief outline of the anatomy of the eye and its functions (Dahl 2021; Kolb 1995; Snell 2013) is provided below and illustrated in Figure 7.15.

- The *orbit* is a cavity in the skull which contains the eyeball, also known as the globe.
- The *globe* is a round structure also known commonly as the eyeball, which sits in the orbit.
- The *sclera* is the white part of the eye that extends around the eye and gives shape to the eye. It is known to be a tough, leather-like tissue.
- *Extraocular muscles* control the movements of the eye. There are six extraocular muscles that attach to the sclera. Two eyes work together to look left, right, up, or down, and also to rotate.
- The *cornea* is a clear and transparent tissue found at the front of the eye which focuses light onto the retina. Transparency of the cornea allows us to visualise the coloured part of the eye which is behind the cornea, called the iris. Contact lenses are typically worn in front of the cornea.
- The *iris* is the coloured part of the eye between the cornea and lens, which controls the amount of light that enters the eye. The iris has a central opening known as the *pupil*. The iris is made of two types of muscles. The first set of muscles are circular, the fibres are arranged in a ring around the pupil

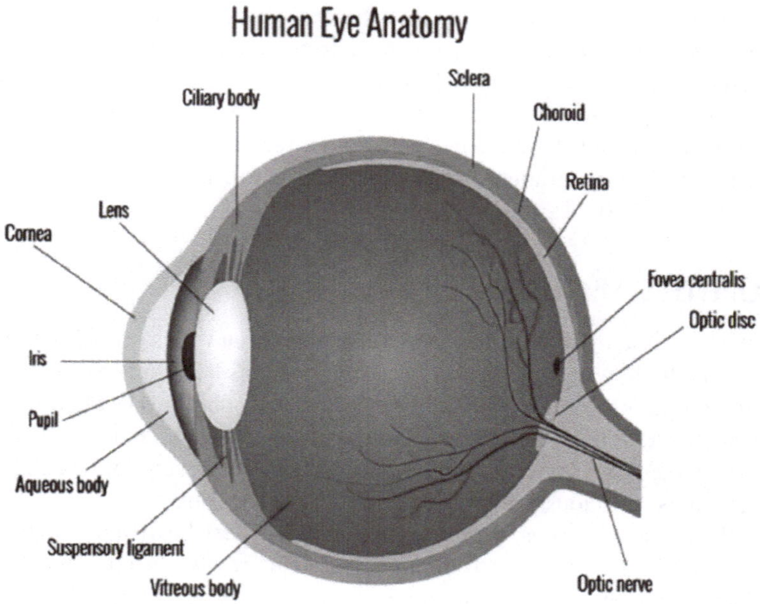

FIGURE 7.15 Anatomy of the eye.

and contract in bright light causing the pupil to constrict (become smaller). The second set of muscles are radial, the fibres radiate outward from the pupil and contract in the dark causing the pupil to dilate (become larger).

- The *lens* is a transparent, sphere shaped structure that is located just behind the iris. It is connected to the *ciliary body* (a ring of muscular tissue) by fine fibres, called zonules. The lens and ciliary body work together to control fine focusing of light. The lens also works with the cornea to focus light onto the retina.
- The *vitreous cavity* is located at the back of the eye and contains a jelly like fluid, known as the vitreous humour. The vitreous humour functions to retain the spherical shape of the eye.
- The *retina* is a nerve fibre layer found at the back of the eye. It is composed of nine distinct layers. The retina functions to process light energy into electrical energy. This electrical energy is transmitted by nerve cells to the optic nerve. The optic nerve transmits these signals to the brain which converts them into images. Further processing of these signals helps us understand the context of the images we see. The two main types of cells found in the photoreceptor layer of the retina are the rods and cones. The rods are accountable for vision at low light levels (scotopic vision) and do not have the ability to provide colour vision. On the other hand, cones are active at higher light levels (photopic vision) and provide us with colour vision.
- The *macula* is a small area located at the middle of the retina which provides us with central vision. The macula contains a high volume of cones which are responsible for colour vision.

- The *choroid* is a vascular layer that lies between the retina and the sclera which nourishes the retina.
- The *optic nerve* connects the eye and brain. It contains millions of nerve fibres, which are responsible for carrying nerve signals to the brain. These nerve signals are then processed by the brain.

7.6.1 Biomaterials

In ophthalmology, biomaterials that have been used in medical textiles are used in making contact lenses, intraocular implants, glaucoma drainage implants, and orbital implants. Whilst not necessarily used as a textile, future development may see considerable overlap with the textile field as advances are made, and for this reason this section has been included within the textbook.

7.6.2 Contact Lens

A contact lens is a small, clear plastic disc worn in front of the cornea to provide good vision. It is preferable over traditional glasses for cosmetic purposes. It is commonly used to correct vision in conditions like myopia (short sightedness), hypermetropia (long sightedness), astigmatism, and keratoconus (5). It can also be used to improve the aesthetic appearance of the eye if the cornea is disfigured due to trauma or infection. A recent advancement in contact lenses is drug-loaded contact lenses, which provide sustained delivery of drugs to the eye in conditions such as advanced glaucoma (raised intraocular pressure) (Alvarez-Lorenzo et al. 2002, 2182–2192; Kolb 1995; Singh et al. 2020).

Contact lenses are made of various types of polymers such as silicone hydrogel, polymethyl methacrylate (PMMA), hydroxyl ethyl methacrylate (HEMA), and polyvinyl alcohol (PVA). Silicone hydrogel is the most commonly used material these days (Musgrave and Fang 2019, 261). The desired properties of contact lenses include easy handling, comfort for extended hours of use, durability, and high oxygen permeability. They are commonly classified as hard or soft based on their properties.

- Hard contact lenses are rigid, durable, and gas permeable and may be referred to as rigid gas permeable (RGP) contact lenses. The gas permeable nature allows the cornea to receive oxygen. These lenses are usually made from a combination of a plastic with another material. They hold their shape firmly which is important in conditions like keratoconus and astigmatism where the aim is to reshape the cornea and provide sharper vision (Downie and Lindsay 2015, 299–311).
- Soft contact lenses are made from an oxygen-permeable, flexible material which has a high-water absorbing capacity allowing it stay hydrated for extended periods of time (Musgrave and Fang 2019, 261). The benefit of the soft contact lens is that its flexibility allows the lens to fit the shape of the cornea much faster than the rigid lens.

7.6.3 Keratoprosthesis

Keratoprosthesis is a surgical procedure undertaken to treat corneal blindness. Corneal blindness may be due to multiple causes such as Steven Johnson syndrome (SJS), chemical injury, failed grafts, or ocular pemphigoid. The procedure itself involves the removal of the full thickness of abnormal cornea and replaces it with an artificial corneal transplant made of biomaterials. It is recommended for patients who have had one or more failed donor corneal transplants. Biomaterials used in this procedure include plastics like polymethylmethacrylate (PMMA) and metals like titanium, platinum, tantalum, and gold (Khan, Dudenhoefer, and Dohlman 2001, 282–287; Nonpassopon, Niparugs, and Cortina 2020, 1189).

7.6.4 Intraocular Implants

A cataract develops when the natural transparent lens of the eye becomes cloudy and obscures vision. Cataracts are very common with age and are the leading cause of blindness in the world. Cataract surgery is the mainstay of treatment and involves the removal and replacement of the clouded lens with an artificial intraocular lens (IOL) (Allen and Vasavada 2006, 128–132).

Intraocular lenses are made of a variety of different types of plastics, for example, PMMA, acrylic, and silicone. The most commonly used plastic today is PMMA (Kretz, Scholtz, and Auffarth 2014). This is because of its excellent ability to allow high penetration of light, its biocompatible nature with the body, and its hydrophobic surface. The lipophilic biomaterial is vital in reducing the risk of anterior and posterior capsular clouding (opacification) (Zemaitiene et al. 2008, 936). Importantly, it is also fairly inexpensive. The disadvantage is that PMMA is not very flexible and thus a bigger surgical incision is required to implant it into the eye. This can leave the patient with post-operative astigmatism (change in the corneal shape) (Kretz, Scholtz, and Auffarth 2014).

To combat this, foldable lenses that are flexible have been developed. These are made of various materials like silicone, rubber, hydrogel, and acrylic. These lenses can be inserted through small incisions using single-use applicators. This can make the procedure much quicker and easier. In addition, it also reduces the risk of ocular infection and post-operative astigmatism (Kretz, Scholtz, and Auffarth 2014).

7.6.5 Scleral Buckle in Retinal Detachment Surgery

Retinal detachment is when a break in the retinal layer allows fluid from the vitreous cavity to seep through and cause a separation in the layers of the retina. This can result in sudden painless loss of vision (Fraser and Steel 2010). Scleral buckling surgery is a procedure used in the treatment of large retinal detachments. It works by suturing a silicone or sponge buckle to the sclera which aims to press the sclera towards the torn retina. The buckle will hold the retinal tear in place and allow it to heal.

7.6.6 Orbital Implants

Orbital implants are often used after removal of the eyeball; this is known as enucleation or evisceration. Enucleation/Evisceration can be performed for multiple reasons including malignancy, infections, or severe trauma. An orbital implant is used as a substitute for the globe to help maintain the orbit, facilitate motility, and provide an aesthetic to the socket. Orbital implants can be porous or non-porous. Traditionally, they have been non-porous and consist of materials such as silicone, acrylic, glass, and polymethyl methacrylate (PMMA) (Wladis et al. 2018, 311–317), but porous materials have become more popular because porous materials, in theory, allow tissue growth into the implant and thus increase the stability of the implant within the orbit. The porous materials used include polyethylene, aluminium oxide, and hydroxyapatite (Su and Yen, 2004, 274–280). The difficulty with porous materials is thought to be that their rough surface may result in friction and thus degradation of the surface. Therefore, some surgeons are using wrapped, or polymer-coated, implants. The optimal biomaterial for orbital implants is still debated and has not yet been conclusively determined, so there may be an opportunity for textile materials to become involved.

7.6.7 Viscoelastic Substances (VES)

Viscoelastic substances are also referred to as ophthalmic viscosurgical devices (OVDs) and are substances used during intraocular surgeries to protect and improve visibility of the cornea, maintain the space within the eye to facilitate manipulation of intraocular tissues, and control intraocular bleeds. Most commonly they are used in cataract surgery, ocular trauma, corneal grafting, glaucoma, and anterior and posterior segment surgeries. Viscoelastic substances are made of various materials like sodium hyaluronate, chondroitin sulphate, or hydroxypropyl methylcellulose. The properties required of OVDs include transparency, non-toxic, easy to infuse and remove, and should not interact with instruments. The main drawback is that incomplete removal of the substance can lead to increased pressure in the eye post-operatively. However, the raised ocular pressure is transient – lasts up to 72 hours (Liesegang 1993, 127–147).

7.7 RESORBABLE SCAFFOLDS FOR CELL GROWTH

The scaffold-based approach for cell regeneration is also known as the top-down approach. A temporary scaffold is made onto which cells are seeded and that assembly is then allowed to mature in a bioreactor, where the transplanted cells adhering to the scaffold proliferate. Thus, scaffolds can be seen to serve as a substitute for the native extracellular matrix and to play a pivotal role in tissue regeneration by providing temporary support for cells whilst natural extracellular matrix forms. Scaffolds have been used to generate a range of cells and they may be made from natural fibres, such as collagen, elastin, silk, or alginate, or from synthetic fibres, such as polylactic acid, polycaprolactone, or polyether polyurethane (Jafari et al. 2017, 431–459).

The choice of synthetic polymers is limited by their biodegradability and cytotoxicity to human cells. Resorbable scaffolds used to provide temporary support during cell growth are particularly interesting; both the surface topographic features, such as roughness and hydrophilicity, and the scaffold microstructures, such as pore size, porosity, pore interconnectivity, and pore/fibre architectures influence the cell–scaffold interactions, and architecture also plays a pivotal role.

A scaffold needs to meet certain criteria for tissue regeneration. For example, it needs to have a surface and internal structure that support cellular behaviours, have mechanical properties similar to the native tissue being repaired, biocompatibility, and a degradation that matches tissue regeneration. Scaffolds need to be prepared and tailored to suit the target tissue, for example, for skin regeneration a flat scaffold is desired whereas for a vascular graft a hollow tubular scaffold should be made. It has been confirmed that skin cells attach, grow, and organise better on nanofibrous structures even though cell diameter is larger than that of the fibre (Mohamed and Xing 2012, 29). Moreover, Sun et al. reported that fibre diameter needs to be below 10 μm for fibroblast adhesion and migration, and fibroblasts are not capable of bridging inter-fibre distances greater than 200 μm (Sun et al. 2007, 1318–1328). Therefore, for skin-tissue engineering, the ideal scaffold capable of promoting skin regeneration with biological and mechanical properties similar to the healthy skin will need to be both nanoscale in size and in nanofibrous form.

Scaffolds can be created in a number of ways, such as stereolithography (Song et al. 2017), selective laser sintering (XiaoHui et al. 2015, 15–25), gas foaming (Moghadam et al. 2017, 115–127), solvent casting (Rai et al. 2017, 326–335), solvent casting and particulate leaching (Revati et al. 2017, 752–759), freeze drying (Ghorbani, Zamanian, and Norjehdehian 2017, 159–172), extrusion-based systems (Jiang and Chen 2014, 1947–1953), laser drawing (Suzuki and Aoki 2008, 2499–2505), template assisted (Raoufi et al. 2016, 1059–1066), thermally induced phase separation (Ma and Xue 2014), molecular self-assembly (Takeuchi et al. 2016, 279–288), electrospinning (Grande et al. 2017, 129–137), and three-dimensional printing (Guo et al. 2015, 85–95). Of course, the manufacturing technique of scaffolds depends on the target tissue to be regenerated; however, a technique capable of producing three-dimensional construct/scaffold is highly desirable, so the advent of electrospinning of nanofibres has been pivotal in the development of scaffolds (see Chapter 3, Section 3.3.3). Nanofibres are more attractive than other nanostructured materials mainly due to their high aspect ratio and enormous surface area per unit mass. Tuneable porosity, malleability to conform to a wide variety of sizes and shapes, and the ability to control the nanofibre composition to achieve the desired results are some of the other benefits (Bhardwaj and Kundu 2010, 325–347). Although most electrospinning units are suitable for fabricating either two-dimensional structures of porous fibres consisting of random orientated mats or aligned fibrous arrays or yarns, it is possible to get three-dimensional structures by multilayering electrospinning, post-processing after electrospinning, or by using modified collector shapes. Whilst electrospun scaffolds typically possess a high porosity, they lack the appropriate mechanical properties for load-bearing capability (Vaquette and Cooper-White 2013, 4599–4608) and pore size can also be problematic; if the pores are too small, vascular ingrowth is restricted. One modification to solve some of these 'problems' is to combine nanofibres with fibres or filaments of a larger scale produced by wet spinning, melt spinning, microfluidic spinning, and fibre bonding (Khorshidi et al. 2016, 715–738). Scaffolds and regenerative medicine are very much a new area of medicine and there is still much scope for development.

7.8 TESTING OF IMPLANTABLE MEDICAL TEXTILES

Implantable medical textile devices have some of the highest levels of regulatory burden, and these have been tightened further with recent concerns regarding certain implants, for example, implantable mesh. Under EU regulations, implants may be Class IIb or Class III; the main criteria are that they are invasive and remain in the body for more than 30 days.

Chapter 6 provides more comprehensive guidance on the possible tests required. Unlike other devices, many implants carry additional mandatory clinical studies. Some of the tests required include the following, which is not an exhaustive list.

- Biocompatibility: Tests and studies as dictated by the ISO 10993 family.
- Performance testing: Tests as dictated by the performance requirements contained within the product specification. Any software will need to be tested too, and this also includes machine code on chipsets.
- Clinical evaluation (validation and verification in the USA): Conducted as per MEDDEV 2.7.1/4 and the new Medical Devices Regulations guidelines.
- Electrical safety: For any device containing any form of electrical power and components, safety, ingression, and electromagnetic compatibility (EMC) – testing to ISO 60601 will be required.

REFERENCES

Ahmad, M. H., S. Pathak, K. D. Clement, and E. H. Aly. "Meta-analysis of the use of sterilized mosquito net mesh for inguinal hernia repair in less economically developed countries." *British Journal of Surgery Open* 3, no. 4 (2019): 429–435.

Allen, David, and Abhay Vasavada. "Cataract and surgery for cataract." *British Medical Journal* 333, no. 7559 (2006): 128–132.

Alvarez-Lorenzo, Carmen, Haruyiki Hiratani, Jose Luis Gomez-Amoza, Ramón Martínez-Pacheco, Consuelo Souto, and Angel Concheiro. "Soft contact lenses capable of sustained delivery of timolol." *Journal of Pharmaceutical Sciences* 91, no. 10 (2002): 2182–2192.

Ambler, Graeme K., and Christopher P. Twine. "Graft type for femoro-popliteal bypass surgery." *Cochrane Database of Systematic Reviews* 2 (2018).

Amri, Amna, Gaetan Laroche, Nabil Chakfe, and Frederic Heim. "Fibrous composite material for textile heart valve design: In vitro assessment." *Biomedical Engineering/Biomedizinische Technik* 63, no. 3 (2018): 221–230.

Awad, Samir S. "Adherence to surgical care improvement project measures and post-operative surgical site infections." *Surgical Infections* 13, no. 4 (2012): 234–237.

Barrows, T. H. "Degradable implant materials: A review of synthetic absorbable polymers and their applications." *Clinical Materials* 1, no. 4 (1986): 233–257.

Baylón, Karen, Perla Rodríguez-Camarillo, Alex Elías-Zúñiga, Jose Antonio Díaz-Elizondo, Robert Gilkerson, and Karen Lozano. "Past, present and future of surgical meshes: A review." *Membranes* 7, no. 3 (2017): 47.

Ben Abdessalem, Saber, Faten Debbabi, Hanen Jedda, Saber Elmarzougui, and Sofiene Mokhtar. "Tensile and knot performance of polyester braided sutures." *Textile Research Journal* 79, no. 3 (2009): 247–252.

Ben Abdessalem, S., B. Durand, S. Akesbi, N. Chakfe, and J. G. Kretz. "Numerical simulation of blood flow in a curved textile vascular prosthesis." *Journal of the Textile Institute* 96, no. 2 (2005): 117–122.

Bhardwaj, Nandana, and Subhas C. Kundu. "Electrospinning: A fascinating fiber fabrication technique." *Biotechnology Advances* 28, no. 3 (2010): 325–347.

Bhende, Shubhangi, Stephen Rothenburger, Daniel J. Spangler, and Melanie Dito. "In vitro assessment of microbial barrier properties of Dermabond® topical skin adhesive." *Surgical Infections* 3, no. 3 (2002): 251–257.

Bilsel, Yilmaz, and Ilker Abci. "The search for ideal hernia repair; mesh materials and types." *International Journal of Surgery* 10, no. 6 (2012): 317–321.

Brewster, David C., John E. Jones, Thomas K. Chung, Glenn M. Lamuraglia, Christopher J. Kwolek, Michael T. Watkins, Thomas M. Hodgman, and Richard P. Cambria. "Long-term outcomes after endovascular abdominal aortic aneurysm repair: The first decade." *Annals of Surgery* 244, no. 3 (2006): 426.

Brown, Brian, Judith Tanner, and Wendy Padley. "'This wound has spoilt everything': Emotional capital and the experience of surgical site infections." *Sociology of Health & Illness* 36, no. 8 (2014): 1171–1187.

Brown, C. N., and J. G. Finch. "Which mesh for hernia repair?." *The Annals of The Royal College of Surgeons of England* 92, no. 4 (2010): 272–278.

Carr, D. J., A. G. Heward, R. M. Laing, and B. E. Niven. "Measuring the strength of knotted suture materials." *The Journal of the Textile Institute* 100, no. 1 (2009): 51–56.

Centre of Disease Control and Prevention. "Surgical site infection event (SSI)." 2021. Accessed January 5, 2021. https://www.cdc.gov/nhsn/pdfs/pscmanual/9pscssicurrent.pdf.

Chamberlain, Connie S., Jae-Sung Lee, Ellen M. Leiferman, Nicholas X. Maassen, Geoffrey S. Baer, Ray Vanderby, and William L. Murphy. "Effects of BMP-12-releasing sutures on Achilles tendon healing." *Tissue Engineering Part A* 21, no. 5–6 (2015): 916–927.

Chen, Xiaojie, Qian Zhang, Dandan Hou, Jing Lin, Jing Gao, and Lu Wang. "Fabrication and characterization of novel antibacterial silk sutures with different braiding parameters." *Journal of Natural Fibers* (2018).

Chen, Ying, Xin Ding, Yuling Li, Martin W. King, Jie Gao, and Xueqian Zhao. "A bilayer prototype woven vascular prosthesis with improved radial compliance." *Journal of the Textile Institute* 103, no. 1 (2012): 106–111.

Dahl, A. "Anatomy and Physiology of the Eye." 2021. Accessed April 25, 2021. https://www.emedicinehealth.com/anatomy_of_the_eye/article_em.htm.

Damme, H. Van, Manuel Deprez, Etienne Creemers, and Raymond Limet. "Intrinsic structural failure of polyester (Dacron) vascular grafts. A general review." *Acta Chirurgica Belgica* 105, no. 3 (2005): 249–255.

De la Fuente, Carlos, Carlos Cruz-Montecinos, Helen L. Schimidt, Hugo Henríquez, Sebastián Ruidiaz, and Felipe P. Carpes. "Biomechanical properties of different techniques used in vitro for suturing mid-substance Achilles tendon ruptures." *Clinical Biomechanics* 50 (2017): 78–83.

Demyttenaere, Sebastian V., Peter Nau, Matthew Henn, Catherine Beck, Jeffrey Zaruby, Michael Primavera, David Kirsch et al. "Barbed suture for gastrointestinal closure: A randomized control trial." *Surgical Innovation* 16, no. 3 (2009): 237–242.

Deutsch, Manfred, Johann Meinhart, Peter Zilla, Norbert Howanietz, Michael Gorlitzer, Alexander Froeschl, Andreas Stuempflen, Deon Bezuidenhout, and Martin Grabenwoeger. "Long-term experience in autologous in vitro endothelialization of infrainguinal ePTFE grafts." *Journal of Vascular Surgery* 49, no. 2 (2009): 352–362.

Downie, Laura E., and Richard G. Lindsay. "Contact lens management of keratoconus." *Clinical and Experimental Optometry* 98, no. 4 (2015): 299–311.

Eklund, Arne, Agneta Montgomery, Leif Bergkvist, and Claes Rudberg. "Chronic pain 5 years after randomized comparison of laparoscopic and Lichtenstein inguinal hernia repair." *British Journal of Surgery* 97, no. 4 (2010): 600–608.

EU Hernia Trialists Collaboration. "Repair of groin hernia with synthetic mesh: Meta-analysis of randomized controlled trials." *Annals of Surgery* 235, no. 3 (2002): 322.

Fraser, Scott, and David Steel. "Retinal detachment." *BMJ Clinical Evidence* 2010 (2010).

Freitas, A. F. D. P., M. D. de Araujo, W. W. Zu, and R. M. E. Fangueiro. "Development of weft-knitted and braided polypropylene stents for arterial implant." *The Journal of the Textile Institute* 101, no. 12 (2010): 1027–1034.

Freudenberg, Sebastian, Daman Sano, Edgar Ouangre, Christel Weiss, and Torsten J. Wilhelm. "Commercial mesh versus Nylon mosquito net for hernia repair. A randomized double-blind study in Burkina Faso." *World Journal of Surgery* 30, no. 10 (2006): 1784–1789.

Fu, Shaoju, Yao Lu, and Peihua Zhang. "Comparison of polyglycolic acid acupoint catgut embedding therapy monofilaments for a juvenile pseudo-myopia surface modified by two processing methods." *Textile Research Journal* 89, no. 19–20 (2019): 4071–4082.

Fu, Shaoju, Dongchao Yang, Cunyi Zhao, and Peihua Zhang. "Ultrasonic modification of polylactic acid and polyglycolic acid acupoint catgut embedding monofilaments for juvenile pseudomyopia." *Textile Research Journal* 89, no. 17 (2019): 3556–3566.

Fu, Shaoju, and Peihua Zhang. "Design and optimization of a novel chitosan coating system for acupoint catgut embedding materials." *Textile Research Journal* 89, no. 8 (2019): 1557–1572.

Fu, Shaoju, and Peihua Zhang. "Surface modification of polylactic acid (PLA) and polyglycolic acid (PGA) monofilaments via the cold plasma method for acupoint catgut-embedding therapy applications." *Textile Research Journal* 89, no. 18 (2019): 3839–3849.

Fu, Shao-ju, and Pei-hua Zhang. "A study of the chitosan coating method on polyglycolic acid and polylactic acid embedding monofilaments." *Textile Research Journal* 89, no. 3 (2019): 270–280.

Gabrielli, Fabrizio, Clemente Potenza, Pietro Puddu, Francesco Sera, Cinzia Masini, and Damiano Abeni. "Suture materials and other factors associated with tissue reactivity, infection, and wound dehiscence among plastic surgery outpatients." *Plastic and Reconstructive Surgery* 107, no. 1 (2001): 38–45.

Gao, Hongding, Jes Sandermann, J. Prag, L. Lund, and Jes S. Lindholt. "Prevention of primary vascular graft infection with silver-coated polyester graft in a porcine model." *European Journal of Vascular and Endovascular Surgery* 39, no. 4 (2010): 472–477.

Ghorbani, Farnaz, Ali Zamanian, and Hanieh Nojehdehian. "Effects of pore orientation on in-vitro properties of retinoic acid-loaded PLGA/gelatin scaffolds for artificial peripheral nerve application." *Materials Science and Engineering: C* 77 (2017): 159–172.

Giordano, Giovanni G., and Miguel E. Refojo. "Biomaterials in ophthalmology." In *Human Biomaterials Applications*, 301–317. Totowa, NJ: Humana Press, 1996.

Glazener, Cathryn M.A., Suzanne Breeman, Andrew Elders, Christine Hemming, Kevin G. Cooper, Robert M. Freeman, Anthony RB Smith et al. "Mesh, graft, or standard repair for women having primary transvaginal anterior or posterior compartment prolapse surgery: Two parallel-group, multicentre, randomised, controlled trials (PROSPECT)." *The Lancet* 389, no. 10067 (2017): 381–392.

Gori, Tommaso, Alberto Polimeni, Ciro Indolfi, Lorenz Räber, Tom Adriaenssens, and Thomas Münzel. "Predictors of stent thrombosis and their implications for clinical practice." *Nature Reviews Cardiology* 16, no. 4 (2019): 243–256.

Goto, Saori, Takashi Sakamoto, Riki Ganeko, Koya Hida, Toshi A. Furukawa, and Yoshiharu Sakai. "Subcuticular sutures for skin closure in non-obstetric surgery." *Cochrane Database of Systematic Reviews* 4 (2020).

Grande, Daniel, Julien Ramier, Davy Louis Versace, Estelle Renard, and Valérie Langlois. "Design of functionalized biodegradable PHA-based electrospun scaffolds meant for tissue engineering applications." *New Biotechnology* 37 (2017): 129–137.

Grant, Sheila, and Bruce Ramshaw. "Progress in synthetic prosthetic mesh for ventral hernia repair." In *Management of Abdominal Hernias*, 173–178. Cham: Springer, 2018.

Guo, R., A. R. Merkel, J. A. Sterling, J. M. Davidson, and S. A. Guelcher. "Substrate modulus of 3D-printed scaffolds regulates the regenerative response in subcutaneous implants through the macrophage phenotype and Wnt signaling." *Biomaterials* 73 (2015): 85–95.

Gurusamy, Kurinchi Selvan, Clare D. Toon, Victoria B. Allen, and Brian R. Davidson. "Continuous versus interrupted skin sutures for non-obstetric surgery." *Cochrane Database of Systematic Reviews* 2 (2014).

Hansen, Katrina J., John T. Favreau, Jacques P. Guyette, Ze-Wei Tao, Spencer T. Coffin, Anny Cunha-Gavidia, Brian D'Amore et al. "Functional effects of delivering human mesenchymal stem cell-seeded biological sutures to an infarcted heart." *BioResearch Open Access* 5, no. 1 (2016): 249–260.

Hassan, Shoaib, Anjana Haridas, and Venki Sundaram. "Adjustable versus non-adjustable sutures for strabismus." *Cochrane Database of Systematic Reviews* 3 (2018).

Hastings, J. C., W. V. Winkle, E. Barker, D. Hines, and W. Nichols. "Effect of suture materials on healing wounds of the stomach and colon." *Surgery, Gynecology & Obstetrics* 140, no. 5 (1975): 701–707.

Heim, F., and Bhupender S. Gupta. "Textile heart valve prosthesis: The effect of fabric construction parameters on long-term durability." *Textile Research Journal* 79, no. 11 (2009): 1001–1013.

Heim, Frederic, Bernard Durand, and Nabil Chafke. "Textile heart valve prosthesis: From fabric design criteria to early in-vivo performances." *The Journal of Heart Valve Disease* 22, no. 3 (2013): 361–367.

Heim, Frederic, Bernard Durand, and Nabil Chakfe. "Textile heart valve: Novel shaping process and material performances." *Materials and Manufacturing Processes* 26, no. 10 (2011): 1303–1309.

Henriksen, Nadia A., Eva B. Deerenberg, Linas Venclauskas, Rene H. Fortelny, Josep M. Garcia-Alamino, Marc Miserez, and Filip E. Muysoms. "Triclosan-coated sutures and surgical site infection in abdominal surgery: The TRISTAN review, meta-analysis and trial sequential analysis." *Hernia* 21, no. 6 (2017): 833–841.

HerniaSurg Group. "International guidelines for groin hernia management." *Hernia* 22 (2018): 1–165.

Hibino, Narutoshi, Edward McGillicuddy, Goki Matsumura, Yuki Ichihara, Yuji Naito, Christopher Breuer, and Toshiharu Shinoka. "Late-term results of tissue-engineered vascular grafts in humans." *The Journal of Thoracic and Cardiovascular Surgery* 139, no. 2 (2010): 431–436.

Iliadis, Dimitrios Ph, Dimitrios N. Bourlos, Dimitrios S. Mastrokalos, Efstathios Chronopoulos, and George C. Babis. "LARS artificial ligament versus ABC purely polyester ligament for anterior cruciate ligament reconstruction." *Orthopaedic Journal of Sports Medicine* 4, no. 6 (2016): 2325967116653359.

Jackson, Mark R., Todd P. Belott, Timothy Dickason, William J. Kaiser, J. Gregory Modrall, R. James Valentine, and G. Patrick Clagett. "The consequences of a failed femoropopliteal bypass grafting: Comparison of saphenous vein and PTFE grafts." *Journal of Vascular Surgery* 32, no. 3 (2000): 498–505.

Jafari, Maissa, Zahrasadat Paknejad, Maryam Rezai Rad, Saeed Reza Motamedian, Mohammad Jafar Eghbal, Nasser Nadjmi, and Arash Khojasteh. "Polymeric scaffolds in tissue engineering: A literature review." *Journal of Biomedical Materials Research Part B: Applied Biomaterials* 105, no. 2 (2017): 431–459.

Jedda, Hanen, Saber Ben Abdessalem, Mohamed Ragoubi, and Faouzi Sakli. "Contribution to the optimisation of artificial ligament mechanical properties." *Journal of the Textile Institute* 99, no. 3 (2008): 273–280.

Jiang, Cho-Pei, and Yo-Yu Chen. "Biofabrication of hybrid bone scaffolds using a dual-nozzle bioplotter and in-vitro study of osteoblast cell." *International Journal of Precision Engineering and Manufacturing* 15, no. 9 (2014): 1947–1953.

Jones, Huw G., Michael Rees, Omar M. Aboumarzouk, Joshua Brown, James Cragg, Peter Billings, Ben Carter, and Palanichamy Chandran. "Prosthetic mesh placement for the prevention of parastomal herniation." *Cochrane Database of Systematic Reviews* 7 (2018).

Joseph, John, Aarya G. Krishnan, Aleena M. Cherian, Balasubramoniam Rajagopalan, Rajesh Jose, Praveen Varma, Vijayakumar Maniyal, Sivanarayanan Balakrishnan, Shantikumar V. Nair, and Deepthy Menon. "Transforming nanofibers into woven nanotextiles for vascular application." *ACS Applied Materials & Interfaces* 10, no. 23 (2018): 19449–19458.

Karthikesalingam, A., P. J. E. Holt, R. J. Hinchliffe, I. M. Nordon, I. M. Loftus, and M. M. Thompson. "Risk of reintervention after endovascular aortic aneurysm repair." *British Journal of Surgery* 97, no. 5 (2010): 657–663.

Kettle, C., T. Dowswell, and K. Ismail. "Absorbable stitches for repair of episiotomy and tears at childbirth." The Cochrane Library, Published Online: June 16 (2010).

Khan, Bilal, Eric J. Dudenhoefer, and Claes H. Dohlman. "Keratoprosthesis: An update." *Current Opinion in Ophthalmology* 12, no. 4 (2001): 282–287.

Khorshidi, Sajedeh, Atefeh Solouk, Hamid Mirzadeh, Saeedeh Mazinani, Jose M. Lagaron, Shahriar Sharifi, and Seeram Ramakrishna. "A review of key challenges of electrospun scaffolds for tissue-engineering applications." *Journal of Tissue Engineering and Regenerative Medicine* 10, no. 9 (2016): 715–738.

Kingsnorth, Andrew, and Karl LeBlanc. "Hernias: Inguinal and incisional." *The Lancet* 362, no. 9395 (2003): 1561–1571.

Kolb, H. "Gross anatomy of the eye." In *Webvision: The Organization of the Retina and Visual System*. Salt Lake City, UT: University of Utah Health Sciences Center, 1995.

Kretz, Florian, Sibylle Scholtz and Gerd Auffarth. "A Brief History of IOL Materials." 2014. Accessed April 25, 2021. https://theophthalmologist.com/subspecialties/a-brief-history-of-iol-materials.

Lacour, M., C. Ridereau Zins, C. Casa, A. Venara, V. Cartier, S. Yahya, J. Barbieux, and C. Aubé. "CT findings of complications after abdominal wall repair with prosthetic mesh." *Diagnostic and Interventional Imaging* 98, no. 7–8 (2017): 517–528.

Lavoie, Pauline, Jennifer Fletcher, and Nicolas Duval. "Patient satisfaction needs as related to knee stability and objective findings after ACL reconstruction using the LARS artificial ligament." *The Knee* 7, no. 3 (2000): 157–163.

Lee, Hye Sun, So Hyun Park, Jin Hyung Lee, Bong Yong Jeong, Sang Kook Ahn, Young Muk Choi, Doo Jin Choi, and Jeong Ho Chang. "Antimicrobial and biodegradable PLGA medical sutures with natural grapefruit seed extracts." *Materials Letters* 95 (2013): 40–43.

Li, Gang, Yanping Liu, Ping Lan, Yi Li, and Yuling Li. "A prospective bifurcated biomedical stent with seamless woven structure." *Journal of the Textile Institute* 104, no. 9 (2013): 1017–1023.

Liesegang, Thomas J. "Viscoelastics." *International Ophthalmology Clinics* 33, no. 4 (1993): 127–147.

Lindholt, Jes S., B. Gottschalksen, Ninna Johannesen, D. Dueholm, H. Ravn, Ebbe Dag Christensen, B. Viddal et al. "The Scandinavian Propaten® trial–1-year patency of PTFE vascular prostheses with heparin-bonded luminal surfaces compared to ordinary pure PTFE vascular prostheses–A randomised clinical controlled multi-centre trial." *European Journal of Vascular and Endovascular Surgery* 41, no. 5 (2011): 668–673.

Liu, Zhenmi, Jo C. Dumville, Gill Norman, Maggie J. Westby, Jane Blazeby, Emma McFarlane, Nicky J. Welton et al. "Intraoperative interventions for preventing surgical site infection: An overview of Cochrane Reviews." *Cochrane Database of Systematic Reviews* 2 (2018).

Lockhart, Kathleen, Douglas Dunn, Shawn Teo, Jessica Y. Ng, Manvinder Dhillon, Edward Teo, and Mieke L. van Driel. "Mesh versus non-mesh for inguinal and femoral hernia repair." *Cochrane Database of Systematic Reviews* 9 (2018).

Lopes, Renato D., Sergio Leonardi, Daniel M. Wojdyla, Amit N. Vora, Laine Thomas, Robert F. Storey, Dragos Vinereanu et al. "Stent thrombosis in patients with atrial fibrillation undergoing coronary stenting in the AUGUSTUS trial." *Circulation* 141, no. 9 (2020): 781–783.

Ma, Haiyun, and Li Xue. "Carbon nanotubes reinforced poly (L-lactide) scaffolds fabricated by thermally induced phase separation." *Nanotechnology* 26, no. 2 (2014): 025701.

Maher, Christopher, Benjamin Feiner, Kaven Baessler, Corina Christmann-Schmid, Nir Haya, and Jane Marjoribanks. "Transvaginal mesh or grafts compared with native tissue repair for vaginal prolapse." *Cochrane Database of Systematic Reviews* 2 (2016).

McKenzie, A. R. "An experimental multiple barbed suture for the long flexor tendons of the palm and fingers: preliminary report." *The Journal of Bone and Joint Surgery*. British volume 49, no. 3 (1967): 440–447.

Medicines and Healthcare products Regulatory Agency. "Regulating medical devices in the UK." 2021. Accessed January 5, 2021. https://www.gov.uk/guidance/regulating-medical-devices-in-the-uk.

Mirensky, Tamar L., Gregory N. Nelson, Matthew P. Brennan, Jason D. Roh, Narutoshi Hibino, Tai Yi, Toshiharu Shinoka, and Christopher K. Breuer. "Tissue-engineered arterial grafts: Long-term results after implantation in a small animal model." *Journal of Pediatric Surgery* 44, no. 6 (2009): 1127–1133.

Moghadam, M. Zahedi, Sh Hassanajili, F. Esmaeilzadeh, M. Ayatollahi, and M. Ahmadi. "Formation of porous HPCL/LPCL/HA scaffolds with supercritical CO_2 gas foaming method." *Journal of the Mechanical Behavior of Biomedical Materials* 69 (2017): 115–127.

Moghe, A. K., and B. S. Gupta. "Small-diameter blood vessels by weaving: Prototyping and modelling." *Journal of the Textile Institute* 99, no. 5 (2008): 467–477.

Mohamed, Aezeden, and Malcolm Mengqiu Xing. "Nanomaterials and nanotechnology for skin tissue engineering." *International Journal of Burns and Trauma* 2, no. 1 (2012): 29.

Mokhtari, F., M. Salehi, F. Zamani, F. Hajiani, F. Zeighami, and M. Latifi. "Advances in electrospinning: The production and application of nanofibres and nanofibrous structures." *Textile Progress* 48, no. 3 (2016): 119–219.

Moreira, Ricardo, Christine Neusser, Magnus Kruse, Shane Mulderrig, Frederic Wolf, Jan Spillner, Thomas Schmitz-Rode, Stefan Jockenhoevel, and Petra Mela. "Tissue-engineered fibrin-based heart valve with bio-inspired textile reinforcement." *Advanced Healthcare Materials* 5, no. 16 (2016): 2113–2121.

Musgrave, Christopher Stephen Andrew, and Fengzhou Fang. "Contact lens materials: A materials science perspective." *Materials* 12, no. 2 (2019): 261.

NICE. "Mesh for vaginal wall prolapse should only be used in the context of research, says NICE." 2017. Accessed March 6, 2021. https://www.nice.org.uk/news/article/mesh-for-vaginal-wall-prolapse-should-only-be-used-in-the-context-of-research-says-nice.

NICE. "Abdominal aortic aneurysm: diagnosis and 1 management, NICE guideline 4, draft for consultation, May 201." 2018. Accessed June 3, 2020. https://www.nice.org.uk/guidance/gid-cgwave0769/documents/short-version-of-draft-guideline.

Nonpassopon, Manachai, Muanploy Niparugs, and Maria Soledad Cortina. "Boston type 1 keratoprosthesis: Updated perspectives." *Clinical Ophthalmology (Auckland, NZ)* 14 (2020): 1189.

Novitsky, Yuri W., and Luis A. Martin-del-Campo. "Prosthetic options: Advantages and disadvantages." In *Surgical Principles in Inguinal Hernia Repair*, 25–30. Cham: Springer, 2018.

Orlandi, Augusto, and Martin Bennett. "Progenitor cell-derived smooth muscle cells in vascular disease." *Biochemical Pharmacology* 79, no. 12 (2010): 1706–1713.

Pashneh-Tala, Samand, Sheila MacNeil, and Frederik Claeyssens. "The tissue-engineered vascular graft—Past, present, and future." *Tissue Engineering Part B: Reviews* 22, no. 1 (2016): 68–100.

Patel, Sunil V., David D. Paskar, Richard L. Nelson, Satyanarayana S. Vedula, and Scott R. Steele. "Closure methods for laparotomy incisions for preventing incisional hernias and other wound complications." *Cochrane Database of Systematic Reviews* 11 (2017).

Pereira, Carlos Eduardo, Maximiano Albers, Marcello Romiti, Francisco Cardoso Brochado-Neto, and Carlos Alberto Braganąa Pereira. "Meta-analysis of femoropopliteal bypass grafts for lower extremity arterial insufficiency." *Journal of Vascular Surgery* 44, no. 3 (2006): 510–517.

Pourdeyhimi, Behnam. "Vascular grafts: Textile structures and their performance." *Textile Progress* 15, no. 3 (1986): 1–30.

Quinn, James, George Wells, Terri Sutcliffe, Mario Jarmuske, Jennifer Maw, Ian Stiell, and Peter Johns. "Tissue adhesive versus suture wound repair at 1 year: Randomized clinical trial correlating early, 3-month, and 1-year cosmetic outcome." *Annals of Emergency Medicine* 32, no. 6 (1998): 645–649.

Rai, Ranjana, Judith A. Roether, Jonathan C. Knowles, Nicola Mordan, Vehid Salih, Ian C. Locke, Michael P. Gordge et al. "Highly elastomeric poly (3-hydroxyoctanoate) based natural polymer composite for enhanced keratinocyte regeneration." *International Journal of Polymeric Materials and Polymeric Biomaterials* 66, no. 7 (2017): 326–335.

Raoufi, Mohammad, Neda Aslankoohi, Christine Mollenhauer, Heike Boehm, Joachim P. Spatz, and Dorothea Brüggemann. "Template-assisted extrusion of biopolymer nanofibers under physiological conditions." *Integrative Biology* 8, no. 10 (2016): 1059–1066.

Revati, R., M.S. Abdul Majid, M. J. M. Ridzuan, M. Normahira, NF Mohd Nasir, and A. G. Gibson. "Mechanical, thermal and morphological characterisation of 3D porous Pennisetum purpureum/PLA biocomposites scaffold." *Materials Science and Engineering: C* 75 (2017): 752–759.

Royal College of Obstetricians and Gynaecologists. "Mesh." 2019. Accessed March 6, 2021. https://www.rcog.org.uk/en/guidelines-research-services/patient-safety/mesh/.

Royal College of Obstetricians and Gynaecologists. "RCOG/BSUG response to NICE guidance on stress urinary incontinence and pelvic organ prolapse." 2019. Accessed March 6, 2021. https://www.rcog.org.uk/en/news/rcogbsug-response-to-nice-guidance-on-stress-urinary-incontinence-and-pelvic-organ-prolapse/.

Scheuerlein, H., J. Erdmann, F. Rauchfuss, Y. Dittmar, K. Jandt, K. D. Jandt, U. Settmacher, and S. Zankovych. "Preparation and in-vitro analysis of a polyethylenimine coating on hernia meshes." *Zentralblatt fur Chirurgie* 140, no. 2 (2013): 170–178.

Schmidtberg, Brian, Jeremiah D. Johnson, Cameron Kia, Joshua B. Baldino, Elifho Obopilwe, Mark P. Cote, and Lauren E. Geaney. "Flexor hallucis longus transfer improves Achilles tendon load to failure in surgery for non-insertional tendinopathy: A biomechanical study." *Journal of Bone and Joint Surgery* 101, no. 16 (2019): 1505–1512.

Singh, Charanpreet, and Xungai Wang. "A biomechanically optimized knitted stent using a bio-inspired design approach." *Textile Research Journal* 86, no. 4 (2016): 380–392.

Singh, Rohan B., Parul Ichhpujani, Sahil Thakur, and Sumeet Jindal. "Promising therapeutic drug delivery systems for glaucoma: A comprehensive review." *Therapeutic Advances in Ophthalmology* 12 (2020): 2515841420905740.

Snell, Richard S., and Michael A. Lemp. *Clinical Anatomy of the Eye*. John Wiley & Sons, 2013.

Song, Xuan, Zhuofeng Zhang, Zeyu Chen, and Yong Chen. "Porous structure fabrication using a stereolithography-based sugar foaming method." *Journal of Manufacturing Science and Engineering* 139, no. 3 (2017).

Stadelmann, Wayne K., Alexander G. Digenis, and Gordon R. Tobin. "Physiology and healing dynamics of chronic cutaneous wounds." *The American Journal of Surgery* 176, no. 2 (1998): 26S–38S.

Stewart, Andrew, Paul S. Eyers, and Jonothan J. Earnshaw. "Prevention of infection in arterial reconstruction." *Cochrane Database of Systematic Reviews* 3 (2006).

Stoeckel, D., C. Bonsignore, and S. Duda. "A survey of stent designs." *Minimally Invasive Therapy & Allied Technologies* 11, no. 4 (2002): 137–147.

Su, Grant W., and Michael T. Yen. "Current trends in managing the anophthalmic socket after primary enucleation and evisceration." *Ophthalmic Plastic & Reconstructive Surgery* 20, no. 4 (2004): 274–280.

Sun, Tao, David Norton, Robert J. McKean, John W. Haycock, Anthony J. Ryan, and Sheila MacNeil. "Development of a 3D cell culture system for investigating cell interactions with electrospun fibers." *Biotechnology and Bioengineering* 97, no. 5 (2007): 1318–1328.

Suzuki, Akihiro, and Keiko Aoki. "Biodegradable poly (l-lactic acid) nanofiber prepared by a carbon dioxide laser supersonic drawing." *European Polymer Journal* 44, no. 8 (2008): 2499–2505.

Takagi, Hisato, Shin-nosuke Goto, Masafumi Matsui, Hideaki Manabe, and Takuya Umemoto. "A contemporary meta-analysis of Dacron versus polytetrafluoroethylene grafts for femoropopliteal bypass grafting." *Journal of Vascular Surgery* 52, no. 1 (2010): 232–236.

Takeuchi, Takahiro, Takahiro Bizenjima, Yoshihito Ishii, Kentaro Imamura, Eiichi Suzuki, Fumi Seshima, and Atsushi Saito. "Enhanced healing of surgical periodontal defects in rats following application of a self-assembling peptide nanofibre hydrogel." *Journal of Clinical Periodontology* 43, no. 3 (2016): 279–288.

Tsukazaki, Satoshi, Toshiyuki Kikuchi, Kyosuke Fujikawa, Tatsuo Kobayashi, and Bahaa B. Seedhom. "Comparative study of the covered area of Leeds–Keio (LK) artificial ligament and radio frequency generated glow discharge treated Leeds–Keio (Bio-LK) ligament with synovial cells." *Journal of Long-Term Effects of Medical Implants* 13, no. 4 (2003): 355–362.

Turki, Samar, Saber Marzougui, and Saber Ben Abdessalem. "Impact of polyurethane yarns on the mechanical properties of braided artificial ligaments." *The Journal of the Textile Institute* 106, no. 9 (2015): 912–918.

Valencia, Raúl A., Manuel J. García, and John Bustamante. "A comparative computational study of blood flow pattern in exemplary textile vascular grafts." *The Journal of the Textile Institute* 109, no. 7 (2018): 858–870.

Vaquette, Cédryck, and Justin Cooper-White. "A simple method for fabricating 3-D multilayered composite scaffolds." *Acta Biomaterialia* 9, no. 1 (2013): 4599–4608.

Viju, S., G. Thilagavathi, and Bhuvanesh Gupta. "Preparation and properties of PLLA/PLCL fibres for potential use as a monofilament suture." *The Journal of the Textile Institute* 101, no. 9 (2010): 835–841.

Vollebregt, A., K. Fischer, D. Gietelink, and C. H. Van der Vaart. "Primary surgical repair of anterior vaginal prolapse: A randomised trial comparing anatomical and functional outcome between anterior colporrhaphy and trocar-guided transobturator anterior mesh." *BJOG: An International Journal of Obstetrics & Gynaecology* 118, no. 12 (2011): 1518–1527.

Wang, Conger, Yanhui Liu, Yuanming Zhang, and Guangting Han. "Study of the mechanical behavior of Z-structure stents produced by poly-L-lactic acid multi-ply strands." *Textile Research Journal* 89, no. 19–20 (2019): 4230–4238.

Wang, Z. X., C. P. Jiang, Y. Cao, and Y. T. Ding. "Systematic review and meta-analysis of triclosan-coated sutures for the prevention of surgical-site infection." *British Journal of Surgery* 100, no. 4 (2013): 465–473.

White, Geoffrey H., Carlos E. Donayre, Russell A. Williams, Rodney A. White, Bruce E. Stabile, and Samuel E. Wilson. "Exertional disruption of axillofemoral graft anastomosis: 'The axillary pullout syndrome'." *Archives of Surgery* 125, no. 5 (1990): 625–627.

Wladis, Edward J., Vinay K. Aakalu, Rachel K. Sobel, Michael T. Yen, Jurij R. Bilyk, and Louise A. Mawn. "Orbital implants in enucleation surgery: A report by the American Academy of Ophthalmology." *Ophthalmology* 125, no. 2 (2018): 311–317.

XiaoHui, Song, Li Wei, Song PingHui, Su QingYong, Wei QingSong, Shi YuSheng, Liu Kai, and Liu WenGuang. "Selective laser sintering of aliphatic-polycarbonate/hydroxyapatite composite scaffolds for medical applications." *The International Journal of Advanced Manufacturing Technology* 81, no. 1 (2015): 15–25.

Xing, Mei-yi, Cheng-long Yu, Yu-fen Wu, Lu Wang, and Guo-ping Guan. "Preparation and characterization of a polyvinyl alcohol/polyacrylamide hydrogel vascular graft reinforced with a braided fiber stent." *Textile Research Journal* 90, no. 13–14 (2020): 1537–1548.

Yeager, Richard A., and John M. Porter. "Arterial and prosthetic graft infection." *Annals of Vascular Surgery* 6, no. 5 (1992): 485–491.

Yousefi, Atieh, Antoine Vaesken, Amna Amri, Lakshmi Prasad Dasi, and Frederic Heim. "Heart valves from polyester fibers vs. biological tissue: comparative study in vitro." *Annals of Biomedical Engineering* 45, no. 2 (2017): 476–486.

Žemaitienė, Reda, Martynas Špečkauskas, Brigita Glebauskienė, and Vytautas Jašinskas. "Comparison of postoperative results after implantation of hydrophilic acrylic or hydrophobic acrylic intraocular lens: Data of one-year prospective clinical study." *Medicina* 44, no. 12 (2008): 936.

Zhang, Wei, Deting Xue, Houfa Yin, Hui Xie, Honghai Ma, Erman Chen, Dongcai Hu, and Zhijun Pan. "Barbed versus traditional sutures for wound closure in knee arthroplasty: A systematic review and meta-analysis." *Scientific Reports* 6 (2016): 19764.

8 Non-implantable Medical Textiles

8.1 INTRODUCTION

Non-implantable medical textiles include dressings and pressure garments such as thromboembolic stockings. The category also includes the various braces, splints, and trusses used for a variety of functions such as protection, augmenting normal anatomy, providing structural support, and enhancing aesthetics.

8.2 WOUND DRESSINGS

The Textile Institute defines wound dressings as 'materials, including textiles, whose functions are to provide protection to a wound against infection, absorb blood and exudate and promote healing' (The Textile Institute 2021). Historically, biological materials such as cobwebs, leaves, seaweed, silver, and honey have all been used as dressings, and whilst surgeon Ambroise Paré stated in the 16th century that 'I dress the wound, God heals it,' in more recent times, there has been more interest directed at the knowledge base behind 'why' and 'how' dressings may aid the healing process (Hakimi et al. 2007, 324–337; Klasen 2000, 131–138; Molan 2006, 40–54).

8.2.1 Desirable Properties in Wound Dressings

It is not the dressing that heals a wound. However, a properly selected dressing will prevent further harm to the wound and also promote healing. In an ideal situation, the wound dressing should prevent microorganisms from reaching the wound and should also maintain a moist environment at the wound interface (Rajendran 2018). A moist environment allows cells to move unhampered by the formation of an eschar (scab) (Balakrishnan 2005, 6335–6342). Other factors to consider when selecting a wound dressing include gas exchange, maintaining appropriate tissue temperature, adherence to the wound, and any debridement action (Dhiyva, Padma, and Santhini 2015). Wounds can be created by a variety of methods: from the surgical knife to trauma or tissue breakdown due to disease. In clinical practice, an acute wound requires different treatment for a chronic wound. As discussed previously in Section 7.3.1, primary closure of a wound differs significantly from allowing a wound to heal by secondary intention, where the wound edges are not approximated.

DOI: 10.1201/9781003170570-8

Dressings may be classified as passive, interactive, or bioactive. Dressings such as gauze are the traditional passive dressings. Interactive products are those that provide a barrier to microbes but are permeable to air and water. Bioactive dressings are those that deliver substances active in wound healing (Paul and Sharma 2004, 18–23) and this field has expanded immensely in the past 30 years due to advances in immunology and the understanding of the science of wound healing (Queen et al. 2004, 59–77); each type of dressing is discussed in turn.

8.2.2 Passive Wound Dressings

Passive wound dressings involve gauzes and secondary wound dressings such as wool and crepe that are used over a smaller wound dressing, often to provide additional padding and compression and may be used post-surgery to prevent haematoma formation. The secondary dressings are often removed around 48–72 hours after surgery.

Gauze dressings consist of loosely woven cotton fabrics or non-woven fabrics where the layers of fibres, often viscose rayon and polyester, pressed so that the surface resembles that of a woven fabric. The non-woven types typically possess the advantage of losing less lint. Whatever the construction of the fabric, the intention is that the dressing provides a barrier between the wound and the environment or external items such as clothing or bedding, thereby providing some protection against bacterial infection. They are also absorbent and aid in absorbing exudate and fluid in a wound, an example is shown in Figure 8.1 (Dhiyva, Padma, and Santhini 2015).

Gauze dressing fabrics can also be finished to be super-hydrophobic and durably antibacterial. For example, cotton gauze was endowed with super-hydrophobic and antibacterial properties by a dip-coating method that involved sequential deposition of positively charged chitosan, negatively charged gallic acid-modified silver

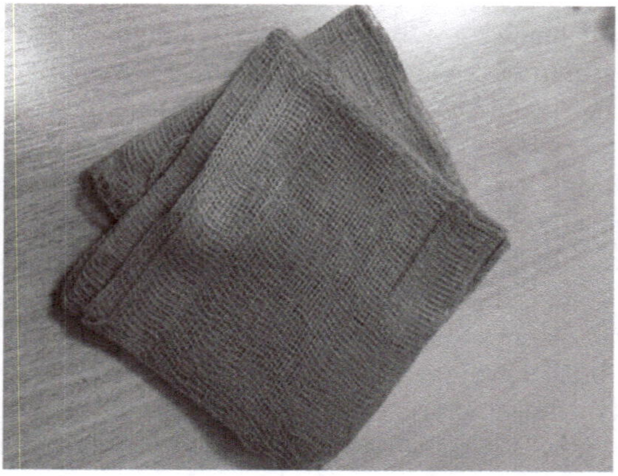

FIGURE 8.1 Sterile gauze. Image kindly provided by Mr Harish Kurup, Orthopaedic Surgeon, UK.

nanoparticles, and 1H,1H,2H,2H-perfluorodecanethiol (PFDT). The wettability of the gauze surface was converted from super-hydrophilic to super-hydrophobic with a water-contact angle (CA) of $158 \pm 2.2°$ and sliding angle (SA) of $5.2 \pm 1.8°$, exhibiting water repellency plus anti-fouling ability as well as bacterial-anti-adhesive action. The coated fabric exhibited antibacterial activity against both *E. Coli* and *S. Aureus*, which was mainly attributed to the synergistic effect of contact-killing by the chitosan together with continuous release of Ag^{+}. In addition, it was found that the outer PFDT deposition could act as a barrier to prevent leaching of the silver nanoparticles during laundry, enhancing the durability of the antibacterial activity (Liu et al. 2019, 1383–1397).

Impregnated gauzes are commonly used in surgery on incisions and traumatic wounds. These typically consist of a fine or open mesh gauze that is impregnated with a petroleum emulsion, an example is shown in Figure 8.2. This allows the dressing to be non-adherent and this prevents disruption of the incision site at dressing change. Such impregnated gauzes can often be used to help maceration of exudative wounds as they transfer exudate to the outer layer (Hanna and Giacopelli 1997, 2–14). Gauzes may also be impregnated with antiseptics, such as iodine to create bactericidal dressings which are of particular use in wounds that are contaminated or superficially infected.

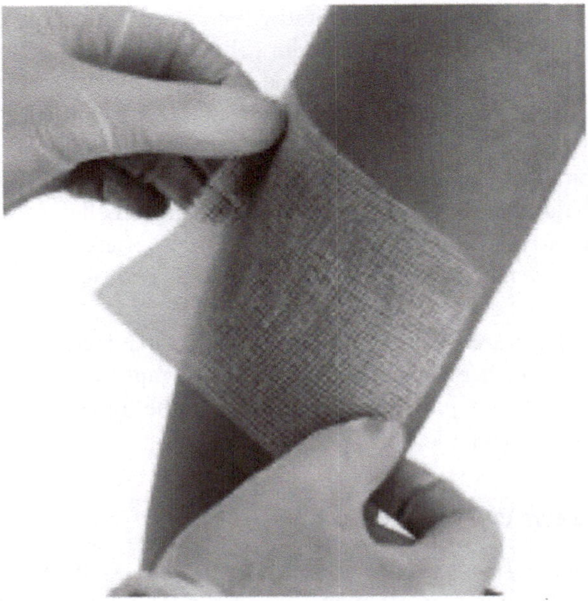

FIGURE 8.2 A example of an impregnated gauze – Jelonet. Reproduced with kind permission granted by Smith and Nephew, USA, 2021.

Bandages may be used to cover a wound or to provide support to underlying dressings, to apply pressure to control bleeding or to support a limb that has been injured. There are three main types of bandages: roller bandages, tubular bandages, and triangular bandages.

(i) *Roller bandages* can broadly be divided into two groups – elastic bandages that apply compression and cotton bandages that are used to cover gauze dressings, for example during post-operative wound care. Typically provided in sterile packages in a variety of lengths and widths those of the most suitable dimensions can therefore be used directly depending on the task at hand.
(ii) *Tubular bandages* are often used on fingers and toes as these areas can be challenging to bandage with traditional gauze.
(iii) *Triangular bandages* may be manufactured from disposable paper or re-usable cotton and can be used to make a sling to support, elevate or immobilise upper limbs or folded to provide a compress that can be used to reduce swelling.

Plasters can be used to cover scrapes and cuts, assist in stemming bleeding and to provide protection to wounds to prevent infection. They are available commercially in a variety of shapes depending on the area, and in various colours and designs to appeal to the paediatric market, and may be made out of fabric or washproof plastic film. Blue plasters are used in the hospitality sector as it is then obvious if they are lost into foodstuffs. Blister plasters contain gel padding which deforms to prevent exerting too much pressure on the blister and protect it from further irritation.

Lint is a historical dressing that may be still be used as either a primary wound dressing due to its excellent absorption properties, or a secondary wound dressing to assist absorption of exudate or to protect and cushion the wound. It may be manufactured from natural fibres such as cotton or regenerated cellulose, such as viscose rayon. Available as rolls or in pre-cut sizes allows for a variety of uses. In addition, it can be used as a base fabric onto which ointments and creams can be added to before being placed next to the skin.

Wadding bandages are traditional wound dressings that are often used over other dressings and held in place with a bandage that overwraps them, most commonly to provide some level of compression after surgery on the limbs as they can assist in preventing a wound haematoma.

8.2.3 Interactive Wound Dressings

Interactive wound dressings may be classified on the basis of their composition.

Transparent film dressings are made of a self-adhesive polyurethane film and are semi-permeable. These allow gas and water vapour exchange but prevent the absorption of wound exudates. As they are occlusive to fluids, they are used on drier wounds where they may help to provide a moist environment and prevent dessication of underlying tissue, though maceration may result if a film dressing is used on wounds with a moderate amount of drainage. They may promote autolysis of necrotic tissue (Hanna and Giacopelli 1997, 2–14). Initially, film dressings were manufactured from nylon derivatives with an adhesive polyethylene frame (Dhiyva, Padma, and Santhini 2015). Transparent films tend to conform and cling well to the surface of the wound and thus reduce friction and shear and blister formation on inflamed surrounding skin (Hanna and Giacopelli 1997, 2–14). They also have the advantage that the skin can be viewed through the dressing.

Semi-permeable foam dressings are manufactured by combining hydrophobic and hydrophilic foams; an example is shown in Figure 8.3. The hydrophobic outer layer protects the wound from liquid but allows gaseous exchange. The foam in the dressing can absorb varying quantities of exudate making semi-permeable foam dressings ideal for ulcer care (Dhiyva, Padma, and Santhini 2015).

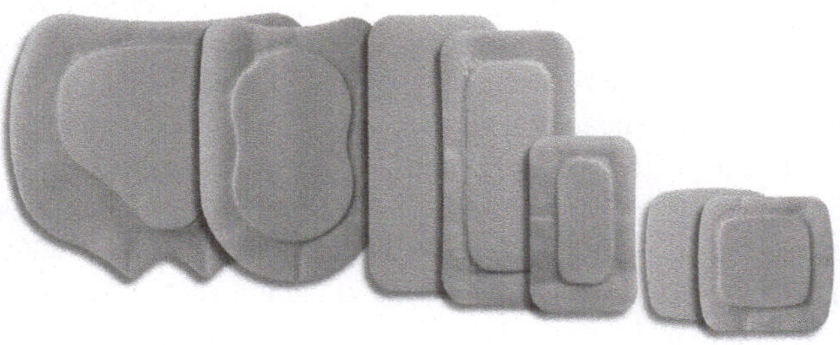

FIGURE 8.3 Semi-permeable foam dressings. Aquacel® Foam dressing. Reproduced with kind permission granted by Convatec, UK, 2021.

Semi-permeable film dressings are thin, flexible dressings made from a transparent polyurethane film with an adhesive backing to enable them to adhere to the skin. They are permeable to oxygen and carbon dioxide as well as water vapour but they do not allow the passage of water or bacteria. Semi-permeable film dressings are most often used when a wound is healing by primary intention as they do not absorb exudate.

Janus fabric dressings have the potential to fulfil similar requirements to those of semi-permeable foam dressings. The characteristic of a Janus fabric is that it possesses very different properties on each side (hence the name) and their potential has been known for some time (Liu, Xin, and Choi 2012, 17426–17434). A useful example as a wound dressing to suppress blood flow consists of a super-hydrophobic outer surface and a super-hydrophilic inner (Zhu et al. 2018). It is also possible to include silver nanoparticles or chitosan into the textile to confer antibacterial properties (Liang et al. 2016, 3958–3968; Matica et al. 2019, 5889) or quaternary ammonium nanoparticles for multifunctional effects including antibacterial performance and rendering the dressing both interactive and bioactive (Xia et al. 2020, 115–296).

Spacer fabrics, because of their structure, which in general terms consists of two adjacent woven or knitted layers connected by threads or yarns which hold the layers separate, have an open central region which offers the prospect of being able to absorb wound exudates. Given sufficiently stiff fibres or filaments connecting the two layers, which may be woven, warp-knitted, or weft-knitted, the spacer fabric also has the potential to offer some cushioning effect. Their resistance to pressure can be adjusted and depends on the type of connecting fibres, their angle in the structure, and the stitch density (Qin 2015, 61; Rajendran 2018). Consequently, they have been considered as possibly useful for heavily exudative wounds, and in particular two types of three-layer spacer fabrics have been proposed as suitable (Yang and Hu, 2017, 1469–1480; Yang and Hu 2017, 1481–1493).

Hydrogel dressings are available in the form of a gelatinous sheet or an amorphous wound filler. They can be used to fill wound defects, such as loss of tissue creating a cavity, and also conform well to wound surfaces. They are non-adhesive, permeable to gases and have a high-water content which aids granulation and also provides a cooling and thus soothing effect. As they provide little absorption, they should be used on a dry or lightly exudative wound to maintain a moist surface; indeed, burns appear to heal quicker with hydrogel dressings than with standard care (Wasiak et al. 2013). Use on a heavily draining wound may lead to maceration and bacterial overgrowth (Hanna and Giacopelli 1997, 2–14; Persin et al. 2017, 444–459).

Hydrocolloids are occlusive dressings that are composed of two layers. The inner layer is a wafer of a gum-like substance (carboxymethylcellulose, gelatin, or pectin) that adheres to the wound surface. The outer layer is a water-resistant film or foam that allows patients to bathe with the dressing in place and prevents bacterial overgrowth. They adhere and conform well to the wound and do not require a further dressing. As the wound produces exudate, it interacts with the inner wafer and forms a gel-like substance. The gel then helps to keep the wound surface moist and provides protection against microbes and any further trauma. The dressings can absorb a moderate amount of exudate before maceration of the underlying tissue becomes a problem.

Alginate dressings are made from the sodium and calcium salts of mannuronic and guluronic acid derived from seaweed. They are absorbent and biodegradable and accelerate wound healing by activating the immune system to produce inflammatory signals. When applied to the wound, ions in the alginate are exchanged with blood and it forms a protective film. Because alginate dressings have the potential to dehydrate the wound, they require to be used together with a secondary dressing (Yang and Hu 2017, 1469–1480).

8.2.4 Bioactive Wound Dressings

Bioactive dressings are manufactured from biomaterials which promote healing. They are sometimes incorporated with growth factors or antimicrobial agents (Persin et al. 2017, 444–459). The dressings are composed of compounds such as collagen, hyaluronic acid, chitosan, alginate, and elastin (Yang and Hu, 2017, 1469–1480). Gelatin, collagen, silk fibroin, cellulose, alginate, and chitosan have been employed in constructing wound dressings because of their non-cytotoxicity and hydrophilicity. Additional functionalities such as antimicrobial properties, growth-factor or drug-release abilities, and their biodegradability provide the potential to hasten the healing process. Chitosan, the polycationic linear polysaccharide derived from chitin, is currently receiving a great deal of attention, not only in the form of textile products for bioactive wound dressings (Al-Jbour et al. 2019, 272–294), but also in the competing form of sponges (Xia et al. 2020, 115296).

Honey has been regarded as a natural healing agent due to its antimicrobial activity, debriding activity, and anti-inflammatory effects. This is felt to be due to its acidity, which may prevent biofilm formation, lower water content which creates a hostile environment for microbial growth, and presence of antimicrobial substances (Bodeker, Ryan, and Ong 1999, 93–98; Davis and Perez 2009, 502–506; Kwakman et al. 2010, 2576–2582; Sato and Miyata 2000, 468–469). Mānuka honey inhibits the growth of a broad range of microorganisms and prevents biofilm formation at the site. Gram-positive organisms such as Methicillin-resistant *Staphylococcus aureus* (MRSA) and *Streptococcus pyogenes* are inhibited. Gram-negative strains such as *Escherichia coli*, *Proteus mirabilis*, *Enterobacter cloacae*, and *Pseudomonas aeruginosa* are inhibited (Bulman et al. 2017, 954). Indeed, a Cochrane review demonstrated high-quality evidence to support honey dressings in healing partial thickness burns at a faster rate than conventional dressings, though it was unclear if there was a difference in rates of adverse events or infection. Furthermore, honey heals infected post-operative wounds more quickly than antiseptic washes and heals pressure ulcers at a faster rate than saline soaks (Jull et al. 2015). Animal trials comparing a honey dressing, milk dressing, combined honey and milk dressing, and 5% sulfadiazine dressing showed that the combination of honey with milk proved the most effective followed by the 5% sulfadiazine (Hosseini et al. 2020, 915). Mānuka honey has been incorporated in an electrospun membrane of silk fibroin and demonstrated to show antibacterial activity against both gram-positive and gram-negative bacteria (Yang et al. 2017, 76–84).

Chitosan, as discussed in Chapter 4, exhibits antimicrobial activity and can be electrospun to create a variety of nanofibrous structures that can be incorporated into wound dressings. The ability to manufacture nanofibrous webs by electrospinning also allows for the incorporation of other molecules, such as antibiotics, through their addition to the spinning solution. Antibiotics can also be incorporated into nanofibres or nanofibrous yarns or webs during fabric finishing, for example by soaking the textile in a solution or by coating the textile rather than incorporating the molecule as mentioned above, at the spinning stage (Rajendran 2018).

Silver and its antimicrobial properties are long established. Silver can be incorporated into fabrics by physical treatments, chemical treatments such as ion exchange, or by the blending of fibres (Rajendran 2018). There is a wide range of silver dressings already in clinical use and the more recent move towards the incorporation of silver nanoparticles into fibres has gained popularity as a result of the emergence of resistance of some bacteria towards antibiotics (Hebeish et al. 2014, 509–515). Work has also been undertaken into the topical delivery of silver for controlling wound infections, for example, using a bilayer chitosan wound dressing (Mi et al. 2002,

438–449). At present, a Cochrane review has concluded that there is insufficient evidence to establish whether silver-containing dressings or topical agents promote wound healing or prevent wound infection (Storm-Versloot et al. 2010). More recent work demonstrates the narrow therapeutic window and potential for toxicity to cells (Nesporova 2020, 1-4).

Wet wraps may be used as a treatment option in the management of skin conditions such as childhood eczema. The traditional wet wrap technique involves application of a corticosteroid ointment and emollient followed by a two-layer mummy-style wrap using roll gauze and vinyl wrap. The method is time consuming and labour intensive with significant training of the parents required. As such there has been a move towards designing garments that can be worn over the emollients to make life easier for parents (Dhandha and Siegfried 2017, 48–51).

Synthetic skin-substitutes are designed to accelerate wound healing by providing extracellular matrix. They can be used in both acute and chronic wounds; for example, in burns patients where there is a scarcity of donor site availability for a skin graft. Pruitt and Levine detailed the attributes of an ideal skin substitute in 1984; little or no antigenicity, tissue compatibility, lack of toxicity, permeability to water vapour, impenetrability to microorganisms, rapid and persistent adherence to a wound surface, porosity for ingrowth of fibrovascular tissue from the wound bed, malleability, elasticity, structural stability, and sufficient tensile strength to maintain its structural integrity (Pruitt and Levine 1984, 312–322).

A variety of products are available which may be classified according to the composition of the source materials (e.g., human vs animal, synthetic vs biological), the intended duration (permanent vs temporary), the intended tissue to be replaced (epidermal vs dermal), or the number of layers (single vs bilaminate) and composites are also made with the intention of more closely mimicking the characteristics of skin, but in general terms, these bioengineered products all aim to promote wound closure.

8.3 PRODUCTS USED FOR HAEMOSTASIS

Haemostasis, simply put, is the cessation of blood flow. Haemostatic textiles are adjuncts to, or facilitators of, haemostasis – the body's method of stopping or reducing blood loss. Electrospinning and the ability to combine conventional fibres with nanofibres have driven an expansion into research into haemostatic textile-based products. Large haemostatic dressings have a role in trauma surgery and in pre-hospital resuscitation to ensure that exsanguination does not occur en route to the emergency room.

> 'All bleeding stops eventually.'

Bleeding can stop in several ways

1. Tamponade – The application of pressure (to a bleeding area).

2. Clotting – A complex cascade of events ultimately leading to the formation of a scaffold or web of fibrin. This subsequently 'catches' the various cellular components of blood involved in clotting and forms an organised plug or seal.
3. Exsanguination – Where the flow of blood is greater than the rate at which it can clot or be stopped, and/or replaced; eventually a sufficient volume of blood may leave the body such that the flow rate is conducive to clot formation. Significant volumes of blood loss are life threatening or fatal.

A number of textile devices exist which facilitate the above processes and may exert their action actively or passively, that is to influence or promote the speed at which clotting occurs or contribute to tamponade and clotting by providing a surface onto which blood components might exert their actions. Some haemostatic textiles are absorbable, lending themselves to internal usage, whereas others are non-absorbable and can be safely removed once a clot has been established.

Textiles in otorhinolaryngology are an essential tool in the surgical armamentarium, owing to their ability to line a small cavity, orifice, or wound. These orifices are typically difficult places to reconstruct or stitch, hence there is a reliance on hydrophilic materials, water tension, adhesion, and haemostasis. Impregnating the textiles with prothrombotic, chemotherapeutic, bacteriostatic, bactericidal, and anti-inflammatory agents has been utilised by some companies to improve surgical outcomes with the ultimate aim of improving quality of life by restoring sensory function to the operated organ.

As such, versatility in structure and function is essential in promoting sound wound healing and minimising surgical complications such as bleeding, infection, and seroma (tissue fluid) formation. Some surgeons may adulterate the textiles with additional medication, e.g., steroid suspension to facilitate drug delivery to a body cavity or orifice for a desired therapeutic effect.

Carboxymethyl cellulose is a commonly used, plant cell-wall-based polymer used primarily as a scaffold rather than as a true tamponade agent in its own right. In woven form, it is used to provide a non-adhesive coating to tamponade devices for epistaxis (nosebleeds), which can also double up as a matrix for clot formation, thus facilitating haemostasis. Unlike other nasal packing material, its hydrophilic, non-adherent nature means that emergency insertion and planned removal of the nasal tampon is a less painful experience for the patient, despite the overall experience being potentially distressing and unpleasant throughout.

Gelatin is an animal-based matrix formed of proteoglycans, glycoproteins, and glycosaminoglycans. It is typically available to surgeons in the form of a dehydrated, soluble, foam to enable lining of cavities, scaffolding, and as a vector for liquid medications. In otorhinolaryngology, it is typically used in ear surgery as a scaffold, but without tamponade effect which might displace a carefully sited, or precarious, graft. Its hydrophilic properties encourage, in the author's experience, free tissue grafts to adhere to, and ultimately integrate with, the recipient site by utilising water tension. The similarities to human tissue fluid and proteinaceous exudate make it readily absorbable thus avoiding the need for removal and causing minimal inflammation, thus reducing the risk of infection.

Decellularised collagen may originate from a variety of animal sources including bovine, equine, and porcine. Acellular bovine collagen is most commonly used in skull base and neurological surgery to repair the dura mater, the tough outermost fibrous layer housing the brain. Its porcine counterpart offers similar properties; however, the equine equivalent is also impregnated with recombinant human thrombin, facilitating haemostasis as well as offering a scaffold.

The lack of cellular material again reduces inflammation and prevents a foreign body reaction by the host but the similarity of collagen compounds across different species means the implanted textile is integrated into during the healing process.

Hydroxylated polyvinyl acetate is deployed as a dehydrated foam which, when saturated with liquid, expands to tamponade. It is commonly used post-operatively but may also be used for managing acute haemorrhage from the nose. Once soaked in blood, a clot will form and harden in situ, hence its removal requires prior rehydration so as to make the removal process less uncomfortable.

It is available in a smaller form for acutely infected ears to facilitate the delivery of antibiotic containing ear drops when, for example, the surrounding tissue has become oedematous, swollen, and prevents drops alone reaching the nidus of infection. As with any non-absorbable foreign body, failure to remove the tampon in a timely fashion can result in colonisation with bacteria and can lead to acute sinusitis in the short term, or toxic shock syndrome.

Calcium alginate may be combined with silver, and as a woven dressing, it is used as a soft wick or absorbent pack in bleeding or infected wounds where antimicrobial effects are desired in addition to haemostasis.

8.4 PRESSURE GARMENTS

Pressure garments that provide external pressure to the human form may be used in medicine for a range of purposes including to prevent venous thromboembolism and venous ulceration, in the treatment of burns and in the management of fractures or other soft tissue injuries.

8.4.1 Desirable Properties in Pressure Garments

Pressure garments must exert the desired pressure comfortably. As they are often worn next to the skin, they must be non-irritant and not cause maceration of the underlying skin. As such, breathability, water permeability, and the thermal behaviour of the garment are all important factors. In addition, the ability to launder and allow reuse is an advantageous property.

8.4.2 Engineering the Pressure Garment

A considerable amount of work has been undertaken to improve understanding about essentials in the engineering of pressure garments, not least in relation to being able to model, predict, and measure the pressure actually being exerted at the intended point(s) on the body, with focus on making choices or adjustments to provide the desired pressure at the correct location. The materials most commonly used in the compression garments contain the elastomeric spandex yarns, sometimes called elastane yarns, (polymeric materials consisting of at least 85% segmented polyurethane), for their rubber-like elasticity and a range of standard fabric constructions can be used (warp knitting, weft knitting, or weaving).

There are several possible approaches to designing and modelling the properties and performance of the compression garments. Maklewska et al. put forward a model for designing knitted compression garments that would exert a pre-set pressure on the human body using the Laplace Law (Maklewska, Nawrocki, and Ledwon 2006, 111–113), and Hong et al. worked with the Young's modulus of the fabric and a finite element model in a study of pressures exerted by tight-fitting clothing (Hong et al. 2011, 1307–1319). Whereas Senthilkumar related the stretch and recovery properties of the cotton/elastane knitted fabrics with the elastane linear density, tension on the elastane yarn during knitting, and cotton yarn loop length (Senthilkumar 2012).

Even so, the engineering situation being addressed is somewhat messy for a variety of reasons. First, there is little information regarding the properties of fabrics used in the construction of existing pressure garments within current literature. As the pressure exerted by the pressure garments is not routinely measured with suitable instruments, at least not in UK hospitals, the real pressures exerted by each pressure garment, currently used to treat hypertrophic scars, are not normally known (Anand, Kanchi Govarthanam, and Gazioglu 2013, 668–674). Second, during pressure garment application in the UK hospitals, there is neither awareness of the impact that the various fabric types will have on the different pressures exerted by pressure garments nor is there a standard test method for the evaluation of fabrics for their use in pressure garments. Pressure garments are normally exempt from Conformité Européenne (CE) marking under the Medical Devices Directive because they are custom made and, therefore, fall into a gap in standards legislation (Anand, Kanchi Govarthanam, and Gazioglu 2013, 668–674).

There has been some work into the pressure exerted. Starting with modelling of compression garments following burns (Anand, Kanchi Govarthanam, and Gazioglu 2013, 668–674; Anand, Kanchi Govarthanum, and Gazioglu 2013, 661–667), the Laplace equation was used to model a pattern-cutting chart that was refined to predict the sub-garment pressure more accurately, irrespective of the shape and size of the limb. The model's accuracy was validated by constructing garments for the arms and legs of a male volunteer and measuring the actual pressures by using a Kikuhime pressure-measuring device. Third, comfort or the lack of it with compression garments can be a major issue. The thermo-physiological properties of the compression garment which provide comfort by preserving body temperature and moisture output close to their normal levels, together with the dimensional, mechanical, and thermo-physiological properties of four fabrics intended for pressure exertion applications, were therefore compared to determine their suitability to be utilised for the management of hypertrophic scarring.

One of the desirable properties of compression garments is that the pressure exerted by the garment on the limb should be uniform in all directions; mechanical properties, such as fabric stiffness, extension, and recovery, should be close to isotropic in all directions to prevent the skin from stretching in the direction where the fabric extension is highest, particularly important when the pressure garment is used on areas of limbs with bony protrusions and areas with a small radius of curvature. It was a power net, the bulkiest one of the four fabrics tested (three power nets and one solid warp-knitted fabric) that was found to possess the best properties for the purpose, but it was also found to be capable of improvement (Anand, Kanchi Govarthanam, and Gazioglu 2013, 668–674).

For an investigation into the effects of elastane linear density, thread density, and weave float length on the extensibility, recovery, and compression properties of bi-stretch woven fabrics for compression garments, various fabric samples were produced using elastane core-spun cotton yarns both in the warp and weft. The elastane linear density, fabric thread density, and weave float size were used as input variables while fabric contraction, sub-garment pressure, fabric stretch, and recovery were taken as response variables. The coefficients of determinations (*R*-sq values) of the regression equations showed good prediction ability of the developed statistical models (Maqsood et al. 2016, 307–315).

Following through on that exercise, the compression properties of bi-stretch woven fabrics were compared with knitted fabrics of the same areal density, all constructed from core-spun elastane yarns with cotton as the sheath, to determine their practical suitability in compression garments using a Kikuhime pressure sensor; durability of their performance after washing was also assessed. It was found that the bi-stretch woven fabrics possessed better compression properties before and after washing and retained their durability after repeated use, whereas the knitted stretchable fabrics lost their compression ability after repeated use and the required sub-garment pressure of the knitted structures after 15 washes was almost half that of the woven bi-stretch fabrics. The simplest woven structure, the plain weave, was the fabric which exerted the highest pressure (Maqsood et al. 2017, 522–527). The subsequent action was to undertake a study on the optimisation of the mechanical and comfort properties of the bi-stretch woven fabrics, an appropriate step given that a high proportion of patients may discard the compression garments because of discomfort (Maqsood et al. 2017, 794–802).

Very recently, a new practical engineering approach to modelling, measuring, and predicting the compression from a compression garment used a cut-strip method to develop two new mathematical models based on 'true Young's modulus' and 'engineering Young's modulus.' Through comparison with Hooke's law and Laplace's law and previous models of Leung et al. and Dubuis et al, using linear regression to assess the experimentally measured compression pressure results, it was found that the newly developed models were more precise and accurate than the previous models (Dubuis et al. 2012, 6; Faisal Siddique et al. 2020, 1689–1703; Leung et al. 2010, 716–727).

Taking a more comprehensive view, the effectiveness of the compression garment was rightly considered to depend not only on the correct technical functioning of the compression item, but also on physiology, pathophysiology, and biomechanics (Liu et al. 2016, 1121–1141). Attention has now moved on to anthropometry in an attempt to improve fit by 3D scanning of 208 subjects and cluster analysis enabling the stratification of lower-limb shapes into three morphologies, based upon determined anthropometric landmarks along the lower extremities. Responding to such a stratified shape-led sizing system was thought to allow the possibility of catering better for both shape and size together, hence also the possibility of improving both fit and more accurate compression treatment for the patient (Liu et al. 2018, 2055–2075).

The research group has also addressed the problem with homogeneous compression garments which apply pressure unevenly, cause discomfort, and fail to administer the necessary pressure with any accuracy to the area where it is required. To counteract those problems, a heterogeneous compression bandage/stocking was knitted and pressure measurements on the wearer showed that these heterogeneous compression shells designed for the lower limbs could redistribute skin pressures around the leg cross section and be higher for the muscle-dominated posterior calves where it was intended to be. It was felt that user compliance in practice might improve if heterogeneous compression stockings with such 'bi-axial' pressure profiles for improved compression performance were to be developed (Liu et al. 2018, 1915–1930). The research group has also undertaken work to try to refine the shape profiles for compression stockings by further application of shape measurement, again in the hope that this might help to improve patient compliance with the compression garment requirement (Liu et al. 2019, 1835–1852).

8.4.3 Thromboembolic Devices

A thrombus, or clot, in the venous system may be formed due to an alteration in one of the triad named after German physician Rudolf Virchow (1821–1902). The triad includes

1. Damage to vessel endothelium
2. Hypercoagulability
3. Stasis of blood flow

Venous thromboembolism (VTE) comprises both deep vein thrombosis (DVT) and pulmonary embolism (PE). Hospital-acquired VTE is a common complication and a leading cause of mortality and morbidity in hospitalised surgical patients. Those occurring during hospitalisation or within 3 months after hospitaliation have been shown to underlie more than 50% of all cases of the population burden of VTE (Kahn et al. 2018). Similarly, PE is a serious post-operative complication that represents a source of preventable morbidity and mortality; in the USA, it is responsible for 5–10% of all hospital inpatient deaths (Townsend et al. 2016). Whilst there are other causes of DVT and PE at the perioperative period, and thus treatments to be directed at these, the use of pressure garments to prevent stasis of blood flow remains an accepted practice. Indeed, consideration is also given to hospital inpatients that are not under the surgical directorate, although there are contraindications to their use and, thus, are not suitable for everyone.

Whilst it may appear that the use of compression stockings is beneficial, evidence is conflicting, though large meta-analyses accept that large well-designed trials are still in need (Bain et al. 2014; Di Nisio et al. 2015; Kahn et al. 2018). Indeed, further evidence is required to distinguish whether thigh-length or below-knee stockings proffer the maximum benefit to patients (Sajid et al. 2012). Compression stockings may also be used to prevent venous leg ulceration and there is a small amount of evidence to support its effectiveness, more so for high-compression rather than medium-compression hosiery. However, the rates of patient intolerance to compression hosiery generally were high (Nelson and Bell-Syer 2014).

In the consumer sector, compression stockings have been shown to reduce the incidence of symptomless VTE in airline passengers (Clarke et al. 2016) (e.g. Flightsocks©, Scholl, Reckitt Benckiser, Slough, UK) and there has been uptake in the health and exercise industry as stockings have been shown to improve endurance performance by increasing proprioception muscle coordination and propulsive force (Bringard, Perrey, and Belluye 2006, 373–378). Bandages and stockings may also be used as a retention bandage, to retain dressings in place, or for support, to provide retention and prevent development of a deformity (Rajendran 2018). Of note, there are contraindications to the use of anti-embolism stockings and these include individuals who have suspected or proven arterial disease, peripheral arterial bypass grafting, peripheral neuropathy or sensory impairment, local conditions such as gangrene or recent skin grafts, known allergy to the material of manufacture, or severe leg oedema (NICE 2021).

Medical compression stockings can be manufactured in a variety of ways including circular or flat-bed knitting and using woven fabrics (Liu et al. 2017, 1121–1141). Adjusting the raw fibre, yarn, and knit structure can produce stockings of varying compression. Maleki et al. investigated the influence of stitch length, strain, washing operation, and repeated usage on the pressure behaviour of knitted fabrics, all of which are important factors impacting the stocking (Maleki et al. 2011). Further studies have demonstrated that the elastane yarn count is the most effective parameter on pressure characteristics (Sari and Oglakcioglu 2018, 1083–1096) and that the tensile energy, tensile strain, shearing stiffness, and bending rigidity are all key mechanical properties for compression stockings (Liu et al. 2010, 79).

In clinical applications, it is important to know the pressure profile, dosage of compression, and the pressure distribution of the stocking. As such, compression bandages are classified according to the level of compression that they provide: Class 1 bandages offer light support at 14–17 mm Hg to control varicose veins and mild oedema; Class II medium support at 18–24 mmHg for the treatment of severe varicose veins, mild oedema, and prevention of ulcer recurrence; and Class 3 offering strong support at 25–35 mmHg for severe varicose veins, post-phlebitic limbs, the prevention of ulcer recurrence, and chronic venous insufficiency (Johnson 2002, 67–74).

There is still no universal standard for graduated compression and so there are three classification systems in use in Europe: British, French, and German. For bandages and stockings used other than in the role of VTE prevention, then the bandage may be combined with other dressings or in a multi-layer format. Indeed, there has been interest from the sports industry to assess the effect of number of fabric layers, fabric composition, and fabric direction in sport compression garments (MacRae, Laing, and Partsch 2016, 1–32; Wardiningsih and Troynikov 2019, 882–890).

Of interest, there is also a role for intermittent pneumatic compression devices in reducing the incidence of VTE in hospital patients. There are several different devices available with variations in their design, including the rate and means of compression (Zhao et al. 2012). The devices work by simulating the normal calf pump mechanism by causing external compression of the deep veins and therefore creating a pulsatile blood flow and venous return. In addition to their use as VTE prophylaxis, they have also been used to treat limb swelling, for example, in patients with lymphoedema or venous leg ulcers (Chen et al. 2001, 383–392).

8.4.4 Pressure Garments in the Management of Fractures and Soft Tissue Injuries

The use of casts in fracture management is probably the most worldwide method of managing fractures today and dates back to ancient times where a variety of methods were utilised to stiff bandages. For example, the Egyptians used glue to stiffen bandages to provide support to the cast whilst the Greeks used cerate (Tornetta 2020). Casts may be applied for a variety of reasons: to prevent movement in the short term to provide pain relief, to provide pressure around the fracture site to aid in healing in an optimal position, to protect underlying surgical repair of tendons, or in combination with traction to name but a few (Tornetta 2020). There are a range of different types of casts that may be applied depending upon the reason. For example, total contact casting may be used in the management of neuropathic foot ulcers to offload the foot and these casts are applied in a modified way to the fracture casts that most will commonly imagine (Nabuurs-Franssen 2005, 243–247). Regardless of that, application of a cast is a specialist topic with the British Orthopaedic Association offering comprehensive courses (British Orthopaedic Association 2020).

Sir John Charnley described the three-point fixation method of applying a moulded plaster to hold a fracture in position. The fracture is reduced to the optimal position and then plaster cast subsequently applied. The plaster is then moulded to apply pressure at the site of the fracture and the sites proximal and distal. The optimal positions of moulding are dependent upon the type and location of the fracture (Charnley 1999). All casts are applied in a similar manner whether using the traditional plaster of Paris or more modern fibreglass materials. Slabs or a roll of cast material are applied over a layer of protective stockinette and layers of synthetic wool padding. In addition, foam may be used over bony prominences to prevent skin breakdown. The layer of padding is important as too much permits secondary fracture displacement and too little causes skin problems and an increased risk of compartment syndrome (Tornetta 2020). Examples of materials used are illustrated in Figure 8.4 and Figure 8.5.

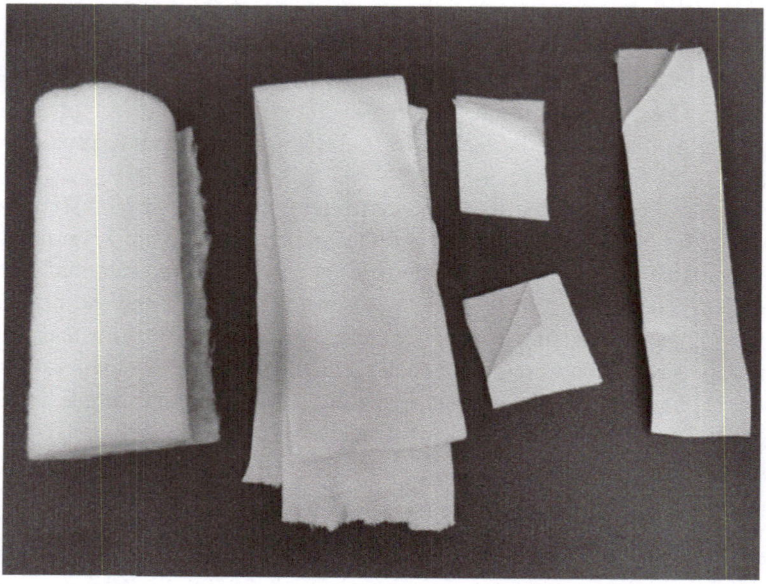

FIGURE 8.4 Commonly used materials for applying a cast to a limb. Image kindly provided by Mr Harish Kurup, Orthopaedic Surgeon, UK.

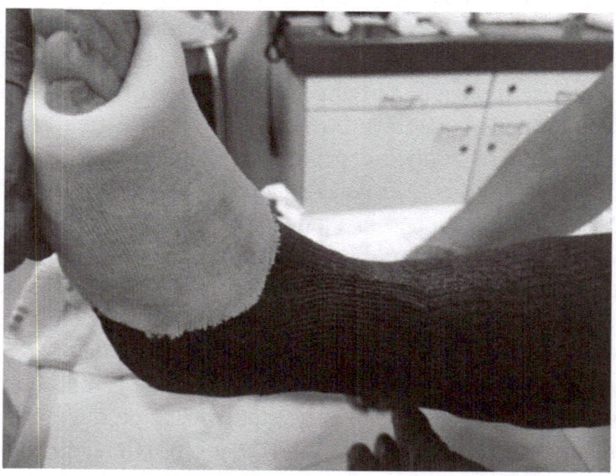

FIGURE 8.5 Example of a fibreglass below-knee cast prior to completion. Image kindly provided by Mr Harish Kurup, Orthopaedic Surgeon, UK.

Plaster of Paris remains the time-honoured material of choice for the treatment of acute fractures. It is named after a large gypsum deposit at Montmartre in Paris and was traditionally used in the construction industry. Its use predates this and it has been found on the insides of pyramids. It was first incorporated into bandages to use in fracture management in the 1850s by two surgeons, Antonius Mathijsen and Nikolai Ivanovich Pirogov (Sharma and Prabu 2013, 107). Plaster of Paris is calcined gypsum ground to a fine powder by milling. When water is added, the more soluble form of calcium sulphate returns to the relatively insoluble form and heat is produced. The big advantage of using plaster of Paris in casting materials is that it allows itself to be moulded (Sharma and Prabu 2013, 107). The plaster of Paris is combined with a woven inextensible bandage and then wrapped in the final layer of the cast around the limb. There are a variety of other materials that can be used in place of plaster of Paris. Some of these are water activated and are stronger and more durable than plaster of Paris. Others are also thermoplastic and can be worked by heating in a water bath or oven and then can be directly moulded to the patient. These tend to be more expensive but have their place (Sharma and Prabu 2013, 107).

Finally, a range of orthotics such as braces, slings, etc. can be used in fracture management and the management of soft tissue injuries and these are discussed in more detail in Section 8.5.4.

Compression garments, such as those illustrated in Figure 8.6, can be used to aid soft tissue recovery. There has been significant interest in this role from sports and exercise science. The rationale for applying compression is to create an external pressure gradient that can theoretically reduce the space available for swelling, haemorrhage (and subsequent haematoma formation). They also provide mechanical support. Within the field of sports science, it has been suggested that compression garments may provide additional benefits by increasing venous return and thus increasing the removal of waste products, such as lactic acid. This allows tissues to return to normal metabolism at a faster rate (Davies, Thompson, and Cooper 2009, 1786–1794; Hsu et al. 2017). A recent systematic review concluded that, whilst studies can demonstrate conflicting results, compression garments demonstrate likely

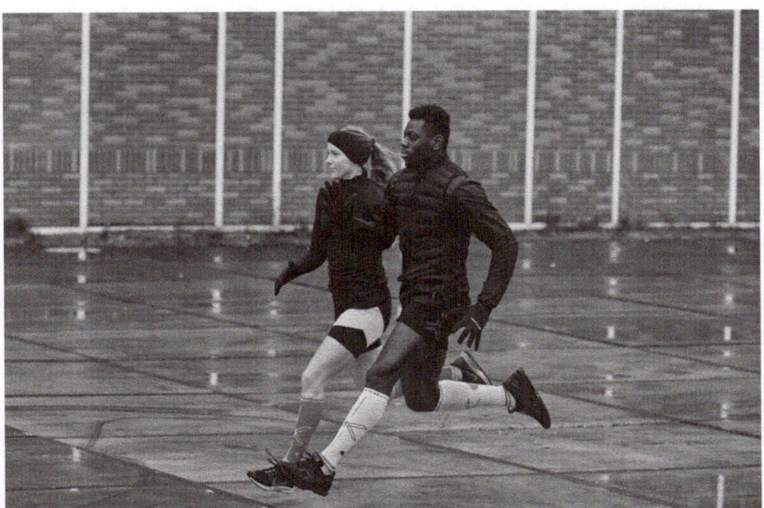

FIGURE 8.6 Compression socks used in fitness injury. Reproduced with kind permission granted by STOX Energy Socks, Amsterdam, 2021.

benefits with strength recovery exercises subject to some of the greatest benefits (Brown et al. 2017, 2245–2267). Other studies have demonstrated that compression garments, when applied after exercise, can reduce delayed onset muscle soreness (DOMS) and inflammatory markers (Kim, Kim, and Lee 2017, 541).

8.4.5 Pressure Garments in the Management of Burns

In 2004, it was estimated that nearly 11 million people worldwide suffered burns severe enough to warrant medical attention (Peck 2011, 1087–1100).

Whilst there have been advances in burn care, abnormal scarring remains one of the most common complications and may occur in up to 70% of cases. Scarring is a healing process of the skin in response to the burn injury. A prolonged inflammatory phase may increase the risk of scarring (Harris et al. 2020) as well as prolonged healing times or abnormal healing patterns.

Jackson produced the burn wound model which divides a burn into zones related to their overall potential for healing.

- Inner zone – dead tissue
- Middle zone – the 'zone of stasis' which is the target of good burns care
- Outer zone – the 'zone of hyperaemia,' a zone of inflammation in response to the injury

Burns are classified according to the components of the skin which are damaged, which in turn reflects the expected time for healing to occur. A superficial burn where the epidermis is burnt but the burn does not extend into the dermis, typified by sunburn, does not require dressing but is treated with emollients and moisturisers. It usually heals in less than 14 days and does not scar. A superficial partial thickness burn, where the epidermis and the superficial part of the dermis are burnt, may require a dressing to absorb fluid and thus prevent maceration, reduce the risk of infection, and prevent secondary deepening of the wound. This also provides an element of pain control. Usually a superficial partial thickness burn heals within 2 weeks, if kept clean and free of infection. It rarely leaves a lasting scar unless a wound complication such as infection occurs. A deeper partial thickness (burn injury extends deeply within the dermis), or full-thickness burn (full-thickness burn injury to epidermis and dermis), often requires a dressing to debride or temporise the remaining tissue prior to surgical debridement and skin grafting unless only a very small area is injured (Douglas and Wood 2017, 94–97).

In deeper burns, dermal appendages are destroyed by the burn injury, so re-epithelialisation occurs primarily from the edges of the burn. Unless very small, these deeper burns take over 2 weeks to heal and are more likely to leave undesirable or pathological scars.

Prolonged healing or genetic predisposition may result in a hypertrophic or a keloid scar. Both are characterised by the deposition of collagen fibres and bundles within the dermis which lack the flexibility or pliability of uninjured skin and are considered pathological scars. Excess collagen is deposited and the scar is thick, non-pliable, itchy, and can be painful. Hypertrophic scars occur within the confines of the original injured skin, usually mature within 2 years or so, and tend not to recur if excised (usually when mature). Keloid scars have a more extended scar-proliferative phase and also extend beyond the original injured skin (Finnerty et al. 2016, 1427–1436).

Pressure garment therapy is considered an effective strategy for the prevention and management of abnormal scarring and to assist with scar maturation by preventing scar contraction and improving scar biomechanics (Kim et al. 2015, 572). It has been the main method of treating hypertrophic scars since the 1970s and can include complicated garments such as gloves (Yu et al. 2013, 269–287). While early usage of compression therapy for burn scars is accepted as standard care, there are no clear guidelines for the timing and duration of compression garment intervention (Tredget, Shupp, and Schneider 2017, 146–147). The garments are designed to exert a pressure of approximately 25 mmHg on the underlying tissue in order to exceed the inherent capillary pressure and a soft, flexible, and extensile fabric with a thickness of 3.81 mm has been recommended previously (Yildiz 2007, 59–64). A number of factors during the manufacturing process can affect the pressure exerted by the garment. Typically, after the patient's body area requiring a pressure garment has been measured, a paper pattern is drawn to the design of the compression garment for that body part. A reduction factor (a predefined percentage reduction in size) is then applied to generate external pressure on the required body part, taking into account the elasticity of the fabric used as well. The pressure exerted could in theory be altered by altering the reduction factor or by double-layering of different fabrics with differing elasticity at the same reduction factor (Leung et al. 2010, 716–727).

Extended use of the garment and use in conjunction with moisturisers and oils may reduce the pressure that the garment exerts (Macintyre, Dahale, and Rae 2016, e365–e373). As well as contact between pressure garments and moisturisers accelerating tension degradation of the fabric, hand washing the pressure garments also seems to reduce the pressure-delivering properties more compared to machine washing the garments (Macintyre, Gilmartin, and Rae 2007, 725–733). Pressure exerted by the garment can also vary if the garment becomes wet e.g., due to sweating or environmental factors. Typically, the pressure exerted by the garment is highest when the garment is dry (Macintyre, Dahale, and Rae 2016, e365–e373). Indeed, heat and associated perspiration has been demonstrated to alter the pressure the garment delivers by the nature of the fibre interacting with moisture. Indeed, fabrics tested in one study all exerted less pressure when wet; the fabrics included a warp-knitted sleeknit made from nylon and elastane, a weft-knitted tubigrip made from cotton with nylon-covered elastodiene, and two different powernet fabrics made from nylon and elastane (Macintyre, Dahale, and Rae 2016, e365–e373). Daily wear (as prescribed by therapists) and repeated laundering also result in a gradual reduction in the pressure exerted by the garments. While this happens universally, some types of fabric are less durable than others and the orientation of the fabric fibres in the garment may affect the duration of maintenance of a therapeutic pressure with long axis fibre orientation parallel to the patient's body part seeming to enhance the degree of and the maintenance of the pressure exerted (Malara et al. 2018, 562–571).

Problems with the garments include increased pain, intolerance to heat, and skin breakdown in some patients (Coghlan et al. 2017, 260–269) and these may impact upon patients' adherence to the treatment plan, with rates of 41–70% reported in the literature. Patient-related treatment experiences with pressure garments following burn injury are both positive and negative. A literature review of patient experiences of wearing pressure garments post burn injury found three common themes amongst patients: concern and frustration with the public's reaction to and treatment of them wearing compression garments; discomfort and irritation while wearing the garment including itching, sweating, skin changes, and activity limitations; and finally, a sense of security and safety whilst wearing the garment. The same study also found gaps in patient education and understanding about why they were wearing pressure garments after their burn injury (Coghlan et al. 2017, 260–269). Another study looked at the reasons for alteration request for pressure garments and found that they mainly related to fit problems. Poorly fitting garments in both circumferential and longitudinal dimensions of the body part as well as incorrect positioning and size of openings for eyes, nose, ears, or mouth and incorrect length or position of zippers were the main reasons for an alteration request. This is useful feedback to the therapist or garment manufacturer (Chi, Lin, and Yang 2008, 965–974). It is also worthwhile noting that the desired pressure requirement that the garment is produced to exert is not always achieved even at the first fitting and that even when it is achieved, it reduces further over time with significant pressure loss by 2 months (Nedelec et al. 2020, 254–262). Pressure garments should be regularly reviewed and refitted and replaced regularly during the therapy process.

A protocol for a Cochrane review to assess the effect of pressure garment therapy in the treatment of burns has recently been published; the outcomes are awaited (Harris et al. 2020). In addition, there has been a call for a formal RCT to be undertaken in this field (Moiemen et al. 2018, 1). Prolonged scar pressure from pressure garments has been shown to alter burn scar biomechanics with less scar contracture, less skin hardness and increased skin strength compared to control scars (Kim et al. 2015, 572). Early cessation of pressure garment therapy (after 17 weeks in one study) also appears to be associated with greater skin graft contraction and more raised, rougher and harder skin grafts (DeBruler et al. 2018, e0197558). The same group also advocate early application of pressure garments after skin graft surgery for burn injury with good results (DeBruler et al. 2019, e310–e321). However, there are differing studies on the effectiveness of pressure garment therapy for burn scars in the literature and a meta-analysis in 2007 concluded that pressure garment treatment did not appear to alter global scar scores but did improve scar height (Anzarut et al. 2009, 77–84). The 'ideal' pressure garment for burn scar therapy remains elusive (Macintyre, Dahale, and Rae 2016, e365–e373).

8.5 ORTHOTICS

An orthosis is defined as an externally applied device, which modifies function by supporting or controlling a body part (Kurup, Clark, and Dega 2012, 79–83).

There are a wide range of orthotics available for all aspects of the body ranging from hernia supports through to hip protectors and,.more recently, exoskeletons. They are made of a range of materials including thermoplastics, polypropylene, subortholen family, acrylic, composite carbon fibres, cork, leather, polyethylene foams, etc.

Modifications of these have made it through to the commercial and consumer markets; for example, the Fitflop™ (London, UK), Masai Barefoot Technology® (Barcelona, Spain), and Earth Shoe® (New York, USA). Mainstream sneaker companies have also been on the forefront of development of customised insoles to address the demand for running adepts to have on-shelf access to shoes addressing over-pronators and supinators. Ethyl-vinyl acetates (EVAs) and silicones have been the materials of predilection here. A few different orthoses will be discussed below.

8.5.1 Desirable Properties in Orthotics

Design of a suitable orthotic begins with determination of the desired treatment objectives. Appropriate materials that can provide mechanical support are critical but rigid braces require a different selection of materials to a flexible insole for a shoe which may have to accommodate foot deformities, support the foot, and also absorb shock and shear forces. Nevertheless, materials must be durable, able to be cleaned or sterilised without degrading, and biocompatible. Breathability is critical as maceration of underlying skin is a potential problem if not.

Products with memory will allow the orthotist to reform and remould the orthosis allowing for correction of shape as deformity minimises. Thermoplastic materials allow the orthotist to mould an orthotic rapidly in clinic to provide treatment without delay.

8.5.2 Hernia Trusses

Hernia trusses have been used for centuries with reports of Sir Astley Cooper using a truss successfully back in the 1820s. They are a mechanical support that assists in maintaining the hernia: ‘a bandage by which ruptures are restrained from lapsing’ (Bynum and Bynum 2017, 1289). Surgery is the only effective treatment, although in patients where surgical risks are excessive, trusses can provide symptomatic relief. A range of trusses are available for patients to maintain a reduced hernia. Trusses are effective in herniae that are completely reducible. A study in the *British Medical Journal* suggested that trusses are not without problems, some of which include discomfort when wearing. The study also reported that poor hernia control can be exacerbated by incorrect truss placement and that a truss increases the probability of complications such as strangulation of the hernia, atrophy of the spermatic cord, and atrophy of the fascial margins (Law and Trapnell 1992, 1092). There is scope for improved designs for the benefit of those not wanting to undergo the surgeon’s knife. Figure 8.7 illustrates a hernia truss.

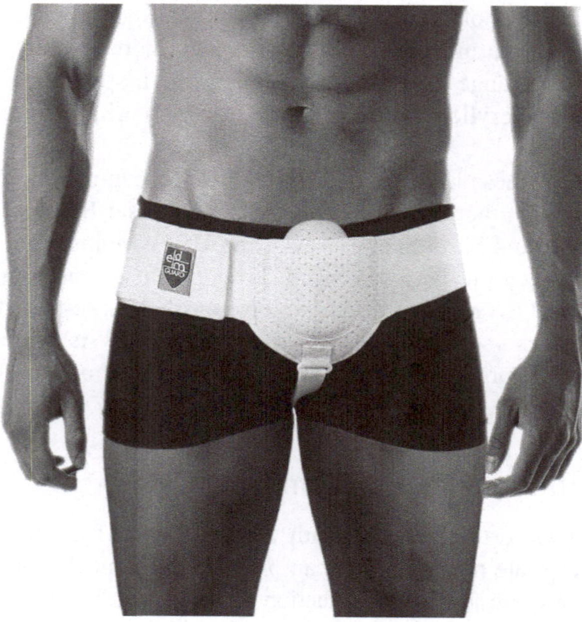

FIGURE 8.7 An example of a hernia truss. Reproduced with kind permission granted by Everyday Medical, Los Angeles, USA, 2021.

8.5.3 Hip Protectors

Hip protectors consist of plastic shields or foam pads fitted in pockets of specially designed underwear that aim to reduce the impact of a fall onto the hip and thus the risk of a hip fracture (Koike et al. 2009, 1613–1620), an example is illustrated by Figure 8.8 and Figure 8.9. Over 700 000 hip fractures occur annually in the UK and the total cost of care is over £2 billion with 10% mortality at 30 days and up to 30% mortality at one year (British Orthopaedic Association 2012). The World Health Organisation still lists hip protectors as an effective means to reduce the incidence of hip fractures (World Health Organization 2018). A Cochrane review found accumulating evidence that casts some doubt on the effectiveness of the provision of hip protectors in reducing the incidence of fragility hip fracture. Many people stop wearing hip protectors because they find them uncomfortable and impractical (Parker, Gillespie, and Gillespie 2005). That said, there are recent publications investigating methods of protecting the hips that may lend themselves to clever design, improved comfort and fit, and higher levels of acceptance (Hughes and Nabhani 2018, 579–584; Wardiningsih, Nawaz, and Troynikov 2019, 924–993; Wardiningsih and Troynikov 2019, 1408–1416; Wardiningsih and Troynikov 2019, 5006–5013).

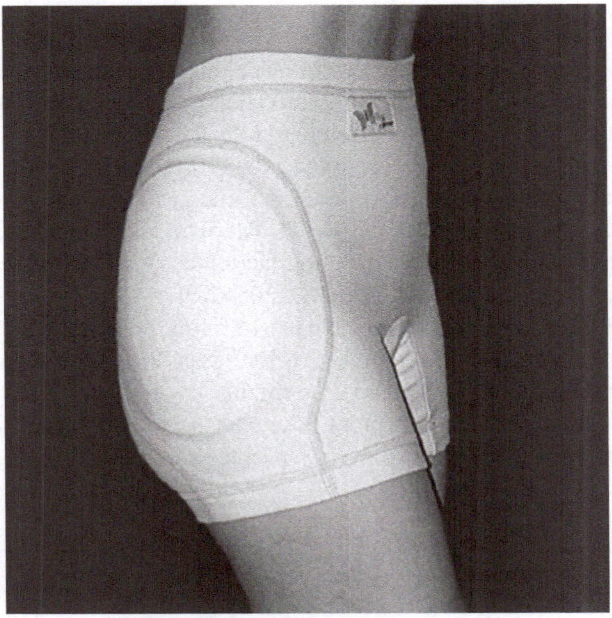

FIGURE 8.8 An example of a hip protector (front view). Reproduced with kind permission granted by Win Health Medical Ltd, Jedburgh, UK.

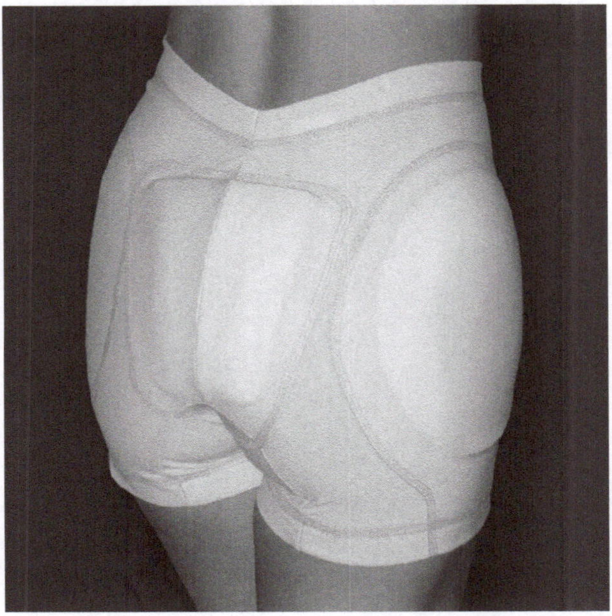

FIGURE 8.9 An example of a hip protector (rear view). Reproduced with kind permission granted by Win Health Medical Ltd, Jedburgh, UK.

8.5.4 Braces and Splints

Braces and splints are common methods of managing many musculoskeletal injuries either as a definitive treatment option, as an adjunct to aid post-operative recovery, or for correcting deformity in the growing child. In recent years, there has been an increasing interest in customising medical and orthopaedic products to provide individual treatment for the patient concerned. Generally speaking, braces may offer protection or assist in protected mobilisation. They can assist in pain relief, improve normal alignment, stretch contractures and facilitate normal movement, and function depending upon their design (Bek 2017, 205–213).

Braces and splints are readily available in two forms: either prefabricated off-the-shelf orthoses or custom-moulded orthoses (Elattar et al. 2018). Customised braces and splints arguably provide a more comfortable fit, lessen the risk of non-compliance, and improve clinical outcomes. They are used in a variety of specialities within medicine and commonly so in orthopaedics as treatment or as an adjunct to

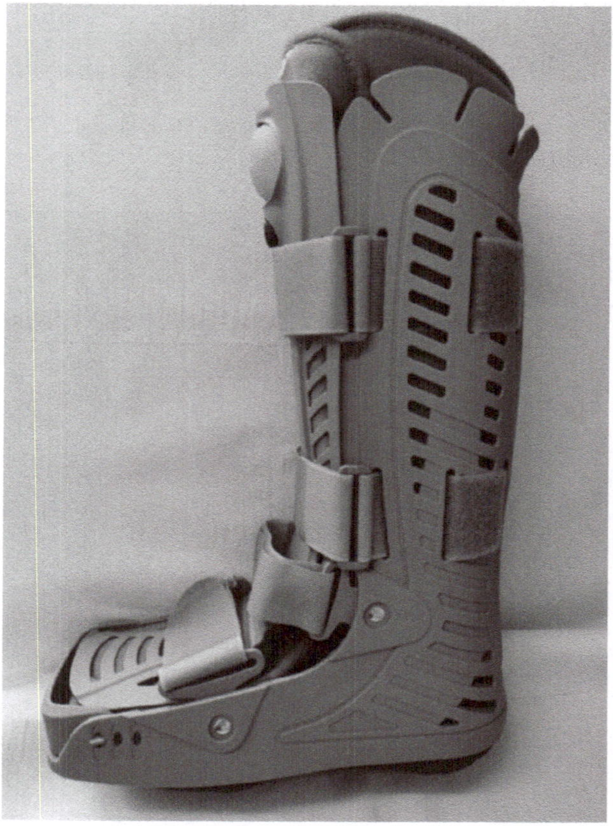

FIGURE 8.10 An example of a below-knee protective boot. Image kindly provided by Mr Harish Kurup, Orthopaedic Surgeon, UK.

aid post-operative recovery. Despite improved design and materials, there are still limitations with using braces and splints (Marinelli et al. 2020, 811–818). Indeed, several Cochrane reviews have been inconclusive as to the benefits of braces and splints in managing a variety of conditions (Duivenvoorden et al. 2015; Hawke et al. 2008; Struiis et al. 2002). That said, they remain a treatment option in the management of acute and chronic orthopaedic issues and the use of thermoplastic materials allows for braces to be quickly and readily manufactured in outpatient clinics for individual patients. Certainly, they have enabled improved early outcomes in the management of Achilles tendon injuries, protected movement following surgical fixation of distal radius, tibial plateau, and ankle fractures. Figure 8.10 and Figure 8.11 provide examples of two commonly available orthoses.

3D printing technology has markedly improved over recent years and several splints and braces have been designed which can be used instead of conventional gypsum plaster. The 3-D-printed casts heal the fracture effectively without casting complications, are patient-specific, ventilated as well as lightweight and feature improved patient comfort, satisfaction, and perceived function. However, the general commercial availability has been hindered by relatively high cost, logistics, and the upskilling required within a clinic set-up to provide this service (Chen et al. 2017, 1–9; Graham et al. 2020, 388–392).

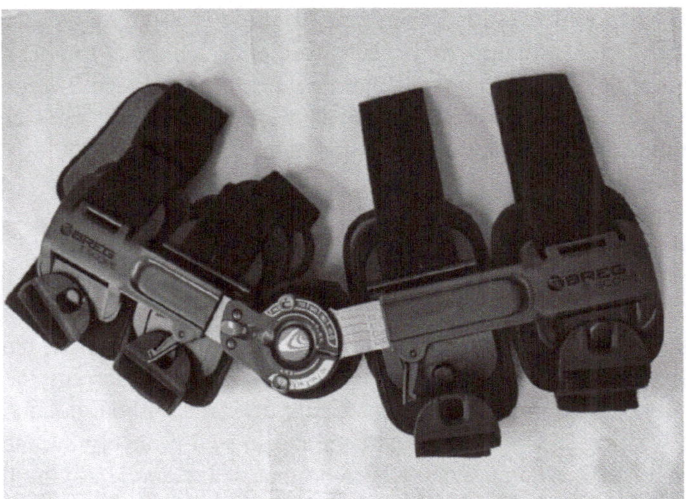

FIGURE 8.11 An example of a knee splint that allows protected range of motion. Image kindly provided by Mr Harish Kurup, Orthopaedic Surgeon, UK. This picture shows a splint used around the knee that allows protected range of motion. A hinge made from two bars sits either side of the leg. These are held in place by straps which have a padded portion to conform to the shape of the leg and Velcro. Image kindly provided by Mr Harish Kurup, Orthopaedic Surgeon, UK.

8.5.5 Scoliosis Braces

Scoliosis is a condition characterised by an abnormal curvature of the spine. Deformities exist in the coronal (AP) and sagittal (lateral) planes and their nature varies based on the underlying subtype of the condition. Beyond the abnormal curves, scoliosis also possesses a rotatory element which compounds the deformity. Once diagnosed, the condition necessitates regular surveillance and appropriate management since, left unchecked, deformity may progress to the extent that it compromises the physiological load capacity of the vertebral column along with function of organs that rely on a straight spine for homeostasis, such as the lungs. Progressive deformity of the thoracic spine, for example, impacts the constitution of the ribcage, itself also deformed as part of the pathophysiological history of progression of the condition; thus interfering with ability of the ribs to facilitate lung inflation.

8.5.5.1 Management of Scoliosis

The essence of scoliosis management involves preventing curve progressions that are at or likely to reach thresholds which will lead to disability. Management revolves around observation, bracing, or surgical correction. It is the magnitude of the curve that dictates which avenue of management best suits a particular patient. There are a number of different curve types that may constitute a scoliosis and whilst classifying them is complex, the general consensus amongst orthopaedic surgeons remains that curves of magnitude greater than 45–50° argue in favour of surgical correction. Those curves of magnitude between 25 and 40° may be amenable to treatment through bracing, the primary mechanism of which seeks to modulate spinal growth as it progresses by applying appropriate external corrective forces opposite to those of the deformity. Because of its dynamic means, bracing is only appropriate in those individuals in whom considerable growth remains (Castro 2003, 1870–1185; Patwardhan et al. 1986, 103–117).

8.5.5.2 Types of Brace

The use of textiles in brace design may be traced as far back as the 1940s, this being the Milwaukee cervico-thoraco-lumbosacral orthosis (CTLSO). Initially used for the treatment of resultant deformity from poliomyelitis, it may be considered primitive by modern standards; nevertheless, it underpins the elements of design from which most modern braces are derived. Without doubt, one of the most negative elements of brace treatment and indeed probably the most significant factor impacting compliance would be that of the social stigma that it portrays. Indeed, many patients favour extensive corrective surgery for this reason (Apter et al. 1978, 156–159).

Advances in textile malleability allowed the evolution of brace design to underarm variants, which became known as thoraco-lumbosacral orthoses or TLSOs. Developed in the 1970s, these allowed the hiding of the brace under clothing and became more attractive to patients as a non-surgical treatment option. Examples of

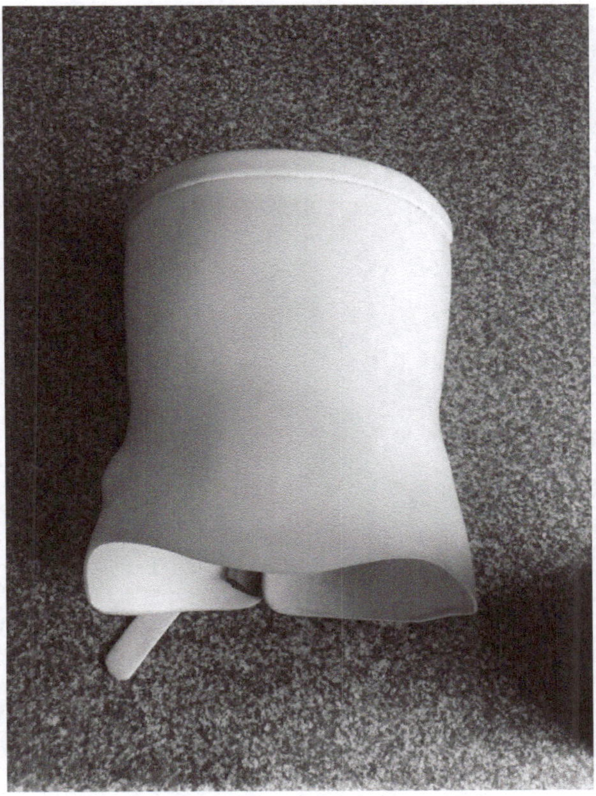

FIGURE 8.12 An example of a brace used to treat scoliosis (front view). Image kindly provided by Mr Wai Weng Yoon, Orthopaedic Surgeon, UK.

these included the Wilmington and Boston braces and indeed the latter of these is still in widespread use today for its applicability, rapidity of manufacture owing to its pre-made fabrication capacity, and corrective efficacy (Emans et al. 1986, 792–801). Figures 8.12 and 8.13 illustrate a Boston brace.

The Wilmington variant affords greater flexibility still, owing to its ability to be custom moulded to a patient to apply multiple deformity corrective forces including de-rotation and then, with the aid of even more modern textiles, facilitate construction of the final brace that is lightweight and closely sculpted, making it an even more desirable choice for patients (Bunnell, et al 1980, 31–38).

The future of even more ergonomic brace manufacture may lie in the ability to marry pre-made fabrication textiles with computer-generated designs (Rigo and Weiss 2008, 303). The composite Rigo System Chêneau is an example of this and has demonstrated considerable success even for curves approaching thresholds that are deemed inappropriate for brace treatment (Weiss et al. 2019, 983–991).

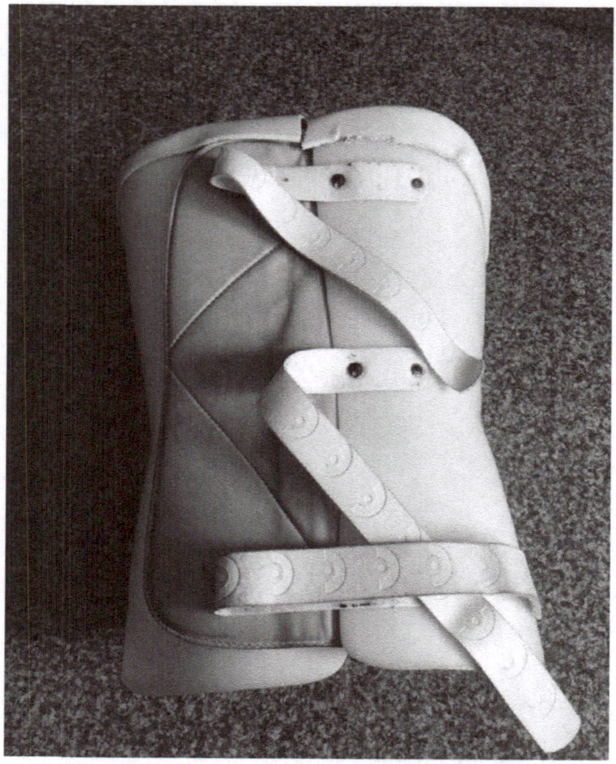

FIGURE 8.13 An example of a brace used to treat scoliosis (rear view). Image kindly provided by Mr Wai Weng Yoon, Orthopaedic Surgeon, UK.

8.5.5.3 Adjuncts to Brace Therapy

A growing body of literature has demonstrated the ability of additional specific exercises to better improve the success of brace treatment. Postural regimes may assist in the improvement of alignment and incorporated breathing exercises ameliorate respiratory function. Several methods have been proposed but irrespective of the one used, there is reasonable suggestion that they provide an effective augment to the realm of non-operative treatment for scoliosis.

8.5.6 Exoskeletons

Exoskeletons are a distinctive kind of robot to be worn as an overall. They effectively support or substitute the owners' own movements (Mikolajewska and Mikolajewski 2011, 227–233).

They can be divided into three broad categories depending upon use.

1. Human performance augmentation
2. Assistive devices for those with disabilities
3. Therapeutic exoskeletons for rehabilitation (Young and Ferris 2016, 171–182)

They may assist all four extremities or just the lower limbs only. The interest in the medical and healthcare use of exoskeletons has been driven by the benefits that the use of a human exoskeleton is closer to 'normal' mobility than using a wheelchair. They have also been perceived as more effective than the traditional assistance and support of therapists and rehabilitative devices (Mikolajewska and Mikolajewski 2011, 227–233). Commercially, the ability to assist the wearer with manual tasks and potentially reduce occupational injuries, for example, to shoulder, back, etc., has driven research into the commercial sector with some of the more advanced exoskeletons using artificial intelligence to power them.

A key driver in the development of exoskeletons is the limited access to rehabilitation clinicians and facilities (Godwin, Wasserman, and Ostwald 2011, 676–684). Body weight-support robot-assisted treadmill training has been shown to lead to comparable or improved functional outcomes in stroke survivors. In the same vein, manually assisted or robot-assisted locomotor training can result in beneficial effects, even for subjects with complete spinal cord injury (Hubli and Dietz 2013, 1–8; Mehrholz and Pohl 2012, 193–199; Van Silfhout et al. 2020, 21). Upper-limb exoskeletons are considered safer than lower-limb exoskeletons because gravity and the potential for falling is eliminated. Another consideration is the risk of fracture from incorrect fitting of exoskeletons that then apply a force to a bone that may have disuse osteopenia (He et al. 2017, 89; Rupal et al. 2017). With the advances in nerve stimulation, the possibility of functioning and life-like exoskeletons/prosthetics that can sense nerve conduction and integrate with the human are also a distinct possibility.

Exoskeletons have also been designed for surgical applications. For example, a passive hand exoskeleton to provide passive assistance (Nishida et al. 2015, 237–243). This may have uses in microsurgery and fine neurosurgical operations where any false movement can have severe consequences.

Prosthetics for amputees are critical in rehabilitation. There have been several advances over the years. There are broad categories: passive devices, body-powered designs, and externally powered designs. Take, for example, the hand. In a hand, the thumb provides approximately 40% of hand function, the index and middle finger 20%, and the ring and little finger 10%. Opposition is critical for normal hand function and the reason why loss of a thumb is so detrimental to hand function. With advances in biomaterials and engineering design, the ability to provide critical grips, such as opposition, three-digit hands, and multi-grasp anthropomorphic hands have seen evolutions in upper-limb prosthetics (Belter, Segil, and SM 2013, 599; Zlotolow and Kozin 2012, 587–593).

Osseo-integration prostheses and innovations have allowed for electrodes to be connected to functioning nerves and hence muscle units. This allows prosthetics to be driven by myoelectric activity and hence mimic the previous limb movements. A recent study reported self-contained, neuromusculoskeletal prosthetic arm (after trans-humeral amputation) that includes sensory feedback from the surface of the prosthetic hand, allowing for intuitive use of the prosthesis in daily life. Implanted electrodes provided bidirectional communication between the prosthesis and electrodes that were implanted in nerves and muscles, thereby creating a self-contained neuromusculoskeletal human–machine interface (Ortiz-Catalan et al. 2020, 1732–1738). Prosthetic fingers can then be covered with materials resembling natural skin. Examples of prosthetics include ProDigits (Optimus Prosthetics, Columbus, OH, USA) and iLIMB (Touch Bionics, Mansfield, MA, USA). Research has been directed at the use of direct brain-wave control for operating prosthetics. Cerebral control has the major advantage that it bypasses the peripheral nervous system in the remaining limb, which may be damaged (da Paz Jr and Braga 2007, 947–951). Another avenue of interest is whether prosthetics can be directly implanted into a stump.

8.6 TESTING OF NON-IMPLANTABLE MEDICAL TEXTILES

Whilst the devices discussed in this chapter are classified as non-implantable, many may still be invasive whilst not meeting the technical definition of an implant (see Chapter 6). In the same manner, some of the devices may be surgically invasive but only transient (less than 60 minutes in place). Regardless of such matters, it is almost certain that many so-called non-implantable items will be in contact with part of the body and, as such, biocompatibility testing will be necessary. If some of the materials chosen have never been used in a medical device before, biocompatibility testing, as per ISO 10993, is necessary, and this is both expensive and time consuming. Over and above that, performance testing will, undoubtedly, be required and carried out in such a way as to meet appropriate testing standards. The performance requirements set must be drawn from the initial product specification and be linked with the associated risk analysis; only in this way will auditors be satisfied.

REFERENCES

Al-Jbour, Nawzat D., Mohammad D. Beg, Jolius Gimbun, and AKM Moshiul Alam. "An overview of chitosan nanofibers and their applications in the drug delivery process." *Current Drug Delivery* 16, no. 4 (2019): 272–294.

Anand, S. C., K. Kanchi Govarthanam, and D. Gazioglu. "A study of the modelling and characterisation of compression garments for hypertrophic scarring after burns. Part 1: Modelling of compression garments." *Journal of the Textile Institute* 104, no. 7 (2013): 661–667.

Anand, S. C., K. Kanchi Govarthanam, and D. Gazioglu. "A study of the modelling and characterisation of compression garments for hypertrophic scarring after burns. Part 2: Characterisation of compression garments." *Journal of the Textile Institute* 104, no. 7 (2013): 668–674.

Anzarut, Alexander, Jarret Olson, Prabhjyot Singh, Brian H. Rowe, and Edward E. Tredget. "The effectiveness of pressure garment therapy for the prevention of abnormal scarring after burn injury: A meta-analysis." *Journal of Plastic, Reconstructive & Aesthetic Surgery* 62, no. 1 (2009): 77–84.

Apter, A., G. Morein, H. Munitz, S. Tyano, B. Maoz, and H. Wijsenbeek. "The psychosocial sequelae of the Milwaukee brace in adolescent girls." *Clinical Orthopaedics and Related Research* 131 (1978): 156–159.

Bain, Emily, Agnes Wilson, Rebecca Tooher, Simon Gates, Lucy-Jane Davis, and Philippa Middleton. "Prophylaxis for venous thromboembolic disease in pregnancy and the early postnatal period." *Cochrane Database of Systematic Reviews* 2 (2014).

Balakrishnan, Biji, M. Mohanty, P. R. Umashankar, and A. Jayakrishnan. "Evaluation of an in situ forming hydrogel wound dressing based on oxidized alginate and gelatin." *Biomaterials* 26, no. 32 (2005): 6335–6342.

Bek, Nilgün. "Splints and orthoses." In *The Shoulder*. Springer, Cham, 2017, pp. 205–213.

Belter, Joseph T., Jacob L. Segil, and BS SM. "Mechanical design and performance specifications of anthropomorphic prosthetic hands: A review." *Journal of Rehabilitation Research and Development* 50, no. 5 (2013): 599.

Bodeker, GerardC, TerenceJ Ryan, and Chi-Keong Ong. "Traditional approaches to wound healing." *Clinics in Dermatology* 17, no. 1 (1999): 93–98.

Bringard, A., S. Perrey, and N. Belluye. "Aerobic energy cost and sensation responses during submaximal running exercise-positive effects of wearing compression tights." *International Journal of Sports Medicine* 27, no. 05 (2006): 373–378.

British Orthopaedic Association. Standards for Trauma. "BOAST 1 Version 2 – Patients Sustainaing a Fragility Hip Fracture". 2012. Accessed March 22nd, 2021. https://www.boa.ac.uk/uploads/assets/6750e0bf-4aa3-4680-b1612265704512db/patients%20sustaining%20a%20fragility%20hip%20fracture.pdf.

British Orthopaedic Association. "Casting Courses". 2020. Accessed Mar 23rd, 2021. https://www.boa.ac.uk/learning-and-events/casting-courses.html.

Brown, Freddy, Conor Gissane, Glyn Howatson, Ken Van Someren, Charles Pedlar, and Jessica Hill. "Compression garments and recovery from exercise: A meta-analysis." *Sports Medicine* 47, no. 11 (2017): 2245–2267.

Bulman, Sophie E.L., Giuseppe Tronci, Parikshit Goswami, Chris Carr, and Stephen J. Russell. "Antibacterial properties of nonwoven wound dressings coated with Manuka honey or methylglyoxal." *Materials* 10, no. 8 (2017): 954.

Bunnell, William P., G. D. MacEwen, and S. H. A. N. M. U. G. A. Jayakumar. "The use of plastic jackets in the non-operative treatment of idiopathic scoliosis. Preliminary report." *The Journal of Bone and Joint Surgery*. American volume 62, no. 1 (1980): 31–38.

Bynum, Bill, and Helen Bynum. "Inguinal hernia truss." *The Lancet* 389, no. 10076 (2017): 1289.

Castro Jr, Frank P. "Adolescent idiopathic scoliosis, bracing, and the Hueter-Volkmann principle." *The Spine Journal* 3, no. 3 (2003): 180–185.

Charnley, J. 1999. "The Closed Treatment of Closed Fractures, 4th edition." Cambridge University Press/The John Charnley Trust.

Chen, A. H., S. G. Frangos, S. Kilaru, and B. E. Sumpio. "Intermittent pneumatic compression devices–Physiological mechanisms of action." *European Journal of Vascular and Endovascular Surgery* 21, no. 5 (2001): 383–392.

Chen, Yan-Jun, Hui Lin, Xiaodong Zhang, Wenhua Huang, Lin Shi, and Defeng Wang. "Application of 3D–printed and patient-specific cast for the treatment of distal radius fractures: Initial experience." *3D Printing in Medicine* 3, no. 1 (2017): 1–9.

Chi, Chia-Fen, Chih-Hsiang Lin, and Han-Sheng Yang. "The causal analysis of requested alterations for pressure garments." *Journal of Burn Care & Research* 29, no. 6 (2008): 965–974.

Clarke, Mike J., Cathryn Broderick, Sally Hopewell, Ed Juszczak, and Anne Eisinga. "Compression stockings for preventing deep vein thrombosis in airline passengers." *Cochrane Database of Systematic Reviews* 9 (2016).

Coghlan, Nicole, Jodie Copley, Tammy Aplin, and Jenny Strong. "Patient experience of wearing compression garments post burn injury: A review of the literature." *Journal of Burn Care & Research* 38, no. 4 (2017): 260–269.

da Paz Jr, Aloysio Campos, and Lucia Willadino Braga. "Brain activation in a myoelectric prosthetic hand: The role of the brain in the rehabilitation of amputees." *Journal of Pediatric Orthopaedics* 27, no. 8 (2007): 947–951.

Davies, Vanessa, Kevin G. Thompson, and Stephen-Mark Cooper. "The effects of compression garments on recovery." *The Journal of Strength & Conditioning Research* 23, no. 6 (2009): 1786–1794.

Davis, Stephen C., and Robert Perez. "Cosmeceuticals and natural products: Wound healing." *Clinics in Dermatology* 27, no. 5 (2009): 502–506.

DeBruler, Danielle M., Molly E. Baumann, Britani N. Blackstone, Jacob C. Zbinden, Kevin L. McFarland, J. Kevin Bailey, Dorothy M. Supp, and Heather M. Powell. "Role of early application of pressure garments following burn injury and autografting." *Plastic and Reconstructive Surgery* 143, no. 2 (2019): 310e–321e.

DeBruler, Danielle M., Jacob C. Zbinden, Molly E. Baumann, Britani N. Blackstone, Megan M. Malara, J. Kevin Bailey, Dorothy M. Supp, and Heather M. Powell. "Early cessation of pressure garment therapy results in scar contraction and thickening." *PloS one* 13, no. 6 (2018): e0197558.

Dhandha, Maulik Manharlal, and Elaine C. Siegfried. "Cost-effective, custom-designed wet wrap garments for children: Experience at Cardinal Glennon children's hospital." *SKIN The Journal of Cutaneous Medicine* 1, no. 1 (2017): 48–51.

Dhivya, Selvaraj, Viswanadha Vijaya Padma, and Elango Santhini. "Wound dressings–A review." *BioMedicine* 5, no. 4 (2015).

Di Nisio, Marcello, Frank Peinemann, Ettore Porreca, and Anne W.S. Rutjes. "Primary prophylaxis for venous thromboembolism in patients undergoing cardiac or thoracic surgery." *Cochrane Database of Systematic Reviews* 6 (2015).

Douglas, Helen E., and Fiona Wood. "Burns dressings." *Australian Family Physician* 46, no. 3 (2017): 94–97.

Dubuis, Laura, Pierre-Yves Rohan, Stéphane Avril, Pierre Badel, and Johan Debayle. "Patient-specific FE model of the leg under elastic compression." In 10th International Symposium on Computer Methods in Biomechanics and Biomedical Engineering, p. 6. 2012.

Duivenvoorden, Tijs, Reinoud W. Brouwer, Tom M. van Raaij, Arianne P. Verhagen, Jan A. N. Verhaar, and Sita M. A. Bierma-Zeinstra. "Braces and orthoses for treating osteoarthritis of the knee." *Cochrane Database of Systematic Reviews* 3 (2015).

Elattar, Osama, Tyler Smith, Adam Ferguson, Daniel Farber, and Keith Wapner. "Uses of braces and orthotics for conservative management of foot and ankle disorders." *Foot & Ankle Orthopaedics* 3, no. 3 (2018): 2473011418780700.

Emans, John B., Andre Kaelin, Philippe Bancel, John E. Hall, and M. E. Miller. "The Boston bracing system for idiopathic scoliosis. Follow-up results in 295 patients." *Spine* 11, no. 8 (1986): 792–801.

Faisal Siddique, Hafiz, Adnan Mazari, Antonin Havelka, Zdenek Kus, David Cirkl, and Lubos Hes. "New approach for the prediction of compression pressure using the cut strip method." *Textile Research Journal* 90, no. 15–16 (2020): 1689–1703.

Finnerty, Celeste C., Marc G. Jeschke, Ludwik K. Branski, Juan P. Barret, Peter Dziewulski, and David N. Herndon. "Hypertrophic scarring: The greatest unmet challenge after burn injury." *The Lancet* 388, no. 10052 (2016): 1427–1436.

Godwin, Kyler M., Joan Wasserman, and Sharon K. Ostwald. "Cost associated with stroke: Outpatient rehabilitative services and medication." *Topics in Stroke Rehabilitation* 18 Supplement 1, no. sup1 (2011): 676–684.

Graham, Jack, Mark Wang, Kaela Frizzell, Cynthia Watkins, Pedro Beredjiklian, and Michael Rivlin. "Conventional vs 3-dimensional printed cast wear comfort." *Hand* 15, no. 3 (2020): 388–392.

Hakimi, Osnat, David P. Knight, Fritz Vollrath, and Pankaj Vadgama. "Spider and mulberry silkworm silks as compatible biomaterials." *Composites Part B: Engineering* 38, no. 3 (2007): 324–337.

Hanna, James R., and Joseph A. Giacopelli. "A review of wound healing and wound dressing products." *The Journal of Foot and Ankle Surgery* 36, no. 1 (1997): 2–14.

Harris, Isobel M., Kwang Chear Lee, Jonathan J. Deeks, David J. Moore, Naiem S. Moiemen, and Janine Dretzke. "Pressure-garment therapy for preventing hypertrophic scarring after burn injury." *Cochrane Database of Systematic Reviews* 1 (2020).

Hawke, Fiona, Joshua Burns, Joel A. Radford, and Verona Du Toit. "Custom-made foot orthoses for the treatment of foot pain." *Cochrane Database of Systematic Reviews* 3 (2008).

He, Yongtian, David Eguren, Trieu Phat Luu, and Jose L. Contreras-Vidal. "Risk management and regulations for lower limb medical exoskeletons: A review." *Medical Devices (Auckland, NZ)* 10 (2017): 89.

Hebeish, A., M. H. El-Rafie, M. A. El-Sheikh, Amany A. Seleem, and Mehrez E. El-Naggar. "Antimicrobial wound dressing and anti-inflammatory efficacy of silver nanoparticles." *International Journal of Biological Macromolecules* 65 (2014): 509–515.

Hong, Liu, Chen Dongsheng, Wei Qufu, and Pan Ruru. "A study of the relationship between clothing pressure and garment bust strain, and Young's modulus of fabric, based on a finite element model." *Textile Research Journal* 81, no. 13 (2011): 1307–1319.

Hosseini, Seyed Mehdi, Reza Fekrazad, Hamid Malekzadeh, Parviz Farzadinia, and Mohammadreza Hajiani. "Evaluation and comparison of the effect of honey, milk and combination of honey–milk on experimental induced second-degree burns of Rabit." *Journal of Family Medicine and Primary Care* 9, no. 2 (2020): 915.

Hsu, Wei-Chun, Li-Wen Tseng, Fu-Chun Chen, Li-Chu Wang, Wen-Wen Yang, Yi-Jia Lin, and Chiang Liu. "Effects of compression garments on surface EMG and physiological responses during and after distance running." *Journal of Sport and Health Science* (2017).

Hubli, Michèle, and Volker Dietz. "The physiological basis of neurorehabilitation-locomotor training after spinal cord injury." *Journal of Neuroengineering and Rehabilitation* 10, no. 1 (2013): 1–8.

Hughes, David, and Farhad Nabhani. "Comparison of impact energy absorbance by various combinations of hip protector and flooring material." *Current Orthopaedic Practice* 29, no. 6 (2018): 579–584.

Johnson, Sue. "Compression hosiery in the prevention and treatment of venous leg ulcers." *Journal of Tissue Viability* 12, no. 2 (2002): 67–74.

Jull, Andrew B., Nicky Cullum, Jo C. Dumville, Maggie J. Westby, Sohan Deshpande, and Natalie Walker. "Honey as a topical treatment for wounds." *Cochrane Database of Systematic Reviews* 3 (2015).

Kahn, Susan R., David R. Morrison, Gisèle Diendéré, Alexandre Piché, Kristian B. Filion, Adi J. Klil-Drori, James D. Douketis et al. "Interventions for implementation of thromboprophylaxis in hospitalized patients at risk for venous thromboembolism." *Cochrane Database of Systematic Reviews* 4 (2018).

Kim, Jayne Y., James J. Willard, Dorothy M. Supp, Sashwati Roy, Gayle M. Gordillo, Chandan K. Sen, and Heather M. Powell. "Burn scar biomechanics following pressure garment therapy." *Plastic and Reconstructive Surgery* 136, no. 3 (2015): 572.

Kim, Jieun, Jooyoung Kim, and Joohyung Lee. "Effect of compression garments on delayed-onset muscle soreness and blood inflammatory markers after eccentric exercise: A randomized controlled trial." *Journal of Exercise Rehabilitation* 13, no. 5 (2017): 541.

Klasen, H. J. "A historical review of the use of silver in the treatment of burns. II. Renewed interest for silver." *Burns* 26, no. 2 (2000): 131–138.

Koike, Tatsuya, Y. Orito, Hiroshi Toyoda, M. Tada, R. Sugama, M. Hoshino, Y. Nakao et al. "External hip protectors are effective for the elderly with higher-than-average risk factors for hip fractures." *Osteoporosis International* 20, no. 9 (2009): 1613–1620.

Kurup, H. V., C. I. M. Clark, and R. K. Dega. "Footwear and orthopaedics." *Foot and Ankle Surgery* 18, no. 2 (2012): 79–83.

Kwakman, Paulus H. S., Anje A. te Velde, Leonie de Boer, Dave Speijer, M. J. Christina Vandenbroucke-Grauls, and Sebastian A. J. Zaat. "How honey kills bacteria." *The FASEB Journal* 24, no. 7 (2010): 2576–2582.

Law, N. W., and J. E. Trapnell. "Does a truss benefit a patient with inguinal hernia?." *BMJ: British Medical Journal* 304, no. 6834 (1992): 1092.

Leung, W. Y., D. W. Yuen, Sun Pui Ng, and San-Qiang Shi. "Pressure prediction model for compression garment design." *Journal of Burn Care & Research* 31, no. 5 (2010): 716–727.

Liang, Donghui, Zhong Lu, Hao Yang, Jingting Gao, and Rong Chen. "Novel asymmetric wettable AgNPs/chitosan wound dressing: In vitro and in vivo evaluation." *ACS Applied Materials & Interfaces* 8, no. 6 (2016): 3958–3968.

Liu, Gongyan, Jun Xiang, Qiongfen Xia, Kaijun Li, Tianxiang Lan, and Ling Yu. "Superhydrophobic cotton gauze with durably antibacterial activity as skin wound dressing." *Cellulose* 26, no. 2 (2019): 1383–1397.

Liu, Rong, Xia Guo, Terence T. Lao, and Trevor Little. "A critical review on compression textiles for compression therapy: Textile-based compression interventions for chronic venous insufficiency." *Textile Research Journal* 87, no. 9 (2017): 1121–1141.

Liu, Rong, Xia Guo, Qiujin Peng, Le Zhang, Terence T. Lao, Trevor Little, Jundong Liu, and Eric Chan. "Stratified body shape-driven sizing system via three-dimensional digital anthropometry for compression textiles of lower extremities." *Textile Research Journal* 88, no. 18 (2018): 2055–2075.

Liu, Rong, Yi-Lin Kwok, Yi Li, and Terence-T. Lao. "Fabric mechanical-surface properties of compression hosiery and their effects on skin pressure magnitudes when worn." *Fibres & Textiles in Eastern Europe* 18, no. 2 (2010): 79.

Liu, Rong, Terence T. Lao, Trevor J. Little, Xinbo Wu, and Xiao Ke. "Can heterogeneous compression textile design reshape skin pressures? A fundamental study." *Textile Research Journal* 88, no. 17 (2018): 1915–1930.

Liu, Rong, Jundong Liu, Terence T. Lao, Michael Ying, and Xinbo Wu. "Determination of leg cross-sectional curvatures and application in pressure prediction for lower body compression garments." *Textile Research Journal* 89, no. 10 (2019): 1835–1852.

Liu, Yuyang, John Haozhong Xin, and Chang-Hwan Choi. "Cotton fabrics with single-faced superhydrophobicity." *Langmuir* 28, no. 50 (2012): 17426–17434.

Macintyre, Lisa, Monali Dahale, and Michelle Rae. "Impact of moisture on the pressure delivering potential of pressure garments." *Journal of Burn Care & Research* 37, no. 4 (2016): e365–e373.

Macintyre, Lisa, Sian Gilmartin, and Michelle Rae. "The impact of design variables and aftercare regime on the long-term performance of pressure garments." *Journal of Burn Care & Research* 28, no. 5 (2007): 725–733.

MacRae, Braid A., Raechel M. Laing, and Hugo Partsch. "General considerations for compression garments in sports: Applied pressures and body coverage." In *Compression garments in sports: Athletic performance and recovery*. Springer, Cham, 2016, pp. 1–32.

Maklewska, Elzbieta, Andrzej Nawrocki, J. Ledwoń, and Krzysztof Kowalski. "Modelling and designing of knitted products used in compressive therapy." *Fibres & Textiles in Eastern Europe* 5 (59) (2006): 111–113.

Malara, Megan M., Jayne Y. Kim, J. Alexander Clark, Britani N. Blackstone, Mark A. Ruegsegger, J. Kevin Bailey, Dorothy M. Supp, and Heather M. Powell. "Structural, chemical, and mechanical properties of pressure garments as a function of simulated use and repeated laundering." *Journal of Burn Care & Research* 39, no. 4 (2018): 562–571.

Maleki, Homa, Marzie Aghajani, A. H. Sadeghi, and Ali Asghar Asgharian Jeddi. "On the pressure behavior of tubular weft knitted fabrics constructed from textured polyester yarns." *Journal of Engineered Fibers and Fabrics* 6, no. 2 (2011): 155892501100600204.

Maqsood, Muhammad, Tanveer Hussain, Naseer Ahmad, and Yasir Nawab. "Multi-response optimization of mechanical and comfort properties of bi-stretch woven fabrics using grey relational analysis in Taguchi method." *The Journal of the Textile Institute* 108, no. 5 (2017): 794–802.

Maqsood, Muhammad, Tanveer Hussain, Mumtaz Hasan Malik, and Yasir Nawab. "Modeling the effect of elastane linear density, fabric thread density, and weave float on the stretch, recovery, and compression properties of bi-stretch woven fabrics for compression garments." *The Journal of The Textile Institute* 107, no. 3 (2016): 307–315.

Maqsood, Muhammad, Yasir Nawab, Jawairia Umar, Muhammad Umair, and Khubab Shaker. "Comparison of compression properties of stretchable knitted fabrics and bi-stretch woven fabrics for compression garments." *The Journal of the Textile Institute* 108, no. 4 (2017): 522–527.

Marinelli, Alessandro, Enrico Guerra, Alice Ritali, and Roberto Rotini. "Elbow brace and rehabilitation." In *Surgical Techniques for Trauma and Sports Related Injuries of the Elbow*. Springer, Berlin, Heidelberg, 2020, pp. 811–818.

Matica, Mariana Adina, Finn Lillelund Aachmann, Anne Tøndervik, Håvard Sletta, and Vasile Ostafe. "Chitosan as a wound dressing starting material: Antimicrobial properties and mode of action." *International Journal of Molecular Sciences* 20, no. 23 (2019): 5889.

Mehrholz, Jan, and Marcus Pohl. "Electromechanical-assisted gait training after stroke: A systematic review comparing end-effector and exoskeleton devices." *Journal of Rehabilitation Medicine* 44, no. 3 (2012): 193–199.

Mi, Fwu-Long, Yu-Bey Wu, Shin-Shing Shyu, Jen-Yu Schoung, Yaw-Bin Huang, Yi-Hung Tsai, and Jong-Yun Hao. "Control of wound infections using a bilayer chitosan wound dressing with sustainable antibiotic delivery." *Journal of Biomedical Materials Research: An Official Journal of The Society for Biomaterials, The Japanese Society for Biomaterials, and The Australian Society for Biomaterials and the Korean Society for Biomaterials* 59, no. 3 (2002): 438–449.

Mikołajewska, Emilia, and Dariusz Mikołajewski. "Exoskeletons in neurological diseases-current and potential future applications." *Advances in Clinical and Expimental Medicine* 20, no. 2 (2011): 227–233.

Moiemen, Naiem, Jonathan Mathers, Laura Jones, Jonathan Bishop, Philip Kinghorn, Mark Monahan, Melanie Calvert et al. "Pressure garment to prevent abnormal scarring after burn injury in adults and children: The PEGASUS feasibility RCT and mixed-methods study." *Health Technology Assessment (Winchester, England)* 22, no. 36 (2018): 1.

Molan, Peter C. "The evidence supporting the use of honey as a wound dressing." *The International Journal of Lower Extremity Wounds* 5, no. 1 (2006): 40–54.

Nabuurs-Franssen, Marrigje H., Ron Sleegers, Maya S. P. Huijberts, Wiel Wijnen, Antal P. Sanders, Geert Walenkamp, and Nicolaas C. Schaper. "Total contact casting of the diabetic foot in daily practice: A prospective follow-up study." *Diabetes Care* 28, no. 2 (2005): 243–247.

National Institute for Health and Care Excellence. "Venous Thromboembolism Overview". 2021. Accessed 22nd March, 2021. https://pathways.nice.org.uk/pathways/venous-thromboembolism/reducing-venous-thromboembolism-risk-in-hospital-patients#path=view%3A/pathways/venous-thromboembolism/venous-thromboembolism-overview.xml&content=view-index.

Nedelec, Bernadette, Ana De Oliveira, Valerie Calva, Marie-Andrée Couture, Chantale Poulin, Leo LaSalle, and José A. Correa. "Longitudinal evaluation of pressure applied by custom fabricated garments worn by adult burn survivors." *Journal of Burn Care & Research* 41, no. 2 (2020): 254–262.

Nelson, E. Andrea, and Sally E. M. Bell-Syer. "Compression for preventing recurrence of venous ulcers." *Cochrane Database of Systematic Reviews* 9 (2014).

Nešporová, Kristina, Vojtěch Pavlík, Barbora Šafránková, Hana Vágnerová, Pavel Odráška, Ondřej Žídek, Natálie Císařová, Svitlana Skoroplyas, Lukáš Kubala, and Vladimír Velebný. "Effects of wound dressings containing silver on skin and immune cells." *Scientific Reports* 10, no. 1 (2020): 1–14.

Nishida, Jun, Kei Nakai, Akira Matsushita, and Kenji Suzuki. "Haptic augmentation of surgical operation using a passive hand exoskeleton." In *Haptic Interaction*. Springer, Tokyo, 2015, pp. 237–243.

Ortiz-Catalan, Max, Enzo Mastinu, Paolo Sassu, Oskar Aszmann, and Rickard Brånemark. "Self-contained neuromusculoskeletal arm prostheses." *New England Journal of Medicine* 382, no. 18 (2020): 1732–1738.

Parker, Martyn J., William J. Gillespie, and Lesley D. Gillespie. "Hip protectors for preventing hip fractures in older people." *Cochrane Database of Systematic Reviews* 3 (2005).

Patwardhan, Avinash G., Wilton H. Bunch, Kevin P. Meade, Ray Vanderby Jr, and Gary W. Knight. "A biomechanical analog of curve progression and orthotic stabilization in idiopathic scoliosis." *Journal of Biomechanics* 19, no. 2 (1986): 103–117.

Paul, Willi, and Chandra P. Sharma. "Chitosan and alginate wound dressings: A short review." *Trends Biomater Artificial Organs* 18, no. 1 (2004): 18–23.

Peck, Michael D. "Epidemiology of burns throughout the world. Part I: Distribution and risk factors." *Burns* 37, no. 7 (2011): 1087–1100.

Peršin, Zdenka, Matej Ravber, Karin Stana Kleinschek, Željko Knez, Mojca Škerget, and Manja Kurečič. "Bio-nanofibrous mats as potential delivering systems of natural substances." *Textile Research Journal* 87, no. 4 (2017): 444–459.

Pruitt, Basil A., and Norman S. Levine. "Characteristics and uses of biologic dressings and skin substitutes." *Archives of Surgery* 119, no. 3 (1984): 312–322.

Qin, Yimin, ed. *Medical Textile Materials*. Woodhead Publishing, 2015.

Queen, Douglas, Heather Orsted, Hiromi Sanada, and Geoff Sussman. "A dressing history." *International Wound Journal* 1, no. 1 (2004): 59–77.

Rajendran, Subbiyan, ed. *Advanced Textiles for Wound Care*. Woodhead Publishing, 2018.

Rigo, Manuel, and H. Weiss. "The Chêneau concept of bracing-biomechanical aspects." *Studies in Health Technology and Informatics* 35 (2008): 303.

Rupal, Baltej Singh, Sajid Rafique, Ashish Singla, Ekta Singla, Magnus Isaksson, and Gurvinder Singh Virk. "Lower-limb exoskeletons: Research trends and regulatory guidelines in medical and non-medical applications." *International Journal of Advanced Robotic Systems* 14, no. 6 (2017): 1729881417743554.

Sajid, Muhammad S., Mital Desai, Richard W. Morris, and George Hamilton. "Knee length versus thigh length graduated compression stockings for prevention of deep vein thrombosis in postoperative surgical patients." *Cochrane Database of Systematic Reviews* 5 (2012).

Sarı, Burak, and Nida Oğlakcıoğlu. "Analysis of the parameters affecting pressure characteristics of medical stockings." *Journal of Industrial Textiles* 47, no. 6 (2018): 1083–1096.

Sato, Tomoi, and Go Miyata. "The nutraceutical benefit, part iii: Honey." *Nutrition (Burbank, Los Angeles County, Calif.)* 16, no. 6 (2000): 468–469.

Senthilkumar, Mani. "Effect of spandex input tension, spandex linear density and cotton yarn loop length on dynamic elastic behavior of cotton/spandex knitted fabrics." *Journal of Textile and Apparel, Technology and Management* 7, no. 4 (2012).

Sharma, Hemant, and Dhanasekara Prabu. "Plaster of Paris: Past, present and future." *Journal of Clinical Orthopaedics and Trauma* 4, no. 3 (2013): 107.

Storm-Versloot, Marja N., Cornelis G. Vos, Dirk T. Ubbink, and Hester Vermeulen. "Topical silver for preventing wound infection." *Cochrane Database of Systematic Reviews* 3 (2010).

Struijs, Peter A. A., Nynke Smidt, H. Arola, C. N. Van Dijk, Rachelle Buchbinder, and Willem J. J. Assendelft. "Orthotic devices for the treatment of tennis elbow." *Cochrane Database of Systematic Reviews* 1 (2002).

The Textile Institute. "Wound Dressing Materials; Surgical Dressings." Textile Terms and Definitions; 2021. https://www.ttandd.org/content/textile-terms-and-definitions and Textile Terms and Definitions, 11th edition; Edited by Denton, M. J. and Daniels, P. N., p. 397.

Tornetta, P. III. "Rockwood and Green's Fractures in Adults, 9th edition". The Orthopedic Trauma Association, Wolters-Kluwer Health, Philadelphia, USA, 2020.

Townsend, C. "Sabiston Textbook of Surgery, 20th edition." Elsevier, 2016.

Tredget, Edward E., Jeffrey W. Shupp, and Jeffrey C. Schneider. "Scar management following burn injury." *Journal of Burn Care & Research* 38, no. 3 (2017): 146–147.

Van Silfhout, L., M. J. R. Edwards, A. J. F. Hosman, H. Van de Meent, and R. H. M. A. Bartels. "The ability to walk after a spinal cord injury with emphasis on exoskeletons: A review." *Moving Forward* 6, no. 5 (2020): 21.

Wardiningsih, Wiah, Nazia Nawaz, and Olga Troynikov. "Performance relevant to the thermophysiological wear comfort of hip protective garments, Part I: Clothing area factor of hip protective garments in clothing ensembles." *The Journal of the Textile Institute* 110, no. 6 (2019): 924–931.

Wardiningsih, Wiah, and Olga Troynikov. "Interface pressure generated by knitted fabrics of different direction, composition and number of layers in sport compression garments." *The Journal of the Textile Institute* 110, no. 6 (2019): 882–890.

Wardiningsih, Wiah, and Olga Troynikov. "Treated knitted fabric for hip-protective pads for elderly women, Part I: Force attenuation capacity." *Textile Research Journal* 89, no. 8 (2019): 1408–1416.

Wardiningsih, Wiah, and Olga Troynikov. "Treated knitted fabric for hip protective pads for elderly women. Part II. Performance relevant to thermal comfort." *Textile Research Journal* 89, no. 23–24 (2019): 5006–5013.

Wasiak, Jason, Heather Cleland, Fiona Campbell, and Anneliese Spinks. "Dressings for superficial and partial thickness burns." *Cochrane Database of Systematic Reviews* 3 (2013).

Weiss, Hans-Rudolf, Deborah Turnbull, Sarah Seibel, and Alexander Kleban. "First end-result of a prospective cohort with AIS treated with a CAD Chêneau style brace." *Journal of Physical Therapy Science* 31, no. 12 (2019): 983–991.

World Health Organization. "Fall". 2018. Accessed March 22, 2021. https://www.who.int/news-room/fact-sheets/detail/falls.

Xia, Guixue, Dongqing Zhai, Yue Sun, Lin Hou, Xiaofan Guo, Lixia Wang, Zhijian Li, and Feng Wang. "Preparation of a novel asymmetric wettable chitosan-based sponge and its role in promoting chronic wound healing." *Carbohydrate Polymers* 227 (2020): 115296.

Yang, Xingxing, Linpeng Fan, Linlin Ma, Yunyi Wang, Si Lin, Fan Yu, Xiaohan Pan, Gejie Luo, Dongdong Zhang, and Hongsheng Wang. "Green electrospun Manuka honey/silk fibroin fibrous matrices as potential wound dressing." *Materials & Design* 119 (2017): 76–84.

Yang, Yadie, and Hong Hu. "Spacer fabric-based exuding wound dressing–Part I: Structural design, fabrication and property evaluation of spacer fabrics." *Textile Research Journal* 87, no. 12 (2017): 1469–1480.

Yang, Yadie, and Hong Hu. "Spacer fabric-based exuding wound dressing–Part II: Comparison with commercial wound dressings." *Textile Research Journal* 87, no. 12 (2017): 1481–1493.

Yıldız, Nilüfer. "A novel technique to determine pressure in pressure garments for hypertrophic burn scars and comfort properties." *Burns* 33, no. 1 (2007): 59–64.

Young, Aaron J., and Daniel P. Ferris. "State of the art and future directions for lower limb robotic exoskeletons." *IEEE Transactions on Neural Systems and Rehabilitation Engineering* 25, no. 2 (2016): 171–182.

Yu, Annie, Kit Lun Yick, Sun Pui Ng, and Joanne Yip. "Prediction of fabric tension and pressure decay for the development of pressure therapy gloves." *Textile Research Journal* 83, no. 3 (2013): 269–287.

Zhao, Jin Min, Mao Lin He, Zeng Ming Xiao, Ting Song Li, Hao Wu, and Hua Jiang. "Different types of intermittent pneumatic compression devices for preventing venous thromboembolism in patients after total hip replacement." *Cochrane Database of Systematic Reviews* 11 (2012).

Zhu, Tang, Junrong Wu, Ning Zhao, Chao Cai, Zhenchao Qian, Fangfang Si, Heng Luo et al. "Superhydrophobic/superhydrophilic janus fabrics reducing blood loss." *Advanced Healthcare Materials* 7, no. 7 (2018): 1701086.

Zlotolow, Dan A., and Scott H. Kozin. "Advances in upper extremity prosthetics." *Hand Clinics* 28, no. 4 (2012): 587–593.

9 Healthcare, Hygiene, and Personal Protective Equipment (PPE)

9.1 INTRODUCTION

Healthcare hygiene and personal protective equipment (PPE) in the medical textile sector cover a vast range from products used for disinfection such as disposable and reusable cleaning materials, through bed linen, furniture and fittings, patient wear and staff clothing, and protective wear. The environment for which they are intended ranges from the operating theatre and the hospital ward, through to clinics and care homes. The range extends from:

i) Items described as 'linen,' as defined for example by the UK Department of Health in their guidance on decontamination of linen for health and social care (where they take it as meaning all reusable textile items requiring cleaning/disinfection via laundry processing including bed linen (blankets, counterpanes, cot sheets and blankets, duvets, duvet covers, pillowcases, and sheets including those which are woven, knitted, half sheets, draw and slide sheets); bibs; blankets; canvases; curtains; hoist slings; patient clothing (gowns, nightdresses and shirts, pyjama tops and bottoms); staff clothing (coats, scrub suits, tabards, uniforms); and towels) (Department of Health, March 2016).
ii) Other items that fall within the healthcare and hygiene category of medical textiles but are not included by the Department of Health in their definition of 'linen' such as orthotic devices and operating table covers and chair seat coverings.
iii) Sanitary wear such as diapers and female hygiene products.
iv) Wipes and surface cleaning materials.
v) Air conditioning filtration devices intended to reduce the exposure of patients and healthcare personnel to pathogens in the healthcare environment.
vi) PPE such as surgical gowns, surgical masks, filtering facepieces (respirators), and gloves.

The types of fibres most commonly used in medical textiles for healthcare, hygiene and personal protective equipment include polyester, polypropylene, viscose rayon, lyocell, and cotton, and may be woven (for reusable items) or non-woven. From a

DOI: 10.1201/9781003170570-9

study concerning the manufacture of non-wovens including polyester, polypropylene, viscose rayon, raw cotton, mechanically cleaned cotton and scoured and bleached cotton, hydro-entanglement was considered to offer advantages in terms of reducing the microbiological burden to such a level as to offer a good base from which more taxing hygiene requirements can be developed (Hinchcliffe et al. 2014). For environments where it is considered necessary not only to try to minimise escape into the atmosphere of tiny flakes of skin or hair from healthcare personnel by enclosing them in scrubs and PPE but also to try to keep loss of fine fibrils from fibres to a minimum, it is best that the fibres used in the garments are synthetic polymer types. However, there is a compromise to be reached in that fabrics composed solely of those fibre types tend to be uncomfortable to wear.

9.2 HEALTHCARE EQUIPMENT

9.2.1 Desirable Properties in Healthcare Equipment

For preference, healthcare equipment should contribute wherever it can to the hygiene and safety of those in the healthcare environment for which it is intended to be a part, namely the patients, healthcare workers and visitors. If it is not possible for an item to be active against pathogens, it should at least be able to be easily cleaned and disinfected. Just because an item or device is traditionally described in a particular way, does not necessarily mean that it will be adequately or fully effective. For instance, those items which have been treated and are thought to be antimicrobial must be able to demonstrate adequate measurable performance in the type of environment for which they are intended. A surgical gown may have been treated with an antimicrobial agent, but that does not necessarily mean that it will exert any such action in practice, and in fact as will be seen later in Section 9.4, that is hardly ever the case up to the present day.

9.2.2 Furniture, Furnishings, and Coverings

A wide range of textiles are used in healthcare and medical equipment, for example, the coverings of clinic couches and chairs through to the curtains that separate bed spaces upon the ward. Whilst there are specifications for disposable surgeon's gloves, test methods for surgical masks to determine blood penetration and test methods to determine wet bacterial penetration including by rubbing through gowns, clean air suits and surgical drapes, there is nothing for furnishings and furniture other than safety tests for electrically driven items and specification for bed castors (ISO 2021). The omission is surprising given that hygiene and ease of cleaning are key considerations in reducing the risk of transmission of infection, not least that of the padding and coverings of operating tables and of supports used to protect pressure points for the patient; infection transmission needs to be minimised and, in addition, the ability of materials to protect the skin without being causative in a pressure sore is a key requirement. To meet the needs set by scarce resources and concerns about pollution, sheets, and bed coverings on inpatient beds need to be designed to match an increasingly pressing economic and environmental context, so life-cycle assessment of all items should be routinely undertaken. The reduced cost and carbon footprint of laundering high-volume-use items compared with single-use and disposal need to be addressed, especially since the development of economical low-temperature laundry systems such as those which utilise ozone to clean and disinfect and report on the achievement of disinfection after processing each load (JLA 2021). A series of British Standards do exist to which bedding can be designed and these include standards for: Mattress covers: (BS 5223-4:1976. Specification for hospital bedding. *Mattress covers of polyurethane coated nylon*), and Pillows: (BS 5223-3:1976. Specification for hospital bedding. *Flexible polyurethane pillows*) (British Standards Institution 1976).

9.2.3 Hospital Sheets, Pads, and Pillowcases

Sheeting is defined as a medium weight, closely woven, plain weave or 2/2 twill weave fabric made from yarns of medium linear density and used primarily for bed coverings with a typical construction of either:

i) Plain weave: 25 × 23; 35 tex by 33 tex; K = 14.8 + 13.2, or
ii) 2 × 2 twill weave: 24 × 28; 21 × 37 tex; K = 11.0 + 17.0

Where the first sets of numbers are the numbers of threads in the warp and weft directions, and K is the cover factor for each set of threads (The Textile Institute 2021). For institutional use, the yarns chosen are most usually combed cotton/polyester blend fabrics or the 100% polyester equivalent for ease of maintenance and durability; a condenser-spun yarn may be used in the weft. A typical 50/50 polyester cotton sheeting for hospital bed linen has an areal density of 130 g per square metre and the ability to withstand a wash temperature of 71°C to achieve thermal disinfection and pillowcases may be made from the same type of fabric (Interweave 2021). Disposable incontinence underpads may be fitted beneath the bottom sheet on the bed to protect the mattress, items which are also used to protect chairs and other furniture whilst keeping the patient comfortable; their composition is similar to that of a diaper and can be both unobtrusive and reusable if the central layer is composed of superabsorbent in fibre form (SAF™ 2021). For ease of care, the pillow beneath can be wipeable (not washable) by using a flame-retardant polypropylene non-woven fabric cover over a polyester fibre filling which can be particularly helpful when coupled with disposable non-woven pillowcases (eSuppliesMedical™ 2021).

9.2.4 Air Treatment

Before considering the filtration and, in some cases, the sterilisation of incoming air, it is important for the areas taking in and being circulated with the filtered air to be prepared by cleaning, disinfection, and sterilisation.

9.2.4.1 Room Sterilisers

Conventional cleaning and disinfection methods used in hospitals and other healthcare settings depend for their effectiveness on the disinfectant products used and the way they are applied, including allowing sufficient contact time with the disinfectant for the active agent to work. Alternatively, systems intended to eliminate errors in the application of cleaning and disinfection and thereby improve reliability by automated room disinfection may be deployed. The disinfection level achieved by such devices can be high but does not achieve sterility (Otter 2020). The room will be isolated and a room steriliser deploying aerosolised hydrogen peroxide or hydrogen peroxide vapour, ultraviolet-C light or pulsed-xenon ultraviolet, or ozone may be used to treat the room. Examples would be the Ecolab Bioquell BQ-50 (Eco Lab, Saint Paul, MN USA) and the Steris VHP (Steris Life Sciences, Mentor, OH, USA) and ASP Glosair™ (Advanced Sterilisation Products, Irvine, CA USA) which use hydrogen peroxide vapour, the Halomist™ (Halosil International Inc, New Castle, DE USA) which generates an aerosol of hydrogen peroxide with silver ions, ultraviolet radiation systems such as the UV-C type Tru-D Smart UVC (Tru-D Smart UVC Memphis, TN, USA) and the pulsed xenon UV from Xenex (Xenex Disinfection Services Inc. San Antonio, TX USA). Ozone room sanitising devices, such as the JLA Compact Sanitiser and the JLA Cube Sanitiser, are supplied by JLA (JLA Group, Ripponden, W Yorkshire, UK), a member of EUO_3TA.org, the European Ozone Trade Association (EUO_3TA.org 2021).

Despite use of the term 'steriliser,' what is achieved by these systems is perhaps best described as 'high-level' disinfection, even so, it remains a very worthwhile step in the preparation of the area for use, at which point reliance will be turned to effective filtration of the circulated air and any associated air-treatment devices deemed necessary to remove particles and pathogens or render them not infective.

9.2.4.2 Air Filters

In a modern hospital environment, there is an expectation that apart from heating and ventilation, there will also be provision made for filtration of the air being circulated, particularly, but not exclusively, in operating theatres and intensive care units.

Filtration Mechanisms: A useful review of the main physical mechanisms that apply generally to small particles in air filtration (Maduna and Patnaik 2017) lists them as:

- *Direct Interception*, where the particle follows a flow path to within a particle radius of a filter fibre and is captured.
- *Inertial Impaction*, where the (larger) particle does not deviate with the flow so collides with the filter fibre.
- *Diffusion*, where the very fine particles are jostled by collisions with molecules of gas (Brownian motion) and caused to collide with filter fibres and become trapped.
- *Electrostatic Attraction*, which occurs when opposites charge exists or charges are generated between the filter fibres and particles. Particles therefore collect on the fibre surfaces.

A filter's ability to capture particles depends on the particle size passing into its fibre mass as well as the velocity of the flow passing through the filter. In looking at the range of sizes applicable to bacteria and viruses, (all of which would be classified by BS EN ISO 16890 as PM1), the larger particles in the range, that is, particles above 0.4 µm in diameter, will be captured due to both the impaction and interception mechanisms. Medium particles, in the 0.1 to 0.4 µm diameter range, turn out to be the most penetrating, despite being captured by both the diffusion and interception filtration mechanisms. Small particles, below 0.1 µm in diameter, are captured mostly by the diffusion mechanism, but more effectively than those in the medium size in the range (Maduna and Patnaik 2017; TSI 2012) For such as the coronavirus aerosol droplets, which will vary in size, there will be many of a size which will fall within the range 0.1–0.4 µm where the filter is operating at low effectiveness, at least insofar as these physical mechanisms are concerned.

By contrast with the personal protective devices such as surgical masks and respirators, although such filters are described as high-efficiency particle arrestance (HEPA) air filters, they are expected to treat significant volumes of air, many times the amount taken in by a single individual, so they cannot easily achieve the degree of entrapment of most virus-sized particles by mechanical filtration or attraction by charged electret fibres to the extent that would be routinely achieved by an N95, FFP2, or FFP3 respirator. Instead, wherever it is felt necessary to achieve high levels of decontamination of the air passing through the filter, the mechanical filtration provided by melt-blown non-woven fibre webs can be supplemented by UV-C irradiation in units such as the Steriwhite Air M and related units which may be retrofitted (Dr Hönle AG, UV-Technologie, Gräfelfing/MunicH, Germany) or units coupled with a photocatalytic filter consisting of a filter fabric containing TiO_2 nanoparticles as used in photocatalytic self-cleaning fabrics and/or ionisation (Woo et al. 2012) or electrical discharge within the filtration device itself. Some models include activated carbon for removal of volatile organic compounds (VOCs). Appropriately administered, such additional treatments should prove effective, but recent claims that such devices would remove/destroy SARS-Coronavirus2 have had to be withdrawn because the necessary tests had not yet taken place on this particular virus. In some cases, such as for cleanrooms or demanding hospital settings, the HEPA filter will be coupled with devices which bring about a slight reduction in air pressure in the area to help to limit the transfer of contaminants. Details of examples accessible at the Hepacart, Dust Arrest, and Airvia sites span the range, from fixed or large mobile installations for hospitals, through more-mobile but still substantial devices for hospitals, care homes, schools, and factories, and those which may be described as medical but are actually intended for domestic or small-office/reception area use (HEPACART 2021; DUST ARREST 2021; Airvia Medical Air Purifier.co.uk 2021). There are also ultra-low particulate air (ULPA) filters and whereas HEPA filters are designed to remove up to 99.97% of contaminants of sizes down to 0.3 µm, ULPA filters are designed to remove 99.99% of particles down to 0.12 µm in size which does therefore include virus-sized particles. However, the ULPA filters are much more demanding both in terms of maintenance and operating costs, so they are intended to be reserved for specialist treatment areas.

9.2.4.3 Airflow modelling

Even when filtration is highly effective at removing particles including virus-sized pathogens, the positioning of the circulation device containing the filter remains critical. Excellent work is underway in several centres. For example, concerns regarding the possibility of infection during air travel addressed by Qiyang Chen's team at Purdue University led them to assess three types of ventilation arrangements: mixing ventilation, conventional displacement ventilation, and personalised displacement ventilation. Because the personalised ventilation system performed the best in maintaining cabin thermal comfort and could reduce infection risk when the filtered air supply for each individual passenger sweeps upwards through their sitting position this was the system, they recommended for aircraft cabins (You et al. 2019). Positioning of the air supply to the passengers at a low level with a set number of exhausts was shown to be effective in reducing exposure to contaminants. The work serves to illustrate that whilst textile filtration design is an important component in the removal of contaminants, the overall three-dimensional design of the ventilation system within which it is incorporated is also crucial to its effectiveness (and the difficulties can be appreciated from the dramatic visual output from that team's work on modelling the effect of coughing (The Washington Post 2020). Similar modelling work is being undertaken at the University of Leeds in the UK but in this case focused on the hospital ward by the team involved in the 'Hospital Environment Control, Optimisation and Infection Risk Assessment' (HECOIRA) project led by Cath Noakes. The EPSRC project is being carried out in collaboration with St James' University Teaching Hospital in Leeds, Hairmyres Hospital in Lanarkshire, Monaghans and Apex4D. Building on work published in 2015 (Khan et al. 2015), the team has modelled airflow in a hospital ward with different positioning of inlets and outlets and their simulation can be viewed on the HECOIRA website. Again it can be seen that positioning of inlets and exhausts are critical (HECOIRA 2021) and hopefully, in the near future, coupled with effective filtration by the textiles within the filters and disinfection of the emergent air by exposure to far ultraviolet, the patients and healthcare staff will have better protection against infection from airborne pathogens. Devices such as the Airius air purification system based on photo-hydrionisation circulates hydroperoxides, superoxide ions, and hydroxide ions throughout the space, and shows great promise, claiming to neutralise up to 99% of microorganisms including bacteria, viruses, and fungal spores, not just in the air but also on surfaces and can be used to purify them and the air in healthcare environments, public buildings, and enclosed spaces such as the passenger cabins in aircraft, trains, or waiting rooms. Users include some NHS Trusts, aircraft manufacturers, for example, airbus, government and defence organisations, and major retail organisations (Airius 2021) but concerns have recently been expressed about possible health risks of the by-products generated by such ionisation devices and the lack of sufficient peer-reviewed research into their safety and effectiveness (Zeng et al. 2021).

9.3 HYGIENE PRODUCTS

9.3.1 Desirable Properties in Hygiene Products

Sun, in a chapter concerning disposable and reusable medical textiles, directs the reader to seek improved protective performance, low cost, and minimised environmental impact from medical textiles which could be disposable or reusable (Sun 2011) having pointed to the article by Zins indicating that there were disputes about which types to use (Zins 2006). Single-use disposables do have some attractive features and are the sensible choice in certain settings, whilst in others, they have the potential to incur high costs and to make a substantial contribution to pollution. How to make the decision about which type to use was well-addressed by Walton, who recommended that the use of disposables should be reserved for low-volume applications, where it was not going to be economical to equip to be able to decontaminate and sterilise them (Walton 1986). Hygiene products should, of course, be included in the list of high-usage items worthy of reuse alongside protective garments and other items of PPE and the reusable versions should be therefore given preference by purchasers wherever possible. Where levels of use of certain items mean it is not going to be economical to decontaminate and sterilise for reuse within the healthcare unit itself, third-party reprocessing companies offer services which achieve 30–50% savings from reuse without the unit itself having to invest in the reprocessing equipment. Such arrangements are not necessarily popular with the original equipment manufacturers, who may resort to defensive measures such as by making the original device more difficult to reprocess, by the installation of ‘kill switches’ in the original devices to prevent reprocessing (where possible), or the takeover of reprocessing companies to help their own business, rather than engaging in constructive innovation aimed at helping healthcare providers and their patients (Prasad 2020).

The environmental impact of healthcare was recently assessed by an Australian group (Lenzen et al. 2020), and with the aim of helping to provide those working in the healthcare sector to take steps to mitigate negative environmental impacts, it extended consideration beyond greenhouse gas emissions to a more comprehensive set of seven environmental stressors with known adverse feedback cycles:

- greenhouse gas emissions
- particulate matter
- nitrogen oxide air pollutants
- sulphur dioxide as an air pollutant
- malaria risk
- reactive nitrogen in water
- scarce water use

A New Zealand-based organisation, working from that paper, stated that by generating almost 5% of the world’s carbon emissions, healthcare, if it were a country, would be the world’s fifth biggest polluter, and listed, for consideration, six ways of reducing environmental impact and (often) reducing unnecessary expenditure, namely:

i) Reduce the number of flights taken and offset the carbon emissions on all flights
ii) Choose clean energy
iii) Opt for reusable items
iv) Incentivise staff to consider alternative transport options
v) Reduce meat and dairy options
vi) Choose medical devices which can be remanufactured

As can be seen, opting for reusable items, and selecting medical items that can be remanufactured are featured in that list (Medsalv 2021). In Europe, according to Regulation (EU) 2017/745 of 5 April 2017 on medical devices (EU 2017), *remanufactured* 'single-use' medical devices must meet manufacturer standards and receive a CE mark ensuring they are as safe and as effective as the new equipment and are required to be sterilised to the level of the original device. Healthcare units keen to save on resources and address the growing need to generate less waste, but concerned about the expense of decontamination and sterilisation, are now able to find systems and products to help them to achieve those aims. Practice Greenhealth™ (Reston, VA, USA) has developed the business case and step-by-step guidance documents to give practical help in developing a sound basis from which to reach such a decision about what choice to make for the operating room (Practice Greenhealth 2011); for more information, see also Chapter 2 Section 2.1.5. The availability now of new equipment and products can help to tilt the choice in favour of selecting the reusable option, for example, low temperature, low-cost ozone laundry systems for high-level disinfection (JLA 2021) and 50 times launderable incontinence products which incorporate superabsorbent polymer in fibre form as the central layer in diapers and pads, such as SAF™ (SAF™ 2021).

9.3.2 Incontinence Products

Incontinence products such as body-worn pads and diapers and flatform sheets used in the bed are commonly used as methods of dealing with urinary and faecal incontinence. With increasing concerns over sustainability and environmental impact, there has been a drive back towards reusable products (McCarthy 2011). Ultimately the product needs to remove liquid from the surrounding skin, to keep the skin clean and dry, and enclose it safely within the product. The layer that is in direct contact with the skin needs to be non-irritant (Gutshall et al. 2016). The disposable diaper is a composite non-woven article that contains an outer (protective) layer, and an inner covering layer supporting the absorbent layer in the middle part of the diaper; the inner covering layer may be manufactured from a polyester-fibre web or a spunlaid polypropylene-fibre non-woven material (Rigby, Anand and Horrocks 1997) Although the materials in the central layers need to be absorbent, the permeable non-absorbent outer layer or coverstock may be manufactured from polyethylene

(Horrocks and Anand 2016). The methods of construction and manufacture of composite non-wovens such as the Coform Process (Kimberly-Clark, Irving, TX, USA) which mixes melt-blown polypropylene with absorbents such as wood pulp as used for diapers and wipes, were detailed by Das in a review which also includes details about the Spunbond + Melt blown + Spunbond, or SMS Process (Kimberly-Clark, Irving, TX, USA) as used for the manufacture of non-woven composites for protective covers, barrier fabrics, sanitary products, and facemasks (Das et al. 2012). The lengthwise and transverse strength arising from the central melt-blown component whilst not outstanding is good enough to give the necessary support whilst the spunbonded outer layers provide the soft handle suitable for these applications. There is a move towards developing spacer fabrics that may be suitable not only for disposable but also reusable products (Yang and Hu 2017a, b) and the launderability of incontinence products utilising superabsorbent polymers in fibre form, such as SAF™ as the central layer in diapers (SAF™ 2021) shows great promise because the material is durable to 50 laundry cycles and despite requiring longer drying periods, should be able to demonstrate substantial savings compared to their disposable equivalents.

9.3.3 Feminine Hygiene Products

Currently, there are many feminine hygiene options on offer and the industry was worth US$20.9 billion in 2020 and is forecast to grow to US$27.7 billion by 2025 with a compound annual growth rate of 5.8% (MarketsandMarkets 2021) but although it is a lucrative business, 'Period Poverty' is an issue that affects women and girls all over the world. It is the name for the lack of access to sanitary products due to financial constraints. It is estimated that 1 in 10 girls in Africa miss school because of a lack of access to sanitary products and that 12% of menstruating women in India cannot afford period products (Action Aid 2021). The film PadMan is based upon social entrepreneur Arunachalam Muruganananatham who invented the low-cost sanitary pad making machine and is credited for innovating grassroots mechanisms for generating awareness about traditional unhygienic practices around menstruation in rural India (Kannadasan 2018). However, it is not only in developing countries where there are period poverty problems. In the UK, in 2017, it was reported that 1 in 10 girls had been unable to afford sanitary products and had to improvise sanitary wear (Bagness 2020); a move in the right direction took place in 2020 when the 5% value-added tax (colloquially known as the 'Tampon Tax') on sanitary products was scrapped (GOV.UK 2021).

Biodegradable and biocompatible options or reusable options are where the sector is likely headed. Environmental concerns are seeing a move towards non-applicator tampons (which reduces the waste derived from the applicator), silicon menstrual cups and washable, reusable garments such as period panties. The need to manufacture at competitive prices to allow access to those who live in poverty in both developed and developing countries is of the utmost importance.

During the First World War, it was noted that cellulose fibre was more effective at absorbing blood compared to woven cloth bandages, so Kotex manufactured the first cellulose sanitary napkin in 1918 from surplus high-absorption war bandages

(Delaney 1988; Vostral 2008) and by 1921, it was the first successfully mass-marketed sanitary napkin. Modern disposable tampons were patented in 1933 and were often regarded as a healthier alternative to pads due to hygiene concerns about the proximity of pads to faecal bacteria (Sackren 1939, 329). They were already in use in medicine to stop bleeding in deep wounds. Dr Mary Barton published in the *British Medical Journal* to address concerns that tampons would be unbecoming. She pointed out that tampons did not cause abrasions and boils on the vulva unlike sanitary pads (Gardner and Barton 1942, 709–710). However, ongoing hesitancy regarding tampons led to the development of the sanitary belt in 1956. This product featured an adhesive to keep the pad in place and was invented by Mary Beatrice Davidson Kenner (Stanley 1995). Ongoing design work saw the first beltless pads in 1972 and then a range of variations in 1980 of pad design and tampon absorbency.

Toxic shock syndrome (TSS), was first named in 1978 and entered public realms in 1980 due to an outbreak in the USA. Researchers confirmed that TSS was associated with tampons, specifically a tampon manufactured by Proctor and Gamble called Rely. This tampon was manufactured from carboxymethyl cellulose and compressed beads of polyester. It was supposedly more absorbent than other available brands (CDC 2020a; Vostral 2011, 447) which were usually manufactured from cotton and viscose rayon. Before 1976, tampons were not subject to medical testing standards in the USA. Following the TSS outbreak, The Federal Drug and Alcohol Administration of the United States began requiring absorbency standards. In 1989, a link was deduced between synthetic materials, carboxymethyl cellulose, polyester, polyacrylate rayon, and viscose rayon and TSS. The synthetic materials created a fertile environment for the amplification of the toxigenic bacterium *Staphylococcus aureus*. Subsequently, there was phasing out of these materials (Lanes and Rothman 1990, 1379–1385; Tierno and Hanna 1989, S182–S187). The TSS outbreak caused research to be directed to finding more natural polymer alternatives, such as cotton, rayon, or a blend of the two (Tampax® 2020).

As a response to a rise in feminism and an increasing environmentalist movement, reusable menstrual cups, period sponges, and biodegradable options were trialled. In addition, the design of the tampon has altered as the knowledge base on menstruation and anatomy has increased. In the 1990s, major commercial tampon brands moved away from dioxin-producing chlorine gas bleaching methods to chlorine-free bleaching processes. Whilst dioxin levels at even a trace level remain controversial, the FDA now recommends that manufacturers list *any* possible chemical residue on their labelling (FDA 2020a).

9.3.4 Cloths and Wipes

Cloths and wipes made from non-woven fabrics (Das et al. 2012) are commonly used on the ward for cleaning patients, staff, or equipment and typically contain antibacterial and cleaning agents; preferably they would be able to be decontaminated and reused, otherwise, it is thought that they would be better if they were flushable (Kim and Hergeth 2012) and biodegradable (Soukupova et al. 2007). It appears that not all wipes are similarly effective, but also, they do need to be used in a particular manner to work effectively. The efficacies of two types of non-woven wipe have been assessed by dynamic wiping, and it was found that of the two, the hydrophilic wipes (those composed of lyocell) were more consistently effective than those made from polypropylene. Use of a high-density lyocell fabric (150 $g.m^{-2}$), at high pressure (13.8 $kN.m^{-2}$) was considered best practice (Edwards et al. 2019). Antimicrobial agents such as quaternary ammonium compounds are some of the most widely used disinfecting agents and in the case of wipes, it is ready to release rather than adsorption which is required from the impregnated carrier fabric. Quaternary ammonium compounds can be strongly adsorbed on to cotton, but it was shown that whereas raising the alkalinity of their solutions increased the amount of alkyl-dimethyl-benzyl-ammonium chloride (ADBAC) adsorbed onto cotton non-woven fabrics, a more-acidic solution reduced ADBAC adsorption, as did increasing the temperature and concentration of salts in the solution. Non-ionic surfactants or low molecular weight quaternary ammonium compounds reduced ADBAC adsorption onto cotton fabrics in a concentration-dependent manner. Because their adsorption behaviour was dependent on the composition of the solution, incorporation of the additives that promote ADBAC release into the antimicrobial solution was able to be optimised to enable ready release of the ADBAC from the wipe onto the surface required to be disinfected (Hinchliffe et al. 2017a,b).

Successful disinfection of a hard surface can be impeded by the presence of a soil load in the form of protein, fat, or other material, so the use of greige cotton as the non-woven wipe material improved the performance of the disinfecting wipe over other fibre types. It was shown by dynamic wiping assays that successful disinfection of a hard surface was greatly enhanced by a wipe fabric that also effectively removed organic contaminants and was strong enough to resist structural failure, and the use of greige cotton also reduced water wastage when the disinfecting solution was being applied (Hron et al. 2019).

A useful and detailed review of the efficacy of disinfectant-impregnated wipes used for surface disinfection in hospitals has been undertaken recently (Song, Vossbein, and Zille 2019). In the EU, the disinfectant efficacy test is regulated and issued by the European Committee for Normalization (CEN), Technical Committee 216 (TC 216) under the work programme 'Chemical Disinfectants and Antiseptics' and it is Standard EN 16615 that is the most suitable. For the USA, it is the Environmental Protection Agency (EPA) which undertakes that kind of regulation. Even so, yet, there are few test methods for assessing the efficacy of impregnated wipes, the main ones being EN 16615:2015, the modified AOAC international method 961.02 and ASTM E2896–12 and ASTM E2967–15, all of which fall short in terms of variations that may occur during their application and/or the limited range of surfaces embraced by the standard. Also, according to the reviewers (Song, Vossbein, and Zille 2019), several information gaps have to be filled to obtain consistent and exhaustive knowledge about the interaction between textile and substrate, in particular regarding:

i) material compatibility (combination of wipe and disinfectant)
ii) liquor ratio (wipe mass/disinfection solution volume)
iii) contact time (of disinfectant and wipes)
iv) durability to storage

Even so, despite shortcomings, the ASTM test has been adopted (Sattar et al. 2015). A different approach to disinfection is detailed to combat the growing threat of hospital-acquired infections; it relies on a dry non-woven wipe composed of viscose rayon containing sufficient beneficial bacteria or spores which, on wetting and using the wipe, are released, and spread over the wiped surface. The released beneficial bacteria inhibit pathogens by growing and colonising on the wiped surfaces (Dural-Erem et al. 2019).

9.3.5 Dental Floss

The purpose of dental floss is to clean the interproximal areas between teeth, initially to stop uncomfortable and inflammatory food packing, then to mechanically debride the surfaces of teeth to reduce the stagnant build-up of cariogenic bacteria which preferentially produce acidic by-products of sugar metabolism which lead to the development of caries (decay) first within the enamel and then the dentine of the tooth (Worthington et al. 2019).

The effects of interdental toothpicks have been noted on skeletal remains and an ornate toothpick has been found in a Mesopotamian tomb dated 3000BC, however, what we would consider modern dental floss is credited to Levi Spear Parmly (1790–1859) a dentist practising in New Orleans. He stated that caries and the general health of the gums could be controlled by means of a waxed silken thread to be passed between the teeth to dislodge irritating matter, he started to advertise such use in 1815 (Fischman 1997). Waxed silk thread was widely available for use in sewing but it was not until 1882 when the Codman and Schurleff medical supply company started to mass produce unwaxed dental floss. In 1896 Johnson and Johnson patented the idea of waxed dental floss and built a cutter for the silk thread into the dispenser. Their floss was based on their own silk suture material.

Given the development of nylon by DuPont in the late 1930s into the 1940s, silk was replaced by nylon then waxed and in the 1950s developed into tape – more suitable for the tighter contacts between teeth. One of the key problems with floss throughout the 1950s and 1960s was the tendency to 'shred' so binders were used to limit this effect. Both the waxed and unwaxed flosses incorporated binders such as polyethylene and polypropylene. PTFE presented an ideal solution to the shredding problem, being less likely to shred in the first place but also having reduced surface resistance meaning that it could 'slip' easily between teeth. Texturised dental floss, treated with a combination of non-water-soluble polymer and water-soluble polymer to allow for the non-shredding of material but also the dissolving of the polymer which will leave medicaments such as fluoride, xylitol, or flavourings. When texturised filaments are extended, the bulk arising from the loops and twists in the filaments are lost and the filaments can become neatly aligned and as a result, they can be inserted more easily into smaller spaces. Once the tension is removed the textured filaments in the floss open out again into their textured shape, expanding to fill the space and provide more effective cleansing. This feature of textured yarns in dental floss is particularly useful under fixed-bridge work.

The addition of flavourings is intended to make the flossing process more pleasant but also remind the user to 'move on' to a new part of the floss. Xylitol and sorbitol are also added both of which are known to reduce the incidence of dental caries when in the form of chewing gum (Nasseripour et al. 2021) together with fluoride to decrease the risk of dental caries (Jørgensen et al. 1989). There appears to be no detectable difference in efficacy between waxen/unwaxed nylon or PTFE-based flosses (Lamberts, Wunderlich and Cafesse 1982), but instead, the main issue affecting all types of floss is that of user dexterity. Whether held in the fingers or in a plastic holder, floss remains difficult to use effectively. As with the use of all medical textiles, there is some environmental impact, so future developments need to centre not only around improving usability but also on reducing that impact.

9.3.6 Reusability and Disposability of Hygiene Products

Sun, in a chapter concerning disposable and reusable medical textiles, directs the reader to seek improved protective performance, low cost, and minimised environmental impact from medical textiles such as surgical gowns, gloves, drapes, face-masks, dresses, and linens, which could be disposable or reusable (Sun 2011). It could be argued that hygiene products should be included in that list. The environmental impact of healthcare was recently assessed and with the aim of helping to provide those working in the healthcare sector to take steps to mitigate negative environmental impacts extended consideration beyond only greenhouse gas emissions a set of seven environmental stressors with known adverse feedback cycles: greenhouse gas emissions, particulate matter, two air pollutants (nitrogen oxides and sulphur dioxide), malaria risk, reactive nitrogen in water, and scarce water use (Lenzen et al. 2020).

Remanufacture has the potential to reduce cost and environmental impact but there appears to be some reluctance to engage in the process. Within the EU, for example, countries must opt in to accept their scheme, and despite savings of 30 to 50% per device, few opted in immediately. Globally, the use of remanufactured devices saved health systems over €446M in 2019 (Vukelich 2021), and according to the Association of Medical Device Reprocessors (AMDR) in their briefing note '*The Business case for Reprocessing*,,' putting a policy of reprocessing into practice by a 200-bed hospital 'enabled a saving of between $600,000 US and $1million US per annum' in the year 2000 (AMDR 2011). It also directs the reader to 'an extensive body of peer-reviewed literature supporting the safety and lower cost of reprocessed devices' referencing 125 papers about the value and safety of reprocessing (AMDR 2021).

Regarding disposal, in 2015, the European Commission published proposals to amend six EU Waste Directives, including the Waste Framework Directive, the Landfill Directive and the Packaging and Packaging Waste Directive. Known as the Circular Economy Package, the proposal entered into force on July 4, 2018. Beginning in 2020, countries in the EU must send recycling rejects of separately collected material from material recycling facilities' gates to mechanical biological treatment plants for treatment or other treatment facilities instead of landfill and incineration (EU 2018). They are allowed ten years to achieve the requirement.

9.4 PERSONAL AND PROTECTIVE EQUIPMENT

Personal protective equipment is intended to protect both the patient and the healthcare worker. The overriding principle for patient care embedded in the Hippocratic Oath which used to be sworn on entrance into the medical profession, now superseded by the Physician's Pledge in the Declaration of Geneva, is that 'the health and well-being of the patient will be the first consideration' and another part of the Pledge requires the physician to attend to their own 'health, well-being, and abilities in order to provide care of the highest standard' (World Medical Association 2017).

9.4.1 Desirable Properties in Personal and Protective Equipment

In practice, medical practitioners and healthcare workers in general need not only to be equipped with the means to help the patient but also to be provided with adequate personal protection to help them to provide such care effectively no matter where they are working. The requirement was admirably well explained by Janine Jagger, Director of the International Healthcare Worker Safety Center at the University of Virginia, School of Medicine, as follows:

> The basic measures for protecting Health Care Workers from the life-threatening risk of blood-borne pathogen infection should be viewed everywhere as essential and included in the national health priorities of all nations. The resources for this task are unlikely to be forthcoming unless we re-assess the value we place on Health Care Workers. They are not merely a service commodity; they are an invaluable asset to their countries and to the world community. Without them there would be no health care. All of us benefit from protecting their lives and health.. (Jagger 2007)

The design, development, and provision of PPE which will protect both the patient and the healthcare worker, the establishment of adequate test methods able to prove its supposed level of performance in a realistic setting and processes that ensure adequate supplies at times of crisis, are all critical to achieve the mission set down by Janine Jagger. More research and development into PPE is necessary to improve its performance, but it has to be acknowledged that those efforts will be wasted if government officials or healthcare administrators then fail to undertake their responsibilities for ensuring adequacy in its supply.

In a hospital or other healthcare setting, the personal protective equipment used by healthcare workers include everything up to complete protective outfits with independent air supply, face and eye shields, gloves and surgical facemasks or respirators. For the UK, the health and safety regulations that apply in the case of the presence or likely presence of biological agents (such as viruses, bacteria, fungal spores, prions etc.) are those of the Control of Substances Hazardous to Health (COSHH) Regulations 2002, which are designed to provide a framework of actions to control risk from exposure to hazardous substances (Health & Safety Executive 2013).

The central approach in COSSH is one of risk assessment, and in their recent 'Rapid Evidence Review' (Health and Safety Executive 2020) the Health and Safety Executive (HSE) stressed that no PPE is 100% effective. The HSE also stressed that the level of protection offered is dependent on the outcome of a thorough risk assessment based on the inherent characteristics of the hazard, including routes of transmission and the type(s) of activities being performed as well as the correct selection, training, donning, use, doffing, storage, decontamination (of reusable items), and waste disposal. COSHH Regulation 7 and its associated Approved Code of Practice (ACOP) to (Health and Safety Executive 2013) state that where employers cannot prevent exposure to a biological agent, they should take steps to ensure that it is controlled adequately (by consideration of the requirements set out in Regulation 7(3), (4), (6), and (7), Applying Good Practice. The need is stressed to use each requirement where, and to the extent that it is applicable; the assessment carried out under Regulation 6 shows that it will lead to a reduction in risk).

An excellent review of the requirements for adequately functional healthcare workers' clothing contains sufficient detail to provide the information needed to enable textile and apparel specialists to develop their specifications for improved products; this is particularly the case because of a developing need to provide protection in the widening variety of working environments that healthcare personnel are now likely to experience. The review draws attention to the need to address the role that the textiles used in healthcare settings might play in the acquisition and retention of pathogens (e.g., privacy curtains, bedlinen, upholstery, furniture, and furnishings), including the textiles used in uniforms, scrubs, and other apparel. There is also a need to give appropriate consideration to variations in laundering and sterilising practices. The review acknowledges that the textiles employed in healthcare settings can have a significant role in protecting healthcare workers and that there has been limited adoption of available textile technologies such as fluid repellency and antimicrobial action by healthcare institutions, in part because of their failure to recognise the impact such treatments can have on risk reduction, and a failure to become engaged in the necessary research and publication about their effectiveness in healthcare settings (Mitchell, Spencer and Edmiston 2015).

9.4.2 Surgical Gowns, Aprons and Hats

Surgical gowns were introduced primarily as a protective barrier to reduce surgical-site infection and protect the patient from contamination originating with the surgical team. They aim to achieve this by controlling skin flakes and bacteria shed by the user and by preventing the direct transmission of microbes. Finally, a surgical gown must also demonstrate good wearing comfort whilst keeping the surgeon and team comfortable, particularly in longer operations (Aibibu, Lehmann and Offermann 2003; Aslan, Kaplan, and Çetin 2013). Currently, for the UK, there are a series of standards applied to protective clothing items such as surgical gowns namely:

British Standards relating to items and materials:

i) BS EN 13795-1 2019: Surgical clothing and drapes. Requirements and test methods. Surgical drapes and gowns
ii) BS EN 13795-2:2019: Surgical clothing and drapes. Requirements and test methods. Clean air suits

iii) BS 3314:1982: Specification for protective aprons for wet work
iv) BS EN 455-1, 2, 3, 4: 2020, 2015, 2015, 2009: Medical gloves for single use

The latter relate to non-textile latex, nitrile, and vinyl products, so are only included for completeness.

British Standards relating to performance requirements and test methods:

v) BS EN ISO 22610: 2006/2018: *Surgical drapes, gowns and clean air suits, used as medical devices, for patients, clinical staff and equipment. Test method to determine the resistance to wet bacterial penetration*
vi) BS 3546:2001 *Coated fabrics for use in the manufacture of water-penetration resistant clothing*
vii) BS EN 14126:2003**:** *Protective clothing. Performance requirements and test methods for protective clothing against infective agents*
viii) BS EN ISO 11810:2015 *Lasers and laser-related equipment. Test method and classification for the laser resistance of surgical drapes and/or patient protective covers. Primary ignition, penetration, flame spread and secondary ignition*

For the USA, standards from ASTM (ASTM 2017; ASTM 2013), from AATC (American Association of Textile Chemists and Colorists 2019) and from ANSI/AATM.

ASTM International, Standards and Specifications:

i) ASTM F1670/F1670M-17a: *Standard Test Method for Resistance of Materials Used in Protective Clothing to Penetration by Synthetic Blood* (ASTM 2017) *and*
ii) ASTM F1671/F1671M-13: *Standard Test Method for Resistance of Materials Used in Protective Clothing to Penetration by Blood-Borne Pathogens Using Phi-X174 Bacteriophage Penetration as a Test System* (ASTM 2013)

AATCC (American Association of Textile Chemists and Colorists) Test Method:

i) AATCC TM127-2017: *Water Resistance: Hydrostatic Pressure Test* (American Association of Textile Chemists and Colorists 2019)

ANSI/AAMI (American National Standards Institute/Association of the Advancement of Medical Instrumentation) Standard

i) ANSI/AAMI PB70:2012 'Liquid barrier performance and classification of protective apparel and drapes intended for use in health care facilities.'

International standards

i) ISO 16603:2004: *Clothing for protection against contact with blood and body fluids — Determination of the resistance of protective clothing materials to penetration by blood and body fluids — Test method using synthetic blood* (International Standards Organisation 2004a).
ii) ISO 16604:2004: *Clothing for protection against contact with blood and body fluids — Determination of resistance of protective clothing materials to penetration by blood-borne pathogens — Test method using Phi-X 174 bacteriophage* (International Standards Organisation 2004b)

A literature review undertaken in 2015 by the National Health Service Scotland for their *National Infection Prevention and Control Manual* provides a useful context on the range of protective equipment, what evidence there is for its effectiveness and its proper use. The review recommended full-body, fluid-repellant gowns for situations where splashing might occur and pointed out that superiority of plastic gowns has been questioned whilst noting that there was little evidence identified as to when reusable aprons/gowns might be appropriate (NHS National Services Scotland 2015). The NHS Scotland report could provide a useful basis from which textile and apparel specialists might engage in the next phase of product development, not least in terms of improving the prospects for reusability. There is also guidance on infection control measures regarding PPE/healthcare worker's protective clothing and its use, not only from the WHO given the COVID-19 pandemic (World Health Organization 2020), but also through organisations focused on practitioner levels, such as the Association for Perioperative Practice (Association for Perioperative Practice 2020), where there is guidance adapted from *Pandemic Influenza: Guidance for Infection prevention and control in healthcare settings, 2020* issued jointly by the Department of Health and Social Care (DHSC), Public Health Wales (PHW), Public Health Agency (PHA) Northern Ireland, Health Protection Scotland (HPS) and Public Health England as official guidance.

Traditionally, one or more layers of sterile woven cotton cloth were used as an aseptic barrier, however, in 1948, an article in the *Lancet* highlighted a problem with these surgical gowns; when a gown became 'wet,' it acted as a sieve and allowed bacteria to pass through the fabric (Colebrook & Hood 1948). Cotton fabric used at this time had a pore size of 80–100µm, too large to prevent the passage of skin cells and bacteria (Eisen 2011). Further work in this period showed that interposing with a waterproof layer reduced the passage of bacteria (Beck and Collette 1952).

Implant surgery further drove the development of surgical gowns. The pore size in woven fabrics is an important factor of microbial transmission (Maqsood et al. 2016), as is the repellency of the fabric. Testing and modelling showed that more compact structures achieved by shorter thread floats and higher thread densities made the fabrics more water resistant but less permeable to air; the statistical models were thought to be of help in determining the appropriate compromise between protective properties and comfort (Leonas and Jinkins 1997). Well before this work was published, Charnley, the grandfather of modern-day orthopaedic surgery, had developed Ventile® fabric made from long staple cotton in a fabric structure intended to reduce permeability to liquids (Ventile 2020) and had also designed the total body exhaust gown (Charnley and Eftekhar 1969). Whilst not without problems, for example, the total body exhaust gown had to be connected to a power source; when utilised in a laminar flow theatre, the rate of surgical site infection has been shown to be significantly less than when an ordinary gown is used (Lidwell et al. 1982) There has been continual work directed at the ideal fibre, construction of fabric, and construction of the garment and garment design recommendations have been made, particularly related to ease of hygienic doffing (Verbeek et al. 2020), and efforts have been made to help healthcare personnel to make better choices for their protection. For example, in 2003, together with the American National Standards Institute (ANSI), the American Association for the Advancement of Medical Instrumentation (AAMI) developed an FDA-approved classification scheme for gowns, now updated to ANSI/AAMI PB70:2012 which places them in one of four categories depending on the protection they provide (FDA 2021a):

Level 1: *Minimal risk*, to be used, for example, during basic care, standard isolation, cover gown for visitors, or in a standard medical unit. It provides a slight barrier to small amounts of fluid penetration. One type of test is used to determine its effectiveness level by means of water impacting the surface of the gown material to assess barrier protection performance.

Level 2: *Low risk*, to be worn, for example, whilst taking a sample of blood, inserting a suture, in the Intensive Care Unit or a pathology laboratory. It provides a better barrier to larger amounts of fluid penetration through splatter than a Level 1 gown and to fluid exposure through soaking. Two tests are conducted in this case to assess barrier protection performance, water impacting the surface of the gown material as for the Level 1 material and subjecting the material to the possibility of penetration of liquid under hydrostatic pressure.

Level 3: *Moderate risk*, to be used, for example, during arterial blood draw, inserting an intravenous line, in the Emergency Room, or for trauma cases. The same two types of tests are used to determine barrier protection performance as for Level 2 but with more impact force and greater hydrostatic pressure. The Level 3 material provides a barrier to larger amounts of fluid penetration through splatter and greater fluid exposure through soaking than Level 2.

Level 4: *High risk*, to be used, for example, during long, fluid intense procedures, surgery, when pathogen resistance is needed, or infectious diseases are suspected (non-airborne). Requirements are higher for all of the types of tests conducted to determine performance to Levels 1-3 and barrier level performance must be sufficient to prevent all fluid penetration for up to 1 hour and virus penetration for up to 1 hour, the latter being tested with a simulated blood containing a virus/surrogate virus. If no virus/surrogate is found at the end of the test, the gown material has shown the required performance.

Together with the required level of performance of the material, the FDA also specifies which parts of the gown need to exhibit that particular level of barrier protection depending on its intended use, as shown in Figure 9.1.

There are areas to the back of the surgical gown marked 'D' which do not need to demonstrate barrier protection, and nor do the cuffs or seams for the surgical isolation gowns, but all other regions will need to be able to demonstrate barrier performance at an appropriate point on the ANSI/AAMI PB70 scale. Gowns used away from surgery (non-surgical gowns) need to provide all-round protection to the

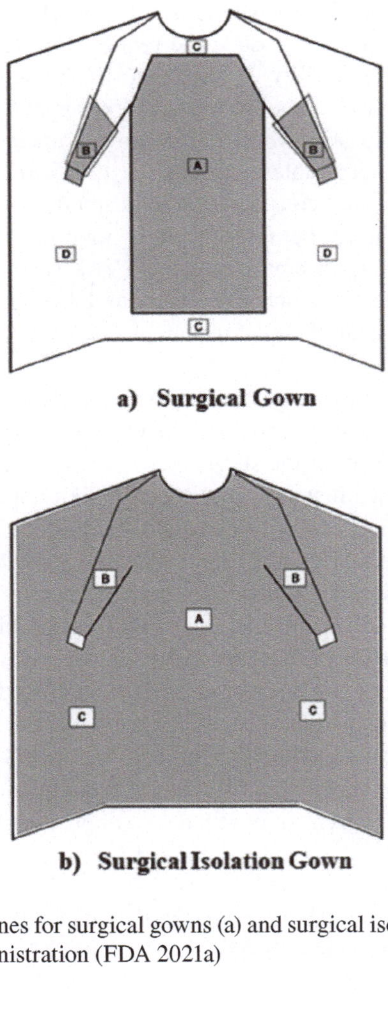

FIGURE 9.1 Critical zones for surgical gowns (a) and surgical isolation gowns (b) Courtesy US Food and Drug Administration (FDA 2021a)

same pattern as the surgical isolation gown at least to the minimum level on the ANSI/AAMI PB70 scale, but again, the level will depend on where it is intended to be worn. The same FDA site (FDA 2021a) guides the reader to ASTM F2407 which it describes as 'the umbrella document of tests' to apply to surgical gowns for tear resistance, seam strength, lint generation, evaporative resistance, and water vapour transmission, and it also provides clear illustrations of the critical zones for both surgical and non-surgical gowns.

A laminated fabric with a nano-finished PET outer layer, a microporous membrane sandwiched between that, and an inner layer made of non-woven viscose rayon was considered to be one way of creating a barrier to the ingress of viruses; tested according to the ASTM F1671: 2003 Viral Penetration Test, it achieved Level 4 protection according to the ANSI/AAMI PB70:2012 classification system. It was also claimed that the applied finish of titanium dioxide/methylene blue exhibited antiviral properties (Parthasarathi and Thilagavathi 2015).

There has been a move towards single-use disposable non-woven gowns that do not require laundering and thus reduce the requirement for access to an in-house or commercial laundering facility. It has been determined, however, that disposable non-woven fabric gowns made from polypropylene or 55/45 cellulose/PET were less comfortable than reusable woven fabric gowns made from micro-fibre polyester reinforced with a permeable membrane or 65/35 PET/cotton (Aslan, Kaplan and Çetin 2013) an important consideration in hospital operating theatres (Xu et al. 2012). The non-woven fabrics being used can be modified by laminating the fabric (Laing 2008) and by using plasma treatments (Virk et al. 2004). Multi-layer fabrics such as those supplied by Gore® (WL Gore and Associates, Newark, Delaware, USA) and Rotecno® (Rotecno® AG, Switzerland) have also been trialled (Gulihar, Taub and Taylor 2009).

Whether the surgical gown is of the disposable or reusable type, it was demonstrated using synthetic blood, isopropanol, and artificial sweat, that wetting by any such liquid from the wearer, or the surgical environment may compromise the barrier properties of the gown material. It was considered that gown replacement protocols should take this into account (Wei and Cloud 2011). The transfer of bacteria through contact between fabrics was found to be aided by the presence of moisture and the application of friction. Of seven different fabrics (cotton, silk, viscose rayon, wool, polyester (PET), polypropylene, and a PET-cotton blend), bacterial transfer was found to be highest for PET followed by viscose rayon, whilst polypropylene showed the least transfer (Varshney et al. 2020). Such studies indicate why it has been considered judicious for antimicrobial agents to have been incorporated into gown fabrics for many years (Morris, Vigo and Welch 1981). Given a rise in antimicrobial resistance in recent years, this line of thought and technique might have become questionable, however, more recent developments in nanotechnology have shown that:

- silver release from treatments to incorporate nanosilver into fabrics is safe to the skin (Lee and Jeong 2005)

- silver incorporated into fabrics can withstand challenge by a variety of chemical agents (such as artificial sweat to represent in-use exposure
- silver incorporated into fabrics can withstand a mimic for landfill leachate to simulate end-of-life exposure)
- silver incorporated into fabrics can maintain high antibacterial efficacy down to levels on fabrics as low as ~10 μg Ag (g fabric)$^{-1}$ under conditions of normal use (below this concentration, efficacy significantly decreases) (Spielman-Sun et al. 2018).

Attractive characteristics such as these have led to the development of improved antibacterial fabrics based on silver release for their effectiveness, for example:

i) a recently reported method for large-scale economic and high-speed production of antibacterial fabrics based on silver applied by liquid flame spray followed by plasma coating, and considered suitable for single-use PPE items in a hospital environment (Brobbey et al. 2020), would now require further testing on-site to determine not only its suitability and performance in the intended environment but also its durability to laundering to enable reuse

ii) durable nanosilver treatments achievable in a variety of ways, for example
   a) by a finishing treatment on cotton fabric, first applying single-walled carbon nanotubes (CNTs) then microwave heating to deposit silver nanoparticles onto the CNTs (Kumar et al. 2019) or
   b) by anchoring silver ions to PET fabric by coordination bond using tannic acid by alternately immersing in an aqueous solution of silver nitrate followed by tannic acid for five cycles. Durability to laundering and residual antibacterial activity was investigated, and the results appeared to be very good. After 30 cycles of accelerated washing, the silver loading was found to have decreased from 5.0 wt% to 2.2 wt% but the remaining coordinated silver ions continued to make the sample highly antibacterial against *S. aureus* (99.99 ± 0.03%), *E. coli* (99.99 ± 0.05%), and *S. albicans* (99 ± 0.14%) (Ou et al. 2019), or
   c) by enhancing its durability by combined finishing with silver nanoparticles and carboxymethyl chitosan binder on a cotton fabric surface through what was described as a 'simple mist modification process.' Durability in terms of bacterial reduction rates against both *S. aureus* and *E. coli* with these remaining at over 95% after 50 wash cycles were attributed to the carboxymethyl chitosan binder being covalently linked to the cotton fabric via esterification and the silver nanoparticles being tightly held onto the fibre surface through coordination with the amine groups on the carboxymethyl chitosan. It was considered to be as a result of these methods of attachment, that the coating of AgNPs on the cotton fabric showed excellent antibacterial properties and laundering durability (Xu et al. 2017).

Clearly, much of the work to date on surgical gowns has been concerned with attempting to reduce the transmission of bacteria (with, it must be said, not as much success as would be hoped), and given the increasing risk of pandemics, it becomes increasingly clear that detailed attention should also be paid to viral transmission, and protection from prions. There has been a search into the elusive 'ideal' surgical gown with research on seam type, the glove-gown interface, and the ideal fabric and design (Lee and Obendorf 2007) and the COVID-19 pandemic has highlighted the importance of robust protection for both the patient and the healthcare professional (Public Health England 2020).

Sun provided a useful list of properties that the 'ideal' surgical gowns and drapes should possess (Sun 2011):

(a) waterproofing to block strike-through of blood or body liquid
(b) comfort during wear, so as to avoid heat stress to wearers
(c) rapid inactivation of a broad spectrum of microorganisms
(d) non-toxicity and a minimised environmental impact
(e) durability to a specified number of washes
(f) possession of a biocidal function that can be easily recharged or refreshed
(g) ability to be eventually disposed of with minimum environmental impact

The need for air- and moisture-vapour permeability in the fabric for the gown is critical to wearer comfort as is its ability to provide a satisfactory barrier function; in terms of the ANSI/AAMI classification system for gowns, Sun states that tests have shown that bacteria can wet penetrate ANSI/AAMI PB 70 Level 3 materials given a short contact time (Sun 2011), so it is only the Level 4 type which would meet the barrier requirement. For the gown itself, safety in donning, doffing, and disposal is of paramount importance as a mistake in any of these steps can have serious negative consequences. For example, one hospital protocol involved not tying the inner tie of the surgical gown, such that the gown could be removed easily with a quick tug and folded in on itself as it was doffed prior to disposal. Other hospitals reported wearing a surgical gown as a 'human skin' simply donning and doffing the aprons worn over the gown from patient to patient, whilst leaving the gown in situ. This had the benefit not only of protecting the user but also of reducing demand on stretched PPE resources. Hats are thought to be useful because of their ability to enclose the hair and prevent its loss contaminating the surgical site, a principle similar to the practice in food manufacturing and food preparation in restaurants which is expected from any design which successfully achieves and maintains enclosure. Standard ANSI/AAMI PB70:2012 'Liquid barrier performance and classification of protective apparel and drapes intended for use in health care facilities' is currently under review (Smit 2018) and it is expected that the protection that can be offered by more items will be defined in a manner similar to that used for surgical gowns and is likely to include barrier and critical area requirements for decontamination garments such as open-back gowns; procedure gowns; hoods and toga ensembles, protective sleeves, aprons, and shoe and boot covers (but only those intended to provide barrier protection and not those such as caps or shoe covers used only for hygiene purposes).

Consequently, it is expected that a revised version of AAMI TIR11:2005/(R)2015: 'Selection and use of protective apparel and surgical drapes in health care facilities' will emerge at the same time.

Other day-to-day scenarios, away from the pandemic, where such permeability becomes increasingly important are in surgeries where radiation is used. Those surgeons are required to wear lead aprons with an interior lining layer of lead (0.5 mm) throughout the period of radiographic work as a routine which can trap a large amount of heat within the gown. There have also been concerns that the shielding apron design has not been improved over time to offer better protection to the wearers (White 2003), and particularly to improve cover for female radiographers, who otherwise suffer an increased risk of breast cancer as shown by the U.S. Radiologic Technologist Health Study 1983–998 (Sigurdson et al. 2003). Some work has been done to reduce apron weight by replacing the lead layer with radiation-absorbent textiles so as to capitalise on the improved flexibility of the textile-based shielding material and enable more opportunity for garment shaping, coverage, and comfort whilst maintaining effective shielding (Maghrabi et al. 2016; Aral, Banu Nergis and Candan 2016; Mirzaei et al. 2019).

9.4.3 Surgical Gloves

Over recent times, the materials from which surgical gloves are manufactured has changed. An important finding was the association between the powder on the gloves and the development of starch peritonitis (Ellis 1990). Furthermore, the increase in latex allergy in healthcare workers during the 1990s has also steered the manufacturing of gloves away from latex (Beezhold and Beck 1992). The range of common glove materials has widened to include not only latex but also synthetic polymers such as neoprene, polyisoprene, and nitrile rubber, a synthetic rubber made by co-polymerising acrylonitrile with butadiene (Hartley 2010).

A subject of interest is that of surgical glove perforation and the associated risk of infection to the healthcare worker or the patient. The risk of perforation has been shown to increase with the duration of operating time (increasingly so after 90 minutes) and with the fit of the glove; a poorly fitting glove is more likely to perforate. Studies have shown that the frequency of glove perforation during surgery ranges from 8% to 50% (Misteli et al. 2009; Partecke et al. 2009). The decision to use an additional layer of glove protection is influenced by a range of factors including 'risk' status of the patient, personal preference, and the surgery involved. For example, orthopaedic surgery is considered to have a higher risk of perforation. From personal experience, double layering of gloves can cause reduced sensation and dexterity to the surgeon which can be a problem when delicate work is required. This is supported in the literature (Novak et al. 1999; Wilson et al. 1996). A Cochrane review has compared single gloving with double gloving and the risk of perforation. It was found that there were more perforations in the single layer of the glove than there were in the inner layer of the double-layered gloves. Interestingly, when pooling data from multiple trials, this was consistent regardless of which type of outer glove was worn (Tanner and Parkinson 2006). A UK trial in orthopaedics found that wearing a knitted outer glove, as opposed to a standard latex glove, significantly reduced the risk of perforation to an inner latex glove ($p < 0.0001$) (Tanner, Wraighte and Howard 2006), whereas, to the contrary, a further trial with an outer glove made from a polyester/stainless steel wire weave glove found no statistical difference in inner layer perforations when compared to an outer latex glove (Louis et al. 1998). The permeation of chemicals through the glove, for example, the glutaraldehyde used to fix histological specimens, can also cause problems. One trial demonstrated that latex gloves showed the quickest permeation rate (less than an hour at 3.4% glutaraldehyde solution) whilst gloves manufactured from butyl rubber had the longest permeation rate (greater than eight hours at 3.4% solution). In addition, neoprene and polyvinyl chloride gloves should not be used with glutaraldehyde because the gloves retain or absorb the solution (Jordan et al. 1996).

The glove-gown interface has been a subject of interest following the 2010 joint registry study in New Zealand which showed increased infection rates with use of the modern surgical helmet systems when compared with conventional gowns (Hooper et al. 2011).

9.4.4 Surgical Masks and Respirators

Surgical masks date back to the late 1800s and in 1897, Radecki described a surgical mask that was composed of a single layer of gauze (Spooner 1967). Following on from a paper published by Hamilton in 1905 which advocated the use of masks by nurses performing dressings and doctors at the time of surgery (Rockwood and O'Donoghue 1960), Weaver in 1918, discussed the value of a facemask in preventing the spread of infectious disease. In subsequent years, different types of masks have been tested including gauze, paper, and filter masks. Currently, most masks are made from layered non-woven polypropylene within which the non-woven filter layer is melt blown to produce fine diameter fibres and this is sandwiched between spunbonded cover layers sometimes containing a support layer (Shen and Leonas 2005). In addition, Kimberly Clark produced a Fluidshield Fog Free Surgical mask (MEDEXSUPPLY.com 2021) with a clear visor to offer protection to the eyes (from personal experience, user application error, and a fogging up of the mask may complicate the 'protection' offered to the eyes). The length of time that a mask provides protection for has also been questioned and in fact, whether a mask needs to be worn at all has also been scrutinised (Rockwood and O'Donoghue 1960; Orr 1981), and a recent Cochrane trial was unclear as to whether wearing a surgical face mask by members of the surgical team had any impact on surgical wound infection rates for those undergoing 'clean' surgery (Vincent and Edwards 2016). The situation is more complicated, however, when masks have to protect the healthcare team from the patient, particularly when there is a likelihood of aerosols or spray being generated.

The terms *Surgical Mask or Facemask* when used in the United States, refer to Food and Drug Administration (FDA)-cleared surgical-, laser-, isolation-, dental-, and medical-procedure masks with or without a face shield. They are approved based on test results for particle filtration efficiency, bacterial filtration efficiency, fluid resistance, differential pressure, and flammability. Used by health care personnel during surgical and non-surgical procedures to protect both the patient and the healthcare worker, the Surgical Mask is intended, to cover the user's nose and mouth and provide a physical barrier to splashes/sprays of large droplets of blood or body fluids. There are, of course, also European Standards for masks (EN 14683:2019+AC: 2019; Medical face masks – Requirements and test methods), approved by CEN, the European Committee for Standardisation and available through many European countries' standards organisations (British Standards Institution 2019).

The need for Filtering Facepiece Respirators (FFRs) with Surgical Mask capabilities such as fluid resistance and flammability, was first addressed by the FDA in 1996 through the introduction of the Surgical N95 Respirator. National Institute for Occupational Safety and Health (NIESH)-approved Surgical N95 FFRs, cleared by the FDA for fluid resistance and flammability and intended to offer the combined protection of both an N95 FFR and a surgical mask to healthcare personnel (CDC & NIESH undated), are recommended in the USA during the care of patients with diseases such as tuberculosis and measles and during aerosol-generating procedures on patients with various infectious diseases such as seasonal influenza, novel influenza A, and Ebola. NIESH tests and certifies the adequacy of performance of FFRs according to requirements outlined in the US Title 42 Code of Federal Regulations (CFR) Part 84; for N95 FFRs; the primary tests are filtration efficiency and airflow resistance (Rengasamy et al. 2015). By contrast, in the European Union, the recommended FFR must meet the requirements of the more demanding European standard for filtering half masks, EN 149:2001+A1:2009, wherein the need is to be able to withstand additional challenge by an oily substance and to demonstrate higher efficiency levels than the N95 respirator. High filtration efficiency is essential, but typically, with higher efficiency comes increased difficulty in drawing the air through the filter as the wearer breathes in, pointing to the need for great care to ensure completeness of fit to ensure that unfiltered air is not drawn in from the sides. Guidance on the use of respirators and facial protection equipment has been developed and published by the Healthcare Infection Society Working Group on Respiratory and Facial Protection (Coia et al. 2013). It has been pointed out that the use of surgical N95 FFRs in both surgical and non-surgical environments increases markedly during outbreaks involving a known or suspected respiratory pathogen, and scarcities of respirators were reported during the spread of SARS in 2003 (Srinivasan et al. 2004) and H1N1 influenza in 2009 (Beckman et al. 2013).

With the advent of a growing number of pandemic threats, such as Ebola (originating in 1976 but still recurring, most recently in West Africa in 2014–2016 and sporadic cases being reported in 2020), SARS-CoV-1 (2003), Influenza A (H1N1) (2009–2010) and Middle East Respiratory Syndrome caused by the MERS Coronavirus (MERS-CoV) (2010-on) there has been interest in finding the 'best mask' to prevent infection amongst healthcare workers. During the 2009 H1N1 influenza pandemic, contradictory recommendations were given by leading authorities. The WHO recommended the use of surgical masks (World Health Organization 2009) whereas the US National Academy of Sciences recommended N95 respirator masks (Institute of Medicine 2009; Li 2011). In 2020, for the case of the COVID-19 pandemic, the USA recommended that those encountering patients in a healthcare setting should use an N95 respirator whereas in Europe, the N95 respirator has not been tested against European Standards and does not carry CE approval and it is the FFP2 respirator which is recommended. The WHO also recommends an FFP2 mask or respirator, whilst in the UK the recommendation is to use an FRSM (Fluid-Resistant Surgical Mask) in the lower risk environments but an FFP3 respirator in high-risk situations, unless there is shortage in supply in which case, according to the UK Health and Safety Executive, an FFP2 can be used instead of an FFP3. Within the UK, such judgements must always be based on a risk assessment rather than the hazard (Health and Safety Executive 2020) whereas the Guidance from America's Occupational Safety and Health Administration (OSHA) were those judgements on the protection to use should be based on a hazard analysis (OSHA 2009). It would seem reasonable to suggest that, rather than pedantically abiding by just one or the other, organisations such as the HSE and OSHA should recommend using both risk and hazard analysis.

Guidance from America's Occupational Safety and Health Administration (OSHA) in the past has been similarly pragmatic to that recently issued by the HSE in the UK, more so than that from other regulatory bodies. It considered FFRs to be one-time-use devices when used in the presence of infected patients but advised employers and employees to reuse FFRs during a pandemic, but only if FFRs were in short supply and the device had not been obviously soiled or damaged (e.g., creased or torn), and retained its ability to function properly. NIESH has provided detailed guidance on 'extended use' and 'limited re-use' (NIESH 2020) and the Centers for Disease Control and Protection (CDC) have given extensive guidance on the decontamination and reuse of filtering facepiece respirators, details of methods available, and their applicability with the focus primarily on N95 respirators (but with attention also paid to three oil-proof P100 types), plus guidance on methods not to apply (CDC 2020b).

The respective EU and American test standards (European standard for filtering half masks EN 149:2001+A1:2009 and NIOSH 42CFR84) detail key requirements as shown below in Table 9.1, where N95 meets the requirements of NIOSH42CFR84, but the FFP2, FFP3 respirators are designed to meet EN149:2001+A1:2009.

Apart from the above data taken from the UK Health and Safety Executive 'Rapid Evidence Review, March 2020' (Health and Safety Executive 2020), useful tables of equivalences between respirators from different countries are also given elsewhere (Talhelm 2021; 3M 2020). The images below in Figure 9.2 show a KN95 respirator, the Chinese equivalent of the American N95 respirator, and for comparison, a surgical mask, also of Chinese origin in this case.

To combat transmission of diseases, respirators need to be able to filter out fine particles. Such particles are classified into three categories PM10 (less than 10μm), PM2.5 (less than 2.5μm), and PM1(less than 1μm) by BS EN ISO 16890 (British Standards Institution 2016), which was based on the 'National Air Quality Standard for Particulate Matter' of the US Environmental Protection Agency (EPA); the main attention of the standard is towards High-Efficiency Particulate Air (HEPA) the efficiency standard for air filters for large spaces. BS EN 149:2001 + A1:2009 on the other hand, is the British Standard to which respiratory protective devices are tested using sodium chloride and paraffin oil at 95 l/min.

TABLE 9.1
Comparison of Key Requirements of N95, FFP2 and FFP3 Respirators (Health and Safety Executive 2020)

Requirement	N95	FFP2	FFP3
Assigned Protection factor (APF)	10	10	20
Filter efficiency	≥95% (85 l/min)	≥94% (95 l/min)	≥99% (95 l/min)
Test agent used	NaCl and Paraffin oil	NaCl	NaCl and Paraffin oil
Total inward leakage (TIL)	N/A	≤ 8%	≤ 2%
Inhalation resistance	≤ 343 Pa (85 l/min)	≤ 240 Pa (95 l/min)	≤ 300 Pa (95 l/min)
Exhalation resistance	≤ 245 Pa (85 l/min)	≤ 300 Pa (160 l/min)	≤ 300 Pa (160 l/min) 4
Re-breathed CO2	N/A	≤ 1%	≤ 1%

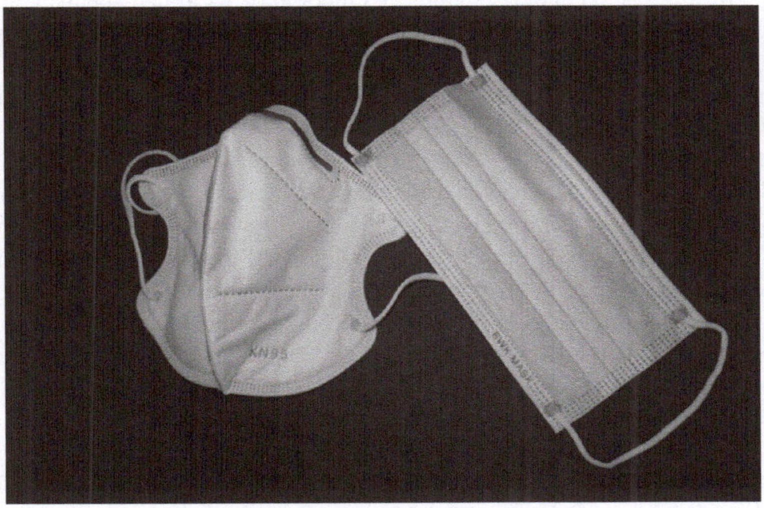

FIGURE 9.2 KN95 Respirator (on the left) and surgical mask (to the right).

Transmission of influenza can occur by sneezing or coughing and the size of the infectious particles, some of which may be aerosols, so size is variable and ranges from 0.1 to 100 μm, the Ebola virus is smaller, with a diameter of 80 nm and the Coronavirus SARS-CoV-2 is about 120 nm in size (3M 2020) but exists primarily in aerosol droplets from 0.05 -16 μm Loeb et al. 2009).

Research to produce a 'better' mask has taken several different avenues. For example, a useful and detailed set of criteria were set down by the Department of Veterans' Affairs project: 'Better Respiratory Equipment using Advanced Technologies for

Healthcare Employees' (BREATHE). A heavyweight Working Group, 'BREATHE' was brought together to design a new and improved respirator specifically for health care personnel, beyond the N95 (and reusable up to ten times), which would be called the B95 (Gosch et al. 2013), but nothing further seems to have emerged from this initiative.

Work has gone ahead however with the intention of improving the performance of the surgical mask. How such a mask is working and its ability to fit closely has been studied, particularly by a group at Shinshu University in Japan, for example by assessing the fitting patterns of masks for closed and open mouths (Morishima et al. 2015). Pleated masks may allow mouth movement but the movement of the mouth can alter the pleats and can still create an air gap, so to allow for the shape variation of the face with the mouth open and to achieve good fitting performance for a larger population, a mask sheet made from knitted fabric was proposed (Morishima et al. 2016), but achieving good mask fit which will also allow for the mouth to open and close still poses problems (Morishima and Mitsuno 2019a), as do the particular requirements in the design of masks for young people (with closed mouth) as explored by researchers from the same group. It proved difficult to achieve good fit for all face shapes (Morishima and Mitsuno 2019b). More recently, a group at the Georgia Institute of Technology in the USA reported work aimed at enhancing both fit and antiviral action in the surgical mask which should improve safety during wear and doffing (Park and Jayaraman 2020), but the underlying design of the surgical mask is such that overall, it is less effective than the tight-fitting surgical respirators such as the N95 and the FFP2 and FFP3.

The presence on the market of sophisticated surgical masks such as the HEIQ Viroblock FFP2 NR illustrates the difficulties facing manufacturers when trying to promote their products. Despite having been tested for its antiviral effectiveness in terms of improved reduction in virus infectivity of the antimicrobial-treated masks compared to untreated control masks for several (specified) viruses, and testing which shows that the HEIQ Viroblock FFP2 NR treatment is durable to up to 30 washes, the wording used on the webpage in describing the effectiveness of the antiviral and antibacterial agent HEIQ Viroblock NPJ03 (HEIQ Viroblock 2021) is very careful to state, in its European version:

> Active healthcare claims on treated articles such as antiviral are not permitted in the USA and require pesticidal device registration. Antiviral claims are permitted in Germany on most treated articles and can be evaluated on a case-by-case basis in other EU territory. Antimicrobial properties built in to protect the product. Product does not protect users or others against pathogens. Always clean the product thoroughly after each use.

The version for the USA is truncated and does not include all the test details or table of results of tests of effectiveness of the treatment against specific viruses and bacteria, and instead the accent in the text is limited to odour control and reduced degradation of the textile. Inability to claim antiviral activity illustrates the importance of being able to demonstrate performance in practice sufficient to secure FDA approval. Even so, it does use the term 'medical fabrics' and claim that they benefit from the antimicrobial treatment:

> Protective medical fabrics, e.g., used for face masks, air filters, medical gowns, curtains, drapes; clothing, upholstery, mattresses; products of all fibre types (especially nonwovens) can benefit from this innovative fabric treatment. Antimicrobial properties built in to protect the product. Product does not protect users or others against bacteria, viruses, germs, or other disease organisms. Always clean the product thoroughly after each use

Regarding research into the construction of masks, the addition of a fluorochemical repellent finish intended for the outer filter layer in masks (Shen and Leonas 2005) and the use of an antimicrobial, nanoparticle covering finish has been reported (Li et al. 2006; HEIQ 2021) as has, most recently, the use of nanofibre webs in the filtration layers to try to improve both filtration effectiveness and comfort (Suen et al. 2020). Attention has also been paid to other ways of helping the filtration material to work more effectively rather than simply by obstruction by the filter fibres; the development of electrets for improving the performance of fibrous filters was reported as early as 1976 (Van Turnhout 1986). Indeed, the feature of N95 and FFP2- and FFP3-type filters which substantially enhances their effectiveness is the incorporation of an electret in the form of polypropylene microfibres charged through exposure by corona charging. Nonpolar polymers such as polyolefins can become even better electret materials for use in air filtration especially if the polymer is loaded with a high-dielectric additive before spinning such as barium titanate (1%) with a particle size mostly below 2.1 μm (Kilic et al. 2015).

Electret filters are used in high-efficiency filtration particularly because they are effective at low-pressure drops, a critical metric in PPE design since it directly affects breathing comfort and the length of time a respirator can be worn. The electret filter as opposed to the mechanical filter displays enhanced ability to capture airborne particles due to coulombic attraction and induced polarisation and therefore tend to exhibit a higher quality factor (QF), i.e., the ratio of relative efficiency to unit pressure drops. Because of their electrical conductivity and low regain values at most humidity levels, polypropylene fibres are very good at retaining their electrical charge; this allows them to continue to attract particles passing into the filter medium even following considerable periods of ageing. It has been shown for example that N95 masks (which do contain an electret layer) retain their performance through storage for periods of at least ten years (Viscusi et al. 2009a).

There is still, however, not only a lack of research in the area of how long a mask remains effective in actual use (critical in surgical applications and infectious disease transmission) but also a problem with acceptance of possible treatments for the decontamination of respirators and a lack of official certification rather than emergency permission to enable their re-use after exposure to viruses, despite useful baseline research conducted ten years ago by Viscusi, Bergman, and co-workers. Various decontamination treatments were explored and reported in 2009 by Viscusi (Viscusi et al. 2009b) and in 2010 by Bergman (Bergman et al. 2010) following the H1N1 outbreak in the USA, because health officials in the USA had expressed concerns about possible shortages of N95 respirators during pandemics such as the H1N1 influenza crisis in 2009. To improve on the information gained earlier by Viscusi (Viscusi et al. 2009b) from successful single application of a number of different decontamination procedures, Bergman (Bergman et al. 2010) investigated three-cycle (3X) processing using eight different methods on six FFR models: ultraviolet germicidal irradiation, ethylene oxide, hydrogen peroxide gas plasma, hydrogen peroxide vapour, microwave-oven-generated steam, bleach, liquid hydrogen peroxide, and moist-heat incubation (pasteurisation). A four-hour 3X submersion of FFR in deionised water was performed for comparison to act as a control. Only the hydrogen peroxide gas-plasma treatment resulted in reduced performance with mean penetration levels > 5% for four of the six FFR models; FFRs treated by the seven other methods and the control samples had expected levels of filter aerosol penetration (< 5%) and filter airflow resistance. However, there was some physical damage to the respirators which varied by treatment method, and it was considered that further research was still needed before any specific decontamination methods could be recommended.

Ten years later, when COVID-19 had been spreading for six months, it was clear that whatever (if any) preparations had taken place to prepare for such a pandemic were seriously inadequate, not just in the USA and the UK, but across the whole of the EU as well, and at that stage in Italy. Responding to that worsening situation, on April 1, 2020, at the height of the COVID-19 epidemic, the Stanford Anaesthesia Informatics and Media Lab in the School of Medicine at Stanford University established a rapidly growing group called N95DECON to create a set of best practices on the decontamination and reuse of N95 respirators; the website is full of guidance and continually updated (N95DECON 2020). Several decontamination methods were put forward, several of which were based on the earlier work published by Viscusi et al. and Bergmann et al. (Viscusi et al. 2009b; Bergman et al. 2010) and some US hospitals such as the Barnes Jewish Hospital in Washington DC (Grossman et al. 2020) were quick off the mark and had already implemented decontamination and reuse procedures for N95 respirators to counteract shortages; they used the system developed by Batelle and reported to the FDA in 2016 (Battelle 2016) which used vaporised hydrogen peroxide generated by a BioQuell Clarus C HPV generator (as used for disinfection of clean rooms, laboratories, equipment and surfaces; Ecolab, Saint Paul, Min, USA). Another approach in place by mid-March at the University of Nebraska Medical Center successfully used ultraviolet irradiation to process used N95 respirators for Nebraska Medicine (Lowe et al. 2020) and a UV-C and high-level disinfection cabinet systems were also explored (Cadnum et al. 2020). A method for use across Europe, involving the reprocessing FFP2 masks was developed, tested, and costed by a Swiss team (Widmer and Richner 2020) and shown to be both effective and cheap to carry out, much more economical than using once and disposing. By mid-April 2020, the FDA had issued several factsheets on decontamination of N95 respirators by various methods. These were put forward based on *Emergency Use Authorisation (EUA)* (FDA 2020b, c). The Stryker decontamination of compatible N95 respirators was approved using the Stryker Sterizone VP4 N95

Respirator Decontamination Cycle in the Sterizone VP4 Sterilizer (compatible N95 respirators are those that do not contain cellulose-based or paper materials, natural rubber, or latex). The device uses vaporised hydrogen peroxide as the decontaminant followed by ozone and this only enabled decontamination for 'single-user reuse up to two times' as was the case for the ASP STERRAD Sterilisation, another hydrogen peroxide vapour system, whereas decontamination with the Sterilucent HC 80TT Vaporized Hydrogen Peroxide (VHP) Sterilizer allowed for a maximum of ten decontamination cycles and a new EUA for Technical Safety Services LLC, Berkeley, CA. which allows decontamination and reuse 20 times was the latest to be issued (June 13, 2020). It is clear from outcomes such as these that blanket approval cannot be given for treatments simply because they make use of the sterilising effects of a particular agent or type of agent. It is the controlled application of the whole treatment procedure that is required to achieve the desired extent of reusability.

The STERIS STEAM Decon Cycle in AMSCO Medium Steam Sterilizers also allowed for a maximum of ten decontamination cycles but the Duke decontamination system, also based on vapour-phase hydrogen peroxide and also allowing for a maximum of ten decontamination cycles, had not been approved by CDC/NIOSH. The best of the methods in the FDA *Emergency Use Authorisation* list, in terms of number of decontamination cycles allowed, was the Battelle Decontamination System for Compatible N95 Respirators, based on exposure to vapourised hydrogen peroxide for 150 minutes, which would allow for up to a maximum of 20 decontamination cycles and was the earliest to be approved under the EUA (29 March 2020) presumably on account of their report to the FDA in 2016 (Battelle 2016). For whatever reasons, the FDA (June 5, 2020) had not yet seen fit to approve Liao et al's preferred system for decontamination and reuse despite it being able to offer 50 cycles of decontamination and reuse (Liao et al. 2020a,b). By April 9, 2021, the FDA in their: "Letter to health care personnel and facilities," was recommending a transition from the use of decontaminated disposable respirators because of increased domestic supply of new respirators (FDA 2021b). What many might consider a far better response with longer term significance, this time based in Canada has been to undertake design and development of a reusable N95 mask to counteract shortages experienced in Manitoba. Precision ADM, a manufacturing company in Winnipeg, won a bid to make 1 million reusable N95 masks for the Manitoba government. The masks, designed by two Manitoba doctors, can be used up to 30 times with disinfecting after each use, says a news release from the province (CBC 2020).

9.4.5 Healthcare Workers' Clothing and Uniforms

Healthcare workers' clothing also requires consideration alongside PPE, and methods have been developed to enable rapid quantitative testing with the real-time polymerase chain reaction (qPCR) to check for the presence of nosocomial pathogens (Rozman et al. 2013). Whilst most of the contamination is from the wearer of the uniform, uniforms have been found to become frequently contaminated below the waist and heavily contaminated after procedures that involve exposure to pathogens

(Speers et al. 1969). Using a plastic apron significantly reduces contamination at the front of the uniform (Babb, Davies and Ayliffe 1983).

Bacterial transfer under dry conditions has also been investigated on the most common reusable fabrics for healthcare professional uniforms (Tencel® and PET/Cotton) (Rogina-Car et al. 2017). A three-layer laminate (PU/PET/PU) for surgical drapes that meets the European Standard for surgical drapes (EN 13795) was used as the reference. The relative performances of each of the other fabrics and their seams in terms of bacterial transfer were checked against this fabric, plus their ability to maintain performance for up to 50 laundering and disinfection cycles which was carried out using hospital laundering and steam-sterilisation services. The PU/PET/PU laminate proved to be the best barrier fabric followed by the Tencel® then the PET/Cotton, barrier performance by the Tencel® improved with repeated laundering and sterilisation. Although, with their greater thickness, bacterial penetration was lower at the seams, the two most commonly used seam types for the manufacture of healthcare uniforms were found not to have a significant influence on microbial barrier efficacy. Having said that, the seam type 1.01.05/504.504.301 was considered more suitable than type 1.01.02/ 301.504, which is more susceptible to gaping on the application of tension to the seam (Rogina-Car et al. 2017); (seam-type terminology here is in line with ISO 4916:1991, Textiles-Seam Types-Classification and Terminology; see (ClothingIndustry 2018) for an illustrated explanation of seam types). Doctors' white coats become progressively more contaminated as they are worn and it is for this reason that hospitals have now made them obsolete on their uniform policy (Wong, Hollis and Nye 1991; Loh, Ng and Holton 2000).

Reference was made earlier (Section 5.5.3) to the need to apply the OECD protocol to tests to determine the effectiveness of treatments aimed at achieving disinfection. From the application of approaches which more closely match the final stage requirements set for OECD 3-Tier testing, evidence is building that indications obtained about antimicrobial efficiency of medical textile workwear obtained by standard test procedures applied in the laboratory may not be demonstrated in the practical setting. Methods which are laboratory based but which more closely match what happens to treated items in the intended area of practice require urgent attention. It is likely that such 'Tier 2' tests will sift out a high proportion of prospective agents/treatments because they do not perform well enough under realistic test regimes. Whereas barrier testing appears to take account of various quite realistic ways that bodily fluids might splash onto or be squeezed into items of PPE, there appears to be a need for Tier 2 test which more closely emulates the conditions to which scrubs, and healthcare workers' uniforms are exposed during the working day. Otherwise, the penalty that is paid is the disappointment of discovering that antimicrobial treatments provide no measurable benefit to patients or healthcare personnel regarding those items:

i) The outcomes of the Antimicrobial Scrub Contamination and Transmission (ASCOT) trial, part of the CDC Prevention Epicenters Program reported in 2017 (Anderson et al. 2017) were negative. Three types of treated polyester/cotton blend scrubs were issued, a control (untreated) set, a set that contained a silver-alloy embedded in its fibres, or scrubs impregnated with an organosilane-based quaternary ammonium and a hydrophobic fluoroacrylate copolymer emulsion. A three-arm, blinded, randomised controlled trial with crossover design was used to determine the efficacy of the antimicrobial-impregnated scrubs in preventing contamination of the healthcare personnel and it showed that those antimicrobial-impregnated scrubs were not effective at reducing contamination, despite the presence in one case of a finish expected to be both antimicrobial and fluid repellent.

ii) A randomised controlled trial with 105 participants (hospital physicians, nurse practitioners, physician assistants, house staff, and nurses working in internal medicine units) was undertaken to compare the extent of bacterial contamination of uniforms and skin when healthcare workers wore 1 of 2 antimicrobial scrubs or standard scrubs. Bacterial colony counts were carried out on cultures taken from the healthcare worker's scrubs and wrists at the end of the working day. There was no evidence that either antimicrobial scrub product decreased bacterial contamination of healthcare workers' uniforms or skin after an eight-hour working day (Burden et al. 2013).

iii) A study undertaken in a veterinary setting suggested that silver impregnation of fabric was ineffective in reducing surface bacterial contamination of surgical scrub tops during use in a veterinary surgical suite. Although silver impregnation appeared to be effective in reducing bacterial contamination on the scrubs during storage, it was found that any bacterial contamination of scrub suits presents when they were first put on could persist through the working day. Rather than assuming that silver impregnation was exerting a positive effect, it was recommended that precautions such as wearing disposable plastic aprons during patient contact, regularly changing surgical scrubs during the working day and strict hand hygiene may be more effective in reducing bacterial contamination than buying supposed 'antibacterial' scrubs (Freeman, Halladay, and Cripps 2012).

iv) Significantly higher bacteria counts were isolated from home-laundered scrubs and unwashed scrubs than from new, hospital-laundered, or disposable scrubs (Nordstrom, Reynolds, and Gerba 2012).

v) A review undertaken at the behest of the Department of Health (England) in 2007 found that there was no robust evidence of a difference in efficacy of decontamination of uniforms/clothing between industrial and domestic laundry processes, or that the home laundering of uniforms provides inadequate decontamination. However, only a small number of relevant studies were found; those found provided limited evidence directly related to the decontamination of uniforms. Studies concerning domestic laundry processes were small scale and largely observational whilst practice current at the time and guidance for laundering uniforms was extrapolated from studies of industrial hospital linen processing (Wilson et al. 2007).

vi) A recent review concluded that a number of studies had indicated that microorganisms survive on textiles for extended periods of time and can transfer on to skin and other surfaces hence raising the possibility that they

> might be transferred through contact between staff or patients and contaminated textiles. A number of case studies linked small outbreaks with inadequate laundering or poor infection-control processes for healthcare laundry. Others demonstrated the survival of potential pathogens during laundering of healthcare textiles, which might possibly increase the risk of infection. Although there are no large-scale epidemiological studies demonstrating a direct link between healthcare-acquired infections and contaminated textiles, evidence of outbreaks given in case studies needs attention. Adequate microbial decontamination of linen and infection control procedures during laundering are required to minimise the risk of infection from healthcare textiles which means that domestic laundering of healthcare worker uniforms is of concern because its lack of control and failure to monitor decontamination may provide a route for potential pathogens to enter the clinical environment. Industrial laundering of healthcare worker uniforms has the potential to provide bettter assurance of decontamination than domestic laundering, due to the ability to monitor the critical laundering parameters (Owen and Laird 2020).

Owen and Laird's review indicates that not much has changed regarding the approach used in conducting research into the development of antimicrobial treatments for uniforms since the DoH (England) report of 2007, and no consensus yet on whether their laundering at home is less effective. What is beginning to show though is that antimicrobial treatments expected to work based on laboratory trials and currently approved test methods are ineffective on workwear, so there remains considerable scope for improvement.

The design of the healthcare workers clothing intended to be used in those situations involving direct contact with a patient is thought to be important in controlling healthcare-acquired infections (HCAIs), with the National Institute for Care Excellence in the UK and Queensland Health in Australia recommending application of a 'Bare Below the Elbows' routine coupled with immediate hand decontamination following patient contact (NICE 2012a; Queensland Health 2017)). Scrubs offer an appropriate design for achieving the routine, but the routine is not universally followed.

As mentioned earlier, the two most commonly used seam types for the manufacture of healthcare uniforms have been tested for their dry-transfer microbial barrier properties using a three-layer textile laminate PET/PU/PET, which meets the European standards for surgical drapes EN 13795 as the reference material alongside PET/cotton blend and Tencel® fabrics. The seams were tested after 1, 10, 20, 30, and 50 hospital laundry washing-and-sterilisation cycles and whilst neither seam choice affected microbial barrier efficiency under dry-transfer conditions, seam type 1.01.05/504.504.301 was considered the more suitable of the two for use in healthcare uniforms.

Laundering of the uniforms and whether this should be undertaken in a professional laundering facility or whether it can be undertaken at home has been considered, primarily because if not carried out conscientiously, there is concern that residual contamination could lead to surgical site infection (SSI). Its incidence depends on the type of procedure carried out, but it is estimated that between 300,000 and 500,000 cases occur annually across the USA (Vera, Umadhay and Fisher 2016) and in the UK, according to NICE, healthcare-associated infections, besides being unsafe for patients, are estimated to cost the NHS approximately £1 billion a year, of which only £56 million is estimated to be incurred after patients are discharged from hospital (NICE 2012b). It has been shown that in a ten-minute wash at 60°C, the addition of either a biological or non-biological detergent was effective in removing MRSA from experimentally contaminated swatches and that low levels of recontamination of uniforms could be effectively removed by (hot) ironing (Lakdawala et al. 2011). Even so, professional laundering should be preferable because its effectiveness can be routinely controlled and monitored (or *potentially* it can be routinely controlled and monitored). Traditionally, healthcare workers' uniforms have been washed industrially in washer-extractors and dried in tunnel driers, rather than by batch continuous washing in tunnel washers and tumble drying. It is thought that this method gives a substantially greater dilution of contamination than either batch or continuous washing machines, though the review was inconclusive (Wilson et al. 2007; Riley, Fergusson and Shen 2017). Heavily contaminated items such as some bedlinen are washed separately from uniform laundry, and that minimises the possibility of cross-contamination. Whereas domestic laundering of uniforms is carried out at temperatures as low as 40°C, commercial laundry tunnel washers for bedlinen typically rely on high temperatures to bring about disinfection. However, low-energy, low-cost wash systems can be very usefully applied for laundering within hospitals, particularly those which generate and use ozone to achieve both decontamination and disinfection such as the OTEX system (JLA 2021).

Whilst little attention generally has been turned to un-scrubbed members of the staff, a substantial reduction in airborne contamination occurs when un-scrubbed staff wear non-woven fabrics. This highlights the importance of the protective barrier that the clothing can offer in terms of preventing contaminants arising from the wearer's body being lost into the working environment during wear. It was found that the efficacy of non-woven clothing was superior to that of woven clothing, even at the end of the day when clothing was showing a frayed appearance. Indeed, as much as a 72% reduction in bacteria dispersal is noted for male surgeons wearing non-woven clothing. When rubber bands were worn over the shirt sleeves of males, the bacterial dispersion was reduced by 35% compared to without demonstrating the importance of axillary dispersion of bacteria in contamination of surrounding environment (Mitchell et al. 1978). With the development of new fabrics and fibres, the potential for development of uniforms expands. Consideration to disposal of used uniforms in an environmental and economic way is also of importance.

9.4.6 Patient Clothing

Consideration should also be given to clothing for patients. Some work has been carried out on clothing for children in the hospital environment (Wong et al. 2000) but it should be expected that the clothing worn by patients could soon play a much more active role in patient care in the future, particularly in the case of 'Electronic Textiles' for monitoring critical functions, garments within which fibres have been engineered to perform particular actions in support of healthcare such as drug delivery from hollow fibres controlled by thermal stimuli (Wai Cheung, Yang and Li 2019) and items made from antimicrobial-treated textiles (given the development of adequate test methods such as those referred to in Section 9.4.7 and Chapter 5 Section 5.3.3)).

9.5 TESTING OF HEALTH AND HYGIENE PRODUCTS

Reference was made in Chapter 5, Section 5.5.3 to the need to apply the OECD protocol to tests to determine the effectiveness of treatments aimed at achieving disinfection (OECD 2008). From the application of approaches which more closely match the final stage requirements set for OECD 3-Tier testing, evidence is building that indications obtained about antimicrobial efficiency of medical textile workwear obtained by standard test procedures applied in the laboratory may not be demonstrated in the practical setting. The negative outcomes of the Antimicrobial Scrub Contamination and Transmission (ASCOT) trial on the ineffectiveness of antimicrobial treatments in the practical setting, as reported in 2017 (Anderson et al. 2017) reinforces that need. Methods which are laboratory based but which more closely match what happens to treated items in practice require urgent attention. It is likely that such 'Tier 2' tests will help by sifting out a very high proportion of what are currently thought to be prospective agents/treatments because they do not perform the expected function under testing regimes that closely simulate those of the real setting (OECD 2019).

Testing regimes where the materials treated with antimicrobial agents involve immersion or long-term contact with moisture simply do not come close to simulating the mostly dry conditions, occasional splashing and pressing against the operating table or patient in the operating theatre, so how the active species from the agent will reach the pathogen, react with it and thereby succeed in disabling it is likely to have to be completely different. Not all of the tests are a waste of time. The barrier tests:

ANSI/AAMI PB70:2012 'Liquid barrier performance and classification of protective apparel and drapes intended for use in health care facilities.'

ISO 16603:2004: *Clothing for protection against contact with blood and body fluids — Determination of the resistance of protective clothing materials to penetration by blood and body fluids — Test method using synthetic blood* (International Standards Organisation 2004a), and

ISO 16604:2004: *Clothing for protection against contact with blood and body fluids — Determination of resistance of protective clothing materials to penetration by blood-borne pathogens — Test method using Phi-X 174 bacteriophage* (International Standards Organisation 2004b)

deserve considerable respect. When suitable test regimes and treatments for scrubs, uniforms, and other general workwear are introduced, they should include the need for the treatment to be durable for up to 50 laundry cycles, and the nature of the cycle to which samples are exposed in the test should be specified to match those which will be used in hospitals or commercial laundries undertaking hospital laundry work. For filter facepieces (respirators), it is not so much a matter of modifying the test method, but more an issue to do with the specification in the first place not including a need for the items to be able to demonstrate their ability to be safely reprocessed and reused, a key performance measure which turns out not to be an impossible task after all (CBC 2020).

9.6 SUMMARY

Healthcare hygiene and personal protective equipment in the medical textile sector cover a vast range from products used for disinfection such as disposable and reusable cleaning materials, through bedlinen, furniture, and fittings such as air filters and air treatment devices, to patient wear and staff clothing and protective wear. The environment for which they are intended ranges from the operating theatre and the hospital ward, through to clinics and care homes. Each item of equipment needs to perform in its own way and, it should be remembered, it should be manufactured in such a way as to suit the requirements set by its intended environment. Many items perform well, but the disposable types take a heavy toll on the environment through greenhouse gas emissions and economically in cost terms. Instead of adopting to use disposables because of habit, directions are given in this chapter on useful sources of information which can be used to help to decide whether to use disposables, remanufactured or reusable items for a particular purpose, and about the improved methods which are becoming available for undertaking decontamination and high-level disinfection. Availability of high-usage items being able to be guaranteed locally and other initiatives to remove the possibility of a return to PPE supply crises such as those which have arisen during the COVID-19 are shown to be important for the future. The example of the 50 times reusable-respirator development in Manitoba during the COVID-19 pandemic demands particular attention. With the exception of the barrier test methods (which are very useful) there is a need to stop mindlessly using traditional test methods more suited to assessing the suitability and effectiveness of antimicrobial agents in implants, wet wipes, or cleaning cloths than for the environmental conditions to which PPE workwear and uniforms are exposed.

Despite an intense level of research work directed at a variety of interesting compounds, most if not all are ineffective in their intended operating environment. Test methods suitable for implanted medical textiles in continuous contact with fluids, and for textiles used in hygiene items and devices involving application of aqueous solutions, are too different from those of the environment which applies to PPE during wear (mostly dry, some splashing, some pressure-transfer of contaminants, some drying out) to give an adequate indication of their likely effectiveness in practice. The value of the more-rigorous OECD ‘Three Tier’ approach should not be ignored. Researchers need to make a new start by following its guidance, rather than adopting easy-to-apply testing regimes not suited to the environment that will be experienced by those wearing the garments.

REFERENCES

3M. "Respiratory Protection for Airborne Exposures to Biohazards: 3M Technical Data Bulletin Release 5 June 2020 #174." 2020. Accessed June 3rd, 2021. https://multimedia.3m.com/mws/media/409903O/respiratory-protection-against-biohazards.pdf.

Action Aid. "Period Poverty." 2021. Accessed May 25th, 2021. https://www.actionaid.org.uk/about-us/what-we-do/womens-economic-empowerment/period-poverty.

Aibibu, Dilibaier, Beata Lehmann, and Peter Offermann. "Barrier effect of woven fabrics used for surgical gowns." *AUTEX Research Journal* 3, no. 4 (2003): 186–193.

Airius. "Air Purification in the PHI cell." 2021. Accessed June 8th, 2021. https://www.airius.co.uk/all-resources/coronavirus-protection-a-simple-solution-that-could-protect-against-the-spread/.

Airvia Medical Air Purifier.co.uk. "High-Performance Air Purifiers by AIRVIA Medical." 2021. Accessed June 3rd, 2021. https://www.airpurifier.co.uk/?gclid=EAIaIQobChMI7cuSlPiU6gIVlfhRCh2IUwGqEAAYASAAEgLKd_D_BwE.

AMDR. "The Business Case for Reprocessing." 2011. Accessed June 3rd, 2021. http://amdr.org/wp-content/uploads/2011/04/Business-Case-for-Reprocessing-for-web-1.pdf.

AMDR. "Peer Reviewed" AMDR Bibliography of Peer-Reviewed Articles and Other Scientific Literature on Reprocessing; AMDR 2021. 2021. Accessed June 3rd, 2021. http://www.amdr.org/news/peer-reviewed/.

American Association of Textile Chemists and Colorists. A"TM127 Test Method for Water Resistance: Hydrostatic Pressure". 2019. Accessed. May 28th, 2020. https://members.aatcc.org/store/tm127/535/.

Anderson, Deverick J., Rachel Addison, Yuliya Lokhnygina, Bobby Warren, Batu Sharma-Kuinkel, Laura J. Rojas, Susan D. Rudin et al. "The antimicrobial scrub contamination and transmission (ASCOT) trial: A three-arm, blinded, randomized controlled trial with crossover design to determine the efficacy of antimicrobial-impregnated scrubs in preventing healthcare provider contamination." *Infection Control & Hospital Epidemiology* 38, no. 10 (2017): 1147–1154.

Aral, Nebahat, F. Banu Nergis, and Cevza Candan. "An alternative X-ray shielding material based on coated textiles." *Textile Research Journal* 86, no. 8 (2016): 803–811.

Aslan, Selçuk, Sibel Kaplan, and Cem Çetin. "An investigation about comfort and protection performances of disposable and reusable surgical gowns by objective and subjective measurements." *Journal of the Textile Institute* 104, no. 8 (2013): 870–882.

Association for Perioperative Practice. "COVID-19: Updated Infection Prevention and Control Guidance". 2020. Acccessed June 3rd, 2021. https://www.afpp.org.uk/news/COVID-19_Updated_Infection_Prevention_and_Control_Guidance.

ASTM. "ASTM F1671 / F1671M-13, Standard Test Method for Resistance of Materials Used in Protective Clothing to Penetration by Blood-Borne Pathogens Using Phi-X174 Bacteriophage Penetration as a Test System." 2013. Accessed June 3rd, 2021. https://www.astm.org/Standards/F1671.htm

ASTM. "ASTM F1670 / F1670M-17a, Standard Test Method for Resistance of Materials Used in Protective Clothing to Penetration by Synthetic Blood." 2017. Accessed June 3rd, 2021. https://www.astm.org/Standards/F1670.htm

Babb, J. R., J. G. Davies, and G. A. J. Ayliffe. "Contamination of protective clothing and nurses' uniforms in an isolation ward." *Journal of Hospital Infection* 4, no. 2 (1983): 149–157.

Bagness, C. "Period Poverty." 2020. Accessed June 3rd, 2021. https://www.rcn.org.uk/clinical-topics/womens-health/promoting-menstrual-wellbeing/period-poverty.

Barton, Mary. "Intravaginal packs." *British Medical Journal* 1, no. 4248 (1942): 709.

Battelle. "Final Report for Bioquell HPV Decontamination for Reuse of N95 Respirator". 2016. Accessed June 3rd, 2021. https://www.fda.gov/media/136386/download.

Beck, Wm C., and Thomas S. Collette. "False faith in the surgeon's gown and surgical drape." *The American Journal of Surgery* 83, no. 2 (1952): 125–126.

Beckman, Stella, Barbara Materna, Suzi Goldmacher, Jennifer Zipprich, Maryann D'Alessandro, Debra Novak, and Robert Harrison. "Evaluation of respiratory protection programs and practices in California hospitals during the 2009–2010 H1N1 influenza pandemic." *American Journal of Infection Control* 41, no. 11 (2013): 1024–1031.

Beezhold, Donald, and William C. Beck. "Surgical glove powders bind latex antigens." *Archives of Surgery* 127, no. 11 (1992): 1354–1357.

Bergman, Michael S., Dennis J. Viscusi, Brian K. Heimbuch, Joseph D. Wander, Anthony R. Sambol, and Ronald E. Shaffer. "Evaluation of multiple (3-cycle) decontamination processing for filtering facepiece respirators." *Journal of Engineered Fibers and Fabrics* 5, no. 4 (2010): 155892501000500405.

British Standards Institution. "Specification for Hospital Bedding" BS 5223–3 and BS 5223-4, 1976." 1976. Accessed June 3rd, 2021. https://shop.bsigroup.com/ProductDetail?pid=000000000000050776.

British Standards Institution. "BS EN ISO 16890; Air filters for general ventilation. Technical Specifications, Requirements and Classification System Based Upon Particulate Matter Efficiency (ePM) (2016)." 2016. Accessed June 3rd, 2021. https://www.iso.org/standard/57864.html

British Standards Institution 2019 "BS EN 14683:2019 Medical face masks. Requirements and test methods. March 2019". Accessed June 3rd, 2021. https://shop.bsigroup.com/ProductDetail/?pid=000000000030401487.

British Standards Institution. "BS. EN 13795-1:2019 Surgical Clothing and Drapes. Requirements and Test Methods. Surgical Drapes and Gowns." 2019. Accessed June 3rd, 2021. https://shop.bsigroup.com/ProductDetail?pid=000000000030358659

Brobbey, Kofi Jocelyn, Janne Haapanen, Mikko Tuominen, Jyrki Mäkelä, Marianne Gunell, Erkki Eerola, Jarkko J. Saarinen, and Martti Toivakka. "High-speed production of antibacterial fabrics using liquid flame spray." *Textile Research Journal* 90, no. 5–6 (2020): 503–511.

Burden, Marisha, Angela Keniston, Maria G. Frank, Carrie A. Brown, Jeff Zoucha, Lilia Cervantes, Diane Weed, Kathy Boyle, Connie Price, and Richard K. Albert. "Bacterial contamination of healthcare workers' uniforms: A randomized controlled trial of antimicrobial scrubs." *Journal of Hospital Medicine* 8, no. 7 (2013): 380–385.

Cadnum, Jennifer L., Daniel F. Li, Sarah N. Redmond, Amrita R. John, Basya Pearlmutter, and Curtis J. Donskey. "Effectiveness of ultraviolet-C light and a high-level disinfection cabinet for decontamination of N95 respirators." *Pathogens and Immunity* 5, no. 1 (2020): 52.

Cao, Wei, and Rinn M. Cloud. "The effect of pre-wetting on liquid penetration performance of surgical gown fabrics." *The Journal of the Textile Institute* 102, no. 7 (2011): 604–611.

CBC. "Shift to Reusable PPE 'An Immediate Need' for Public Health — But Transition Won't be Simple, Experts Say." 2020. Accessed June 28th, 2020. https://www.cbc.ca/news/canada/manitoba/reusable-ppe-covid-19-manitoba-1.5628089

CDC. "Toxic Shock Syndrome: A Lasting Legacy." 2020a. Accessed June 3rd, 2021. https://www.cdc.gov/od/science/wewerethere/toxicshock/index.html

CDC. "Implementing Filtering Facepiece Respirator (FFR) Reuse, Including Reuse after Decontamination, When There Are Known Shortages of N95 Respirators Decontamination and Reuse of Filtering Facepiece Respirators, 30 April 2020." 2020a. Accessed June 3rd, 2021. https://www.cdc.gov/coronavirus/2019-ncov/hcp/ppe-strategy/decontamination-reuse-respirators.html.

Centers for Disease Control and Prevention and the National Institute for Occupational Safety and Health. "Hospital Respiratory Protection Program Toolkit". 2020. Accessed June 3rd, 2021. https://www.cdc.gov/niosh/npptl/pdfs/UnderstandDifferenceInfographic-508.pdf.

Charnley, J., and N. Eftekhar. "Penetration of gown material by organisms from the surgeon's body." *The Lancet* 293, no. 7587 (1969): 172–174.

ClothingIndustry. "Blogspot. Seam Classification and Quality of Seam in Garments". 2018. Accessed June. 20th, 2020. https://clothingindustry.blogspot.com/2018/03/seam-classification-quality-seam.html.

Coia, J. E., L. Ritchie, A. Adisesh, C. Makison Booth, C. Bradley, D. Bunyan, G. Carson et al. "Guidance on the use of respiratory and facial protection equipment." *Journal of Hospital Infection* 85, no. 3 (2013): 170–182.

Colebrook, Leonard, and A. M. Hood. "Infection through soaked dressings." *Lancet* (1948): 682–683.

Das, Dipayan, Arun Kumar Pradhan, R. Chattopadhyay, and S. N. Singh. "Composite nonwovens." *Textile Progress* 44, no. 1 (2012): 1–84.

Delaney, Janice, Mary Jane Lupton, and Emily Toth. *The Curse: A Cultural History of Menstruation*. University of Illinois Press, 1988.

Department of Health. "Health Technical Memorandum 01-04" Decontamination of Linen for Health and Social Care; Guidance for Linen Processors Implementing BS EN 14065. March 2016". 2016. Accessed June 3rd, 2021. https://assets.publishing.service.gov.uk/government/uploads/system/uploads/attachment_data/file/527546/BS_EN14065.pdf

Dural-Erem, Aysin, Per Wessman, Ulrika Husmark, and Vincent Nierstrasz. "Biocontrol of solid surfaces in hospitals using microbial-based wipes." *Textile Research Journal* 89, no. 2 (2019): 216–222.

DUST ARREST. "UV-C Air Purifier with Huge 3'600m3/h Airflow - MAXVAC MEDI 40 Dustblocker Virus Steriliser." 2021. Accessed June 3rd, 2021. https://dustarrest.com/products/maxvac-dustblocker-medi-40-with-uv-c-virus-sterilizer

Edwards, Nicholas W. M., Emma L. Best, Parikshit Goswami, M. H. Wilcox, and Stephen J. Russell. "Factors affecting removal of bacterial pathogens from healthcare surfaces during dynamic wiping." *Textile Research Journal* 89, no. 4 (2019): 580–589.

Eisen, Daniel B. "Surgeon's garb and infection control: What's the evidence?." *Journal of the American Academy of Dermatology* 64, no. 5 (2011): 960–e1.

Ellis, H. "The hazards of surgical glove dusting powders." *Surgery, Gynecology & Obstetrics* 171, no. 6 (1990): 521–527.

eSuppliesMedical™. "Wipe Clean Fluid Proof and Fire Retardant Standard Pillow." 2021. Accessed June 3rd, 2021. https://esuppliesmedical.co.uk/disposables/pillows-pillowcases-incontinence/wipe-clean-fluid-proof-and-fire-retardant-standard-pillow-each.

EU. "Regulation (EU) 2017/745 of the European Parliament and of the Council of 5 April 2017 on medical devices, amending Directive 2001/83/EC, Regulation (EC) No 178/2002 and Regulation (EC) No 1223/2009 and repealing Council Directives 90/385/EEC and 93/42/EEC (Text with EEA relevance.)" 2017. Accessed June 3rd, 2021. https://eur-lex.europa.eu/legal-content/EN/TXT/?uri=CELEX%3A32017R0745.

EU. "Directive (EU) 2018/850 of the European Parliament and of the Council of 30 May 2018 amending Directive 1999/31/EC on the landfill of waste (Text with EEA relevance)". 2018. Accessed June 3rd, 2021. https://eur-lex.europa.eu/legal-content/EN/TXT/?uri=celex:32018L0850

European Ozone Trade Association. 2021. Accessed June 3rd, 2021. https://www.euota.org/.

FDA. "The Facts on Tampons – and How to Use Them Safely". 2020a. Accessed June 3rd, 2021. https://www.fda.gov/consumers/consumer-updates/facts-tampons-and-how-use-them-safely.

FDA. "Decontamination Systems E?UAs for Personal Protective Equipment." 2020b. Accessed June 3rd, 2021. https://www.fda.gov/medical-devices/coronavirus-disease-2019-covid-19-emergency-use-authorizations-medical-devices/decontamination-systems-personal-protective-equipment-euas

FDA. "Letter from Denise M. Hinton, Chief Scientist, Food and Drug Administration to Robert R. Redfield, Director, Centers for Disease Control and Prevention, 28th March 2020". 2020c. Accessed June 3rd, 2021. https://www.fda.gov/media/135763/download.

FDA. "Medical Gowns" Version Current at 13th January 2021. 2021a. Accessed June 3rd, 2021. https://www.fda.gov/medical-devices/personal-protective-equipment-infection-control/medical-gowns.

FDA. "FDA Recommends Transition from Use of Decontaminated Disposable Respirators - Letter to Health Care Personnel and Facilities". 2021b. Accessed June 3rd, 2021. https://www.fda.gov/medical-devices/letters-health-care-providers/fda-recommends-transition-use-decontaminated-disposable-respirators-letter-health-care-personnel-and.

Freeman, A. I., L. J. Halladay, and P. Cripps. "The effect of silver impregnation of surgical scrub suits on surface bacterial contamination." *The Veterinary Journal* 192, no. 3 (2012): 489–493.

Gosch, Megan E., Ronald E. Shaffer, Aaron E. Eagan, Raymond J. Roberge, Victoria J. Davey, and Lewis J. Radonovich Jr. "B95: A new respirator for health care personnel." *American Journal of Infection Control* 41, no. 12 (2013): 1224–1230.

GOV.UK. "Guidance: Women's Sanitary Products (VAT Notice 701/18)." 2021. Accessed June 3rd, 2021. https://www.gov.uk/guidance/vat-on-womens-sanitary-products-notice-70118

Grossman, Julie, Andrew Pierce, Jessica Mody, Jason Gagne, Carol Sykora, Sena Sayood, Susan Cook, Nirah Shomer, Stephen Y. Liang, and Shaina R. Eckhouse. "Institution of a novel process for N95 respirator disinfection with vaporized hydrogen peroxide in the setting of the COVID-19 pandemic at a large academic medical center." *Journal of the American College of Surgeons* 231, no. 2 (2020): 275–280.

Gulihar, A., N. A. Taub, and G. J. S. Taylor. "A randomised prospective comparison of Rotecno versus new Gore occlusive surgical gowns using bacterial air counts in ultra-clean air." *Journal of Hospital Infection* 73, no. 1 (2009): 54–57.

Gutshall, Denise, Shaoying Zhou, Baiyang Wang, Miranda A. Farage, and Anne E. Hochwalt. "Assessing the dermal compatibility of a new female incontinence product line." *Cutaneous and Ocular Toxicology* 35, no. 4 (2016): 287–295.

Hartley, M. "Surgical Gloves". 2010. Accessed June 3rd, 2021. http://www.dermnetnz.org/procedures/surgical-gloves.html

Health and Safety Executive. "Coronavirus (COVID-19) Update. 2020. Accessed May 26th, 2020. https://www.hse.gov.uk/coshh/index.htm.

Health and Safety Executive. "HSE Rapid Evidence Review Publication. 2020. Accessed June 3rd, 2021. https://www.hse.gov.uk/coronavirus/assets/docs/face-mask-equivalence-aprons-gown-eye-protection.pdf

Health & Safety Executive. "The Control of Substances Hazardous to Health Regulations 2002 (as amended), Approved Code of Practice and Guidance; L5 (6th edn) (2013) "Adequate Control of Exposure," Section 91, p29. 2013. Available at: https://www.hse.gov.uk/pubns/priced/l5.pdf.

HECOIRA. "Airflow Simulations". 2021. Accessed June 3rd, 2021. https://hecoira.leeds.ac.uk/real-time-airflow-simulation/.

HEIQ. "HEIQ Viroblock." 2021. Accessed June 3rd, 2021. https://heiq.com/products/functional-textile-technologies/heiq-viroblock/?no_popup=1.

HEPACART. "HEPACART® Infection Control Technologies." 2021. Accessed June 3rd, 2021. https://www.hepacart.com/hepacart-products.

Hinchliffe, Doug J., Anthony De Lucca, Brian Condon, Janet O'Regan, Julie Clemmons, Linghe Zeng, Richard K. Byler et al. "A pilot-scale nonwoven roll goods manufacturing process reduces microbial burden to pharmacopeia acceptance levels for non-sterile hygiene applications." *Textile Research Journal* 84, no. 5 (2014): 546–558.

Hinchliffe, Doug J., Brian D. Condon, Ryan P. Slopek, and Michael Reynolds. "The adsorption of alkyl-dimethyl-benzyl-ammonium chloride onto cotton nonwoven hydroentangled substrates at the solid–liquid interface is minimized by additive chemistries." *Textile Research Journal* 87, no. 1 (2017): 70–80.

Hinchliffe, D. J., B. D. Condon, C. A. Madison, M. Reynolds, and R. J. Hron. "An optimized co-formulation minimized quaternary ammonium compounds adsorption onto raw cotton disposable disinfecting wipes and maintained efficacy against methicillin-resistant Staphylococcus aureus, vancomycin-resistant *Enterococcus faecalis*, and *Pseudomonas aeruginosa*." *Textile Research Journal* 88, no. 20 (2018): 2329–2338.

Hooper, G. J., A. G. Rothwell, C. Frampton, and M. C. Wyatt. "Does the use of laminar flow and space suits reduce early deep infection after total hip and knee replacement? The ten-year results of the New Zealand Joint Registry." *The* Journal of Bone and Joint Surgery. British volume 93, no. 1 (2011): 85–90.

Horrocks, A. R. & Anand, S.C. (eds.) *Handbook of Technical Textiles*, 2nd edition, Volume 2: Technical Textile Applications, Elsevier/Woodhead Publishing/The Textile Institute, 2016, pp. 135–168.

Hron, Rebecca J., Doug J. Hinchliffe, Christopher P. Mattison, and Brian D. Condon. "The effect of cotton fiber inclusion on the hard surface cleaning capacity of nonwoven substrates." *Journal of Engineered Fibers and Fabrics* 14 (2019): 1558925019889620.

Institute of Medicine (US) Committee on Respiratory Protection for Healthcare Workers in the Workplace Against Novel H1N1 Influenza A, Liverman CT, Harris TA, Rogers MEB et al., editors. *Respiratory Protection for Healthcare Workers in the Workplace Against Novel H1N1 Influenza A: A Letter Report.* Washington, DC: National Academies Press (US), 2009. Available from: https://www.ncbi.nlm.nih.gov/books/NBK219944/, doi: 10.17226/12748.

International Standards Organisation. "ISO 16603:2004. Clothing for Protection Against Contact with Blood and Body Fluids – Determination of the Resistance of Protective Clothing Materials to Penetration by Blood and Body Fluids – Test Method Using Synthetic Blood." 2004a. Accessed June 3rd, 2021. https://www.iso.org/standard/32247.html.

International Standards Organisation. "ISO 16604:2004. Clothing for Protection Against Contact with Blood and Body Fluids – Determination of Resistance of Protective Clothing Materials to Penetration by Blood-Borne Pathogens. – Test Methods Using Phi-X 174 Bacteriophage." 2004b. Accessed June 3rd, 2021. https://www.iso.org/standard/32248.html.

International Standards Organisation. "11.140 Hospital Equipment". 2021. Accessed June 3rd, 2021. https://www.iso.org/ics/11.140/x/

Interweave. "Polycotton Flat Sheet Single Bed." 2021. Accessed June 3rd, 2021. https://www.interweavetextiles.com/product/bedding/bed-sheets/polycotton-sheets/polycotton-flat-sheet-single-bed/.

Jagger, Janine. "Caring for healthcare workers: A global perspective." *Infection Control & Hospital Epidemiology* 28, no. 1 (2007): 1–4.

JLA. "Ozone Laundry Disinfection". 2021. Accessed 7th May 2021. https://jla.com/otex/laundry.

Jordan, Susan L. P., Mario F. Stowers, Earl G. Trawick, and Alan B. Theis. "Glutaraldehyde permeation: Choosing the proper glove." *American Journal of Infection Control* 24, no. 2 (1996): 67–69.

Jorgensen, Johnna, M. Shariati, Carol P. Shields, D. P. Durr, and Howard M. Proskin. "Fluoride uptake into demineralized primary enamel from fluoride-impregnated dental floss in vitro." *Pediatric Dentistry Journal* 11, no. 1 (1989): 17–20.

Kannadasan, A. "Meet Muruganantham, the real Pad Man." 2018. Accessed June 3rd, 2021. https://www.thehindu.com/society/the-real-pad-man-muruganantham-before-the-release-of-pad-man/article22658314.ece

Khan, M. Amirul Islam, Nicolas Delbosc, Catherine J. Noakes, and Jonathan Summers. "Real-time flow simulation of indoor environments using lattice Boltzmann method." In *Building Simulation*, vol. 8, no. 4. Springer Berlin Heidelberg, 2015, pp. 405–414.

Kilic, Ali, Eunkyoung Shim, and Behnam Pourdeyhimi. "Electrostatic capture efficiency enhancement of polypropylene electret filters with barium titanate." *Aerosol Science and Technology* 49, no. 8 (2015): 666–673.

Kim, Mun Jung, and Helmut H. Hergeth. "Technology roadmap for flushable nonwoven wipes." *Journal of the Textile Institute* 103, no. 2 (2012): 200–209.

Kumar, Anil, Jasvir Dalal, Sajjan Dahiya, Rajesh Punia, K. D. Sharma, Anil Ohlan, and A. S. Maan. "In situ decoration of silver nanoparticles on single-walled carbon nanotubes by microwave irradiation for enhanced and durable anti-bacterial finishing on cotton fabric." *Ceramics International* 45, no. 1 (2019): 1011–1019.

Lakdawala, N., J. Pham, M. Shah, and J. Holton. "Effectiveness of low-temperature domestic laundry on the decontamination of healthcare workers' uniforms." *Infection Control & Hospital Epidemiology* 32, no. 11 (2011): 1103–1108.

Laing, Raechel M. "Protection provided by clothing and textiles against potential hazards in the operating theatre." *International Journal of Occupational Safety and Ergonomics* 14, no. 1 (2008): 107–115.

Lamberts, David M., Richard C. Wunderlich, and Raul G. Caffesse. "The effect of waxed and unwaxed dental floss on gingival health: Part I. plaque removal and gingival response." *Journal of Periodontology* 53, no. 6 (1982): 393–396.

Lanes, Stephan F., and Kenneth J. Rothman. "Tampon absorbency, composition and oxygen content and risk of toxic shock syndrome." *Journal of Clinical Epidemiology* 43, no. 12 (1990): 1379–1385.

Lee, Hoon Joo, and Sung Hoon Jeong. "Bacteriostasis and skin innoxiousness of nanosize silver colloids on textile fabrics." *Textile Research Journal* 75, no. 7 (2005): 551–556.

Lee, S., and Obendorf, S. K. "Use of electrospun nanofiber web for protective textile materials as barriers to liquid penetration." *Textile Research Journal* 77, no.9 (2007): 696–702.

Lenzen, Manfred, Arunima Malik, Mengyu Li, Jacob Fry, Helga Weisz, Peter-Paul Pichler, Leonardo Suveges Moreira Chaves, Anthony Capon, and David Pencheon. "The environmental footprint of health care: A global assessment." *The Lancet Planetary Health* 4, no. 7 (2020): e271–e279.

Leonas, Karen K., and Renita S. Jinkins. "The relationship of selected fabric characteristics and the barrier effectiveness of surgical gown fabrics." *American Journal of Infection Control* 25, no. 1 (1997): 16–23.

Li, Yuguo. "The secret behind the mask." (2011): 89–91.

Li, Y., P. Leung, L. Yao, Q. W. Song, and E. Newton. "Antimicrobial effect of surgical masks coated with nanoparticles." *Journal of Hospital Infection* 62, no. 1 (2006): 58–63.

Liao, Lei, Wang Xiao, Mervin Zhao, Xuanze Yu, Haotian Wang, Qiqi Wang, Steven Chu, and Yi Cui. "Can N95 respirators be reused after disinfection? How many times?." *ACS Nano* 14, no. 5 (2020): 6348–6356.

Lidwell, O. M., E. J. Lowbury, W. Whyte, R. Blowers, S. J. Stanley, and D. Lowe. "Effect of ultraclean air in operating rooms on deep sepsis in the joint after total hip or knee replacement: A randomised study." *British Medical Journal (Clin Res Ed)*285, no. 6334 (1982): 10–14.

Liverman, Catharyn T. "Respiratory protection for healthcare workers in the workplace against novel H1N1 influenza A: A letter report." (2009).

Loeb, Mark, Nancy Dafoe, James Mahony, Michael John, Alicia Sarabia, Verne Glavin, Richard Webby et al. "Surgical mask vs N95 respirator for preventing influenza among health care workers: A randomized trial." *The Journal of the American Medical Association* 302, no. 17 (2009): 1865–1871.

Loh, W., V. V. Ng, and J. Holton. "Bacterial flora on the white coats of medical students." *Journal of Hospital Infection* 45, no. 1 (2000): 65–68.

Louis, Steven S., Ely L. Steinberg, Orna A. Gruen, Craig S. Bartlett, and David L. Helfet. "Outer gloves in orthopaedic procedures: A polyester/stainless steel wire weave glove liner compared with latex." *Journal of Orthopaedic Trauma* 12, no. 2 (1998): 101–105.

Lowe, J. J. et al. "N95 Filtering Facepiece Respirator Ultraviolet Germicidal Irradiation (UVGI) Process for Decontamination and Reuse". 2020. Accessed June 3rd, 2021. https://www.nebraskamed.com/sites/default/files/documents/covid-19/n-95-decon-process.pdf.

Maduna, Lebo, and Asis Patnaik. "Textiles in air filtration." *Textile Progress* 49, no. 4 (2017): 173–247.

Maghrabi, Huda Ahmed, Arun Vijayan, Pradip Deb, and Lijing Wang. "Bismuth oxide-coated fabrics for X-ray shielding." *Textile Research Journal* 86, no. 6 (2016): 649–658.

Maqsood, Muhammad, Yasir Nawab, Syed Talha Ali Hamdani, Khubab Shaker, Muhammad Umair, and Waqas Ashraf. "Modeling the effect of weave structure and fabric thread density on the barrier effectiveness of woven surgical gowns." *The Journal of The Textile Institute* 107, no. 7 (2016): 873–878.

MarketsandMarkets. "Feminine Hygiene Products Market by Nature (Disposable, Reusable), Type (Sanitary Napkins, Panty Liners, Tampons, Menstrual Cups), Region (Asia Pacific, North America, Europe, Middle East and Africa, South America) - Global Forecast to 2025". 2021. Accessed June 3rd, 2021. https://www.marketsandmarkets.com/Market-Reports/feminine-hygiene-product-market-69114569.html.

McCarthy, Brian J., ed. *Textiles for Hygiene and Infection Control*. Elsevier, 2011.

MEDEXSUPPLY.com. "Kimberly-Clark FLUIDSHIELD Fog-Free Surgical Mask, 100/cs" Accessed June 3rd, 2021. 2021. https://www.medexsupply.com/infection-control-protective-apparel-masks-face-masks-kimberly-clark-fluidshield-fog-free-surgical-mask-100-cs-x_pid-42257.html.

Medsalv. "Saving the Planet: Six Strategies to put your hospital on a Low-Carb (on emissions) diet." 2021. Accessed June 3rd, 2021. https://www.medsalv.com/news/saving-the-planet-six-strategies-to-put-your-hospital-on-a-low-carb-on-emissions-diet

Mirzaei, Majid, Mohammad Zarrebini, Ahmad Shirani, Mohsen Shanbeh, and Sedigheh Borhani. "X-ray shielding by a novel garment woven with melt-spun monofilament weft yarn containing lead and tin particles." *Textile Research Journal* 89, no. 1 (2019): 63–75.

Misteli, Heidi, Walter P. Weber, Stefan Reck, Rachel Rosenthal, Marcel Zwahlen, Philipp Fueglistaler, Martin K. Bolli, Daniel Oertli, Andreas F. Widmer, and Walter R. Marti. "Surgical glove perforation and the risk of surgical site infection." *Archives of Surgery* 144, no. 6 (2009): 553–558.

Mitchell, A., M. Spencer, and C. Edmiston Jr. "Role of healthcare apparel and other healthcare textiles in the transmission of pathogens: A review of the literature." *Journal of Hospital Infection* 90, no. 4 (2015): 285–292.

Mitchell, N. J., D. S. Evans, and Ann Kerr. "Reduction of skin bacteria in theatre air with comfortable, non-woven disposable clothing for operating-theatre staff." *British Medical Journal*, no. 6114 (1978): 696–698.

Morishima, Mika, Yuki Shimizu, Takimaru Fujiyama, and Tamaki Mitsuno. "Analysis of the fitting of patterns of hygiene masks for the closed mouth." *Textile Research Journal* 85, no. 8 (2015): 828–837.

Morishima, Mika, Takimaru Fujiyama, Yuki Shimizu, and Tamaki Mitsuno. "Analysis of fit pattern of a hygiene mask for an opened mouth." *Textile Research Journal* 86, no. 9 (2016): 933–947.

Morishima, Mika, and Tamaki Mitsuno. "A pilot study of the shape of a mask sheet for adult women with their mouths open." In *Proceedings of the International Symposium on Human Factors and Ergonomics in Health Care*, vol. 8, no. 1. Sage CA: Los Angeles, CA: SAGE Publications, 2019, pp. 209–212.

Morishima, Mika, and Tamaki Mitsuno. "Analysis of hygienic face mask patterns for young people." *Textile Research Journal* 89, no. 21–22 (2019): 4670–4680.

Morris, Cletus E., Tyrone L. Vigo, and Clark M. Welch. "Binding of organic antimicrobial agents to cotton fabric as zirconium complexes." *Textile Research Journal* 51, no. 2 (1981): 90–96.

N95DECON. "Resources for N95 Users and Clinical Administrators". 2020. Accessed June 3rd, 2021. https://www.n95decon.org/

NHS National Services Scotland. "Standard Infection Control Precautions (SICPs) Literature Review: Personal Protective Equipment (PPE) –Aprons/Gowns; version 2" (2015). 2015. Accessed June 3rd, 2021. http://www.nipcm.hps.scot.nhs.uk/resources/literature-reviews/standard-infection-control-precautions-literature-reviews/

Nasseripour, Melanie, Jonathon Timothy Newton, Fiona Warburton, Oluwatunmise Awojobi, Sonya Di Giorgio, Jennifer Elizabeth Gallagher, and Avijit Banerjee. "A systematic review and meta-analysis of the role of sugar-free chewing gum on Streptococcus mutans." *BMC Oral Health* 21, no. 1 (2021): 1–11.

NICE. "Effective and Practical Measures to Prevent Infection Outlined by NICE" 28th March 2012". 2012a. Accessed June 3rd, 2021. https://www.nice.org.uk/news/article/effective-and-practical-measures-to-prevent-infection-outlined-by-nice.

NICE. "Healthcare-Associated Infections: Prevention and Control in Primary and Community Care." Clinical Guideline [CG139] Published: 28 March 2012 Last updated: 15 February 2017". 2012b. Accessed June 3rd, 2021. https://www.nice.org.uk/guidance/cg139/chapter/introduction.

NIESH. "Pandemic Planning: Recommended Guidance for Extended Use and Limited Reuse of N95 Filtering Facepiece Respirators in Healthcare Settings, 27 March 2020." 2020. Accessed June 3rd, 2021. https://tools.niehs.nih.gov/wetp/public/hasl_get_blob.cfm?ID=11824.

Nordstrom, Jeanne M., Kelly A. Reynolds, and Charles P. Gerba. "Comparison of bacteria on new, disposable, laundered, and unlaundered hospital scrubs." *American Journal of Infection Control* 40, no. 6 (2012): 539–543.

Novak, Christine B., J. M. Patterson, and Susan E. Mackinnon. "Evaluation of hand sensibility with single and double latex gloves." *Plastic and Reconstructive Surgery* 103, no. 1 (1999): 128–131.

OECD. *Guidance Document on the Evaluation of the Efficacy of Antimicrobial Treated Articles with Claims for External Effects; ENV/JM/MONO(2008)27, 18th November 2008*. 2008. Accessed. June 3rd, 2020. https://www.oecd.org/env/ehs/pesticides-biocides/41692131.pdf.

OECD. "Guidance Document on Use and Development of Tier-2 Laboratory-based Tests Used to Substantiate Claims for Efficacy of Biocide-treated Articles". 2019. Accessed June 3rd, 2021. https://www.oecd.org/officialdocuments/publicdisplaydocumentpdf/?cote=env/jm/mono(2018)20&doclanguage=en

Orr, Neil W. M. "Is a mask necessary in the operating theatre?." *Annals of the Royal College of Surgeons of England* 63, no. 6 (1981): 390.

OSHA. "Factsheet: Respiratory Infection Control: Respirators Versus Surgical Masks". 2009. Accessed June 3rd, 2021. https://www.osha.gov/sites/default/files/publications/OSHA3219.pdf

Otter, J. A., S. Yezli, F. Barbut, and T. M. Perl. "An overview of automated room disinfection systems: When to use them and how to choose them." *Decontamination in Hospitals and Healthcare* (2020): 323–369.

Ou, Junfei, Bo Wu, Mingshan Xue, and Fajun Wang. "Silver ions anchored to fabric via coordination: Evaluation on washing durability and antibacterial activity." *Materials Letters* 237 (2019): 134–136.

Owen, Lucy, and Katie Laird. "The role of textiles as fomites in the healthcare environment: A review of the infection control risk." *PeerJ* 8 (2020): e9790.

Park, Sungmee, and Sundaresan Jayaraman. "From containment to harm reduction from SARS-CoV-2: A fabric mask for enhanced effectiveness, comfort, and compliance." *The Journal of the Textile Institute* (2020): 1–15.

Partecke, Lars Ivo, Anna-Maria Goerdt, Inga Langner, Bernd Jaeger, Ojan Assadian, Claus-Dieter Heidecke, Axel Kramer, and Nils-Olaf Huebner. "Incidence of microperforation for surgical gloves depends on duration of wear." *Infection Control and Hospital Epidemiology* 30, no. 5 (2009): 409.

Parthasarathi, V., and G. Thilagavathi. "Development of tri-laminate antiviral surgical gown for liquid barrier protection." *The Journal of the Textile Institute* 106, no. 10 (2015): 1095–1105.

Practice Greenhealth. "Greening the O.R." 2011. Accessed June 3rd, 2021. https://www.c4spgh.org/HCW1_Presentations/GOR_FullSet_Guidance%20Docs_Web_042711.pdf.

Prasad, Varun. "Competition and Innovation: Evidence from Third-Party Reprocessing in the Medical Device Industry." PhD diss., Department of Economics, Duke University Durham, 2020.

Public Health England. Guidance About Coronavirus (COVID-19) Personal Protective Equipment (PPE). Collection: Coronavirus (COVID-19): Personal Protective Equipment (PPE) hub." 2020. Accessed June 3rd, 2021. https://www.gov.uk/government/collections/coronavirus-covid-19-personal-protective-equipment-ppe.

Queensland Health. "Bare Below the Elbows", 2017. Accessed June. 3rd, 2021. https://www.health.qld.gov.au/__data/assets/pdf_file/0026/680903/bare-below-the-elbows.pdf

Rengasamy, Samy, Deborah Sbarra, Julian Nwoko, and Ronald Shaffer. "Resistance to synthetic blood penetration of National Institute for Occupational Safety and Health-approved N95 filtering facepiece respirators and surgical N95 respirators." *American Journal of Infection Control* 43, no. 11 (2015): 1190–1196.

Rigby, A. J., S. C. Anand, and A. R. Horrocks. "Textile materials for medical and healthcare applications." *Journal of the Textile Institute* 88, no. 3 (1997): 83–93.

Riley, Kate, M. Fergusson, and Jinsong Shen. "Sustainable fabric choice for regularly laundered healthcare uniforms." *The Journal of the Textile Institute* 108, no. 3 (2017): 440–444.

Rockwood, Charles A., and Don H. O'Donoghue. "The surgical mask: Its development, usage, and efficiency: A review of the literature, and new experimental studies." *AMA Archives of Surgery* 80, no. 6 (1960): 963–971.

Rogina-Car, Beti, Ana Budimir, and Drago Katovic. "Microbial barrier properties of healthcare professional uniforms." *Textile Research Journal* 87, no. 15 (2017): 1860–1868.

Rozman, Urška, Sabina Fijan, Sonja Šostar Turk, and Vid Mlakar. "Real-time polymerase chain reaction for quantitative assessment of common pathogens associated with healthcare-acquired infections on hospital textiles." *Textile Research Journal* 83, no. 19 (2013): 2032–2041.

Sackren, H. S. "Vaginal tampons for menstrual absorption." *Clinical Medicine & Surgery* 46 (1939): 327–329.

SAF™. "Washable". 2021. Accessed June 3rd, 2021. https://www.exploresaf.com/washable.

Sattar, S. A., C. Bradley, R. Kibbee, Rebecca Wesgate, M. A. C. Wilkinson, T. Sharpe, and Jean-Yves Maillard. "Disinfectant wipes are appropriate to control microbial bioburden from surfaces: Use of a new ASTM standard test protocol to demonstrate efficacy." *Journal of Hospital Infection* 91, no. 4 (2015): 319–325.

Shen, Hongqing, and Karen K. Leonas. "Study of repellent finish of filtration ability of surgical face masks." *International Nonwovens Journal* 4 (2005): 1558925 005os–1400403.

Sigurdson, Alice J., Michele Morin Doody, R. Sowmya Rao, D. Michal Freedman, Bruce H. Alexander, Michael Hauptmann, Aparna K. Mohan et al. "Cancer incidence in the US radiologic technologists health study, 1983–1998." *Cancer* 97, no. 12 (2003): 3080–3089.

Smit, S. "ANSI/AAMI PB70: Closing the Gap." 2018. Accessed. June 2nd, 2021. https://www.mddionline.com/regulatory-quality/ansiaami-pb70-closing-gap.

Song, Xinyu, Lutz Vossebein, and Andrea Zille. "Efficacy of disinfectant-impregnated wipes used for surface disinfection in hospitals: A review." *Antimicrobial Resistance & Infection Control* 8, no. 1 (2019): 1–14.

Soukupova, Vera, Lydia Boguslavsky, and RaJesh D. AnandJiwala. "Studies on the properties of biodegradable wipes made by the hydroentanglement bonding technique." *Textile Research Journal* 77, no. 5 (2007): 301–311.

Speers Jr, R., R. A. Shooter, H. Gaya, Niranjana Patel, and J. H. Hewitt. "Contamination of nurses' uniforms with *Staphylococcus Aureus*." *The Lancet* 294, no. 7614 (1969): 233–235.

Spielman-Sun, Eleanor, Tatiana Zaikova, Theresa Dankovich, Jie Yun, Margret Ryan, James E. Hutchison, and Gregory V. Lowry. "Effect of silver concentration and chemical transformations on release and antibacterial efficacy in silver-containing textiles." *NanoImpact* 11 (2018): 51–57.

Spooner, John L. "History of surgical face masks." *AORN Journal* 5, no. 1 (1967): 76–80.

Srinivasan, Arjun, Daniel B. Jernign, Laura Liedtke, and Larry Strausbaugh. "Hospital preparedness for severe acute respiratory syndrome in the United States: Views from a national survey of infectious diseases consultants." *Clinical Infectious Diseases* 39, no. 2 (2004): 272–274.

Stanley, Autumn. *Mothers and daughters of invention: Notes for a Revised History of Technology*. Rutgers University Press, 1995.

Stuart, L. Fischman. "The history of oral hygiene products: How far have we come in 6000 years?." Periodontology 2000 15 (1997): 7–14.

Suen, L. K. P., Y. P. Guo, S. S. K. Ho, C. H. Au-Yeung, and S. C. Lam. "Comparing mask fit and usability of traditional and nanofibre N95 filtering facepiece respirators before and after nursing procedures." *Journal of Hospital Infection* 104, no. 3 (2020): 336–343.

Sun, G. "Disposable and reusable medical textiles." In *Textiles for Hygiene and Infection Control*. Woodhead Publishing, 2011, pp. 125–135.

Talhelm, T. "What's the Difference Between N95 and KN95 Masks?". 2021. Accessed June 3rd, 2021. https://smartairfilters.com/en/blog/whats-the-difference-between-n95-and-kn95-masks/

Tampax. "So, What's Really in Tampax Tampons?" 2020. Accessed June 3rd, 2021. https://tampax.com/en-us/tampon-truths/what-tampons-are-made-of/

Tanner, Judith, and Hazel Parkinson. "Double gloving to reduce surgical cross-infection." *Cochrane Database of Systematic Reviews* 3 (2006).

Tanner, Judith, P. Wraighte, and P. Howard. "Knitted outer gloves in primary hip and knee arthroplasty." *Hip International* 16, no. 1 (2006): 62–65.

The Textile Institute. "Textile Terms and Definitions". 2021. https://www.ttandd.org/content/textile-terms-and-definitions and 11th edition; Edited by Denton, M.J. and Daniels, P.N. The Textile Institute, 2002.

The Washington Post. "How Droplets from a Cough Flow Through an Airplane Cabin." 2020. Accessed June 3rd, 2021. www.washington post.com.

Tierno Jr, Philip M., and Bruce A. Hanna. "Ecology of toxic shock syndrome: Amplification of toxic shock syndrome toxin 1 by materials of medical interest." *Reviews of Infectious Diseases* 11 Supplement 1, no. Supplement_1 (1989): S182–S187.

TSI. "Mechanisms of Filtration for High-Efficiency Fibrous Filters-Application". 2012. Accessed June 3rd, 2021.

https://tsi.com/getmedia/d8a4412d-3050-41c8-9e89-bc3a20ffda4d/ITI-041?ext=.pdf.

Van Turnhout, Jan. "Method for the manufacture of an electret fibrous filter." U.S. Patent Application 06/517,937 filed June 3, 1986.

Varshney, Swati, Prashant Pandey, Deepti Gupta, and Shilpi Sharma. "Role of fabric properties, moisture and friction in transfer of bacteria from fabric to fabric." *Textile Research Journal* 90, no. 3–4 (2020): 478–485.

Ventile. "Ventile Specifications". 2020. Accessed June 3rd, 2021. https://ventile.co.uk/wp-content/uploads/2020/10/05-Ventile-Sustainable-Spec-Sheet-1.pdf.

Vera, Christina M. "Laundering methods for reusable surgical scrubs: A literature review." *AANA Journal* 84, no. 4 (2016).

Verbeek, Jos H., Blair Rajamaki, Sharea Ijaz, Riitta Sauni, Elaine Toomey, Bronagh Blackwood, Christina Tikka, Jani H. Ruotsalainen, and F. Selcen Kilinc Balci. "Personal protective equipment for preventing highly infectious diseases due to exposure to contaminated body fluids in healthcare staff." *Cochrane Database of Systematic Reviews* 4 (2020).

Vincent, Marina, and Peggy Edwards. "Disposable surgical face masks for preventing surgical wound infection in clean surgery." *Cochrane Database of Systematic Reviews* 4 (2016).

Virk, Rajpreet K., Gita N. Ramaswamy, Mohamed Bourham, and Brian Lee Bures. "Plasma and antimicrobial treatment of nonwoven fabrics for surgical gowns." *Textile Research Journal* 74, no. 12 (2004): 1073–1079.

Viscusi, Dennis J., Mike Bergman, Edward Sinkule, and Ronald E. Shaffer. "Evaluation of the filtration performance of 21 N95 filtering face piece respirators after prolonged storage." *American Journal of Infection Control* 37, no. 5 (2009): 381–386.

Viscusi, Dennis J., Michael S. Bergman, Benjamin C. Eimer, and Ronald E. Shaffer. "Evaluation of five decontamination methods for filtering facepiece respirators." *Annals of Occupational Hygiene* 53, no. 8 (2009): 815–827.

Vostral, Sharra Louise. *Under Wraps: A History of Menstrual Hygiene Technology*. Lexington Books, 2008.

Vostral, Sharra L. "Rely and toxic shock syndrome: A technological health crisis." *The Yale Journal of Biology and Medicine* 84, no. 4 (2011): 447.

Vukelich, D. "Time to Move Away from Our "Disposable" Health Care Culture." 2021. Accessed June 3rd, 2021. https://www.brusselstimes.com/opinion/163582/time-to-move-away-from-our-disposable-health-care-culture/.

Wai Cheung, Tin, Chenxiao Yang, and Li Li. "An integrated design of self-care textile wearables: Exploration of thermal-stimuli effects and drug delivery function." *Textile Research Journal* 89, no. 13 (2019): 2553–2568.

Walton, J. R. "A new controversy in respiratory equipment management: Reusables versus disposed disposables versus reused disposables." *Respiratory Care* 31, no. 3 (1986): 213–217.

White, J. B. “Rapid response: Lead aprons: Historical & scientific basis for change.” *British Medical Journal* 327 (2003): 371

Widmer, Andreas F., and Gilles Richner. “Proposal for a EN 149 acceptable reprocessing method for FFP2 respirators in times of severe shortage.” *Antimicrobial Resistance & Infection Control* 9, no. 1 (2020): 1–4.

Wilson, J. A., H. P. Loveday, P. N. Hoffman, and R. J. Pratt. “Uniform: An evidence review of the microbiological significance of uniforms and uniform policy in the prevention and control of healthcare-associated infections. Report to the Department of Health (England).” *Journal of Hospital Infection* 66, no. 4 (2007): 301–307.

Wilson, Solomon J., David Sellu, Albert Uy, and Mohammed Ali Jaffer. “Subjective effects of double gloves on surgical performance.” *Annals of the Royal College of Surgeons of England* 78, no. 1 (1996): 20.

Wong, Derek, K. Nye, and Pat Hollis. “Microbial flora on doctors' white coats.” *British Medical Journal* 303, no. 6817 (1991): 1602–1604.

Wong, W. K., Y. L. Kwok, K. Chan, and C. Y. Yeung. “Evaluation of the physical and psychological functions of an existing child patients' garment in a hospital environment in Hong Kong, China.” *Journal of the Textile Institute* 91, no. 1 (2000): 10–19.

Woo, Dong Jin, Nathaniel S. Hansen, Yong Lak Joo, and S. Kay Obendorf. “Photocatalytic self-detoxification by coaxially electrospun fiber containing titanium dioxide nanoparticles.” *Textile Research Journal* 82, no. 18 (2012): 1920–1927.

World Health Organization. Infection Prevention and Control During Health Care When COVID-19 is Suspected: Interim Guidance, 19 March 2020. No. WHO/2019-nCoV/IPC/2020.3. World Health Organization, 2020.

World Health Organization. “Infection Prevention and Control in Health Care for Confirmed or Suspected Cases of Pandemic (H1N1) 2009 and Influenza-like Illnesses.” 2009. Accessed June 3rd, 2021. https://www.who.int/csr/resources/publications/swineflu/swineinfinfcont/en/

World Medical Association. “WMA Declaration of Geneva; Adopted by the 2nd General Assembly of the World Medical Association, Geneva, Switzerland, September 1948 and amended by the 68th WMA General Assembly, Chicago, United States, October 2017.” 2017. Accessed June 3rd, 2021. https://www.wma.net/policies-post/wma-declaration-of-geneva/.

Worthington, Helen V., Laura MacDonald, Tina Poklepovic Pericic, Dario Sambunjak, Trevor M. Johnson, Pauline Imai, and Janet E. Clarkson. “Home use of interdental cleaning devices, in addition to toothbrushing, for preventing and controlling periodontal diseases and dental caries.” *Cochrane Database of Systematic Reviews* 4 (2019).

Xu, QingBo, LiJing Xie, Helena Diao, Fang Li, YanYan Zhang, FeiYa Fu, and XiangDong Liu. “Antibacterial cotton fabric with enhanced durability prepared using silver nanoparticles and carboxymethyl chitosan.” *Carbohydrate Polymers* 177 (2017): 187–193.

Xu, Yin, Rachel H. McQueen, Megan Strickfaden, Annette Aslund, and Jane C. Batcheller. “Establishing thermal comfort: Characterization of selected performance and physical properties of fabrics used in hospital operating room uniforms.” *Journal of the Textile Institute* 103, no. 7 (2012): 698–705.

Yang, Yadie, and Hong Hu. “Spacer fabric-based exuding wound dressing–Part I: Structural design, fabrication and property evaluation of spacer fabrics.” *Textile Research Journal* 87, no. 12 (2017): 1469–1480.

Yang, Yadie, and Hong Hu. “Spacer fabric-based exuding wound dressing–Part II: Comparison with commercial wound dressings.” *Textile Research Journal* 87, no. 12 (2017): 1481–1493.

You, Ruoyu, Chao-Hsin Lin, Daniel Wei, and Qingyan Chen. "Evaluating the commercial airliner cabin environment with different air distribution systems." *Indoor Air* 29, no. 5 (2019): 840–853.

Zeng, Yicheng, Prashik Manwatkar, Aurélie Laguerre, Marina Beke, Insung Kang, Akram S. Ali, Delphine K. Farmer, Elliott T. Gall, Mohammad Heidarinejad, and Brent Stephens. "Evaluating a commercially available in-duct bipolar ionization device for pollutant removal and potential byproduct formation." *Building and Environment* 195 (2021): 107750, ISSN 0360-1323, https://doi.org/10.1016/j.buildenv.2021.107750.

Zins, Howard M. "Environmental, cost and product issues related to reusable healthcare textiles." *Research Journal of Textile and Apparel* (2006).

10 Extracorporeal Devices

10.1 INTRODUCTION

Advances in technology have allowed clinicians to support organ function by using machines and techniques that support or mimic the outcomes of human physiology. Whilst there have been great advances in this field, there is still room for improvement and innovation. In particular, attention needs to be given to the biocompatibility of extracorporeal circuits, as they have a tendency to activate the immune and coagulation systems leading to inflammatory response and coagulopathy. Coagulopathy, in turn, leads to microvascular and macrovascular thrombosis which affects the circuitry and may generate morbidity in the patient.

10.2 EXTRACORPOREAL MEMBRANE OXYGENATION

The cardiovascular and respiratory systems function synergistically. They serve to oxygenate blood, pump the oxygenated blood around the body to organs and tissues in response to demand, and remove the waste products of metabolism. Control of the systems is both central, from signals within the brain, and peripheral, from local tissue signals. The two are a fine-tuned system that allows the human to function within a range of environments and at varying levels of performance.

Extracorporeal membrane oxygenation (ECMO) is a form of extracorporeal life support, with the ability to support the gas exchange function of the lung and cardiovascular systems in the event of reversible cardiovascular or respiratory pathology, refractory to conventional therapies. ECMO is in essence a modification of cardiopulmonary bypass utilised in the theatre environment and, following its first successful utilisation in 1971 (Bonacchi 2016, 213–217), it is now a recognised level of support provided in highly specialised units around the world (the machine is illustrated in Figure 10.1). At its most basic, the principles of an ECMO circuit are to pass blood through an oxygenator where gas exchange takes place. Blood is drained and returned to the patient by means of a pump, which depending on cannula configuration can provide support to the cardiovascular system. The support provided by the ECMO circuit can be defined based on the configuration of the drainage and return cannulae into three main types:

1. Veno-venous (VV-ECMO): Blood is drained from a vein and returned to a vein (respiratory ECMO), supporting the gas exchange properties of the lung.

DOI: 10.1201/9781003170570-10

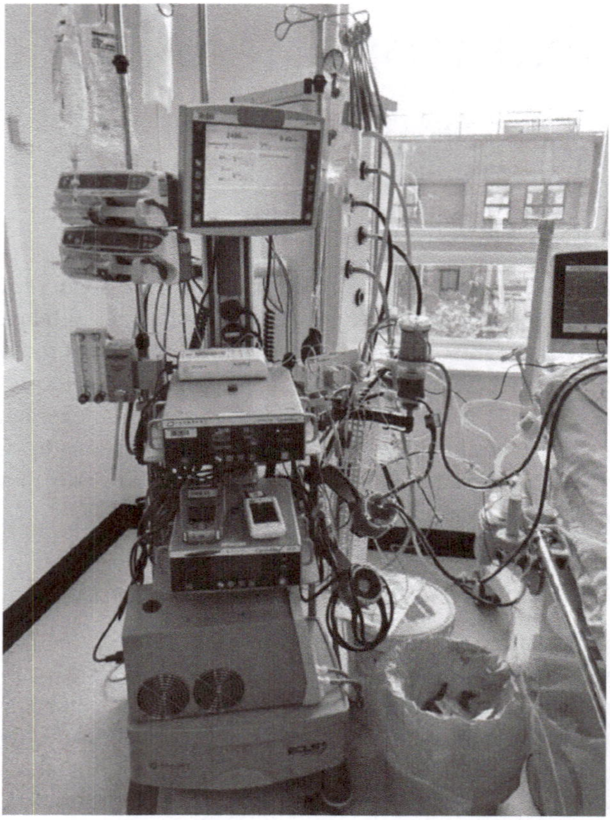

FIGURE 10.1 An example of an ECMO machine used to support gas exchange in the event of reversible cardiovascular or respiratory pathology. Image provided by Dr Matthew Charlton, Consultant Anaesthetist, UK.

2. Veno-arterial (VA-ECMO): Blood is drained from a vein and returned to an artery (cardiac ECMO), supporting the heart and lungs.
3. Arterio-venous (AV-ECMO): Blood is drained from an artery and returned to a vein, utilising the patient's own cardiovascular system as a pump. This configuration is less common and normally used for carbon dioxide clearance only.

Cannulae are commonly placed percutaneously utilising a Seldinger approach. Occasionally they may be placed centrally via a sternotomy for cardiac support post cardiac surgery. In the case of VV-ECMO support, percutaneous venous drainage cannulae are placed in the inferior vena cava via the femoral veins, or the superior and inferior vena cavae utilising a dual-lumen technique via the internal jugular vein. Venous return cannulae are again placed via one of the major accessible veins, with their tip at the level of the right atrium. In peripheral VA-ECMO, venous drainage cannulation is as above. Arterial return cannulae would commonly be placed in either the femoral or subclavian peripheral vessels. For central VA-ECMO support, drainage would be via direct cannulation of the right atrium and aorta respectively. The level of support provided is dependent on the interplay between ECMO flow and the patient's native cardiac output. In the context of respiratory ECMO, flow from the ECMO circuit is pumped back to the right atrium where it mixes with venous blood from the patient before following a normal circulatory path, from the right side of the heart, through the lungs, back to the left side of the heart and on to the systemic circulation. If the patient's cardiac output remains constant in the face of an increased ECMO flow, the amount of oxygenated blood reaching the right atrium will be increased. If the patient's cardiac output is increased in the face of a constant ECMO flow, the amount of oxygenated blood will be decreased. Although ECMO circuitry comes in a number of guises it can be broken down broadly into its key components of cannulae, tubing, pump, oxygenator, and heat exchanger, which are discussed in more detail below.

10.2.1 Tubing

Tubing typically comprises standard medical grade PVC tubing in either 0.64 cm or 1/4" internal diameter for adult and paediatric applications respectively. Tubing should be clear to allow inspection and identification of clots or cracks. It should be as short as possible, to reduce priming volume and to decrease blood exposure to this foreign surface and reduce the risk of thrombus formation, but long enough not to restrict patient movement. Blood flow through 1 m of tubing at 100 mm Hg pressure with an internal diameter of 0.64 cm and 0.95 cm is 2.5 l/min. and 5 l/min. respectively. In an ideal situation, the tubing length should be short enough to keep the priming volume to a minimum but still tolerate the large flows that are required. Paediatric patients and adult patients require different sizes of tubing depending upon the flow that is required. Traditionally for drainage lines, 0.64 cm tubing is used up to selected flows of 1.7 l/min and 0.95 cm tubing for flows above 1.7 l/min. Likewise, for the return line, 0.64 cm tubing can be used up to flows of 2.0 l/min. and 3/8" tubing is used for flows above 2.0 l/min. Some ECMO centres utilise heparin-coated tubing, thereby improving biocompatibility and reducing the risk of thrombosis from activation of the clotting cascade whilst reducing the systemic inflammatory response, but there is, as always, a trade-off between biocompatibility and economic burden.

10.2.2 Pump

The pump forms an integral part of the circuit, driving forward flow through the oxygenator and determining the flow delivered to the patient. Broadly speaking, pumps belong to one of two groups: positive displacement, which includes roller pumps commonly seen on cardiopulmonary bypass circuits, and rotary pumps, of which the centrifugal pump, frequently seen in modern ECMO circuits, is a member of. Centrifugal pumps are the preferred pump type for modern ECMO circuits as they cause less haemolysis and require less anticoagulation, so the remainder of this discussion will focus on the centrifugal pump.

Centrifugal pumps generate flow by means of a spinning rotor (impeller). As the impeller spins, a vortex is generated, creating a negative pressure pre-pump (the drainage limb of the circuit). Blood passing through the pump is then propelled forward creating a positive pressure post-pump. The impeller spins on a small bearing or is magnetically levitated. Bearing free magnetically levitated designs have a number of advantages as they require no direct connection between the pump-head housing and the impeller eliminating heat generation and thrombosis. Flow delivered by a centrifugal pump is not solely determined by the revolutions per minute of the pump-head. The pumps are preload dependent and afterload sensitive. If the preload delivered to the pump is reduced (i.e., if the patient is hypovolaemic), the flow leaving the pump will also reduce, with the impeller motion dissipated as heat energy. Increases in afterload will lead to increased resistance to flow and therefore reduced flow. For these reasons, blood flow through the circuit should be continuously measured, usually by means of an ultrasonic flow meter. Several manufacturers produce pumps, each with their own individual characteristics with regard to static volumes, outlet port size (adult and paediatric compatibility), and the maximum flow rates achievable.

10.2.3 Oxygenator

It is within the oxygenator, the part of the circuit where gas exchange takes place, that the textile material takes pride of place. Historically the process had been facilitated simply by bubbling gas through the blood ('bubble oxygenators'), which had inherent risks of gas embolus amongst other issues. Modern oxygenators employ a membrane which serves to separate the blood and gas phases. Early generation membrane oxygenator devices included flat sheet silicone designs and hollow fibre configurations where the blood ran inside the fibres with the gas surrounding them. The devices were characterised by long blood paths and high-pressure gradients, leading to decreased efficiency and increased haemolysis. Design modification led to changing to having the gas inside the hollow fibres with the blood flowing around them. This led to significant reductions in pressure gradient coupled with increased efficiency, with the hollow fibres providing massive surface area for gas exchange to take place in the surrounding blood. This design is still utilised in modern oxygenators. The first widely used fibre material was microporous polypropylene; however, the lifespan was limited due to plasma leaking into the gas phase side of the membrane, leading to membrane failure. In the early years of this century, polymethylpentene (PMP) fibres became widely available, and its use in place of the polypropylene reduced plasma leakage thereby significantly increasing durability, whilst maintaining efficient gas exchange and low-pressure gradients. PMP membranes are employed in most of the more commonly used oxygenators. Blood is pumped through the oxygenator casing with the PMP fibres submerged within, and it is through this that the gas flows (it is known as sweep gas). The PMP fibre wall forms the interface between blood and gas, and this is where gas exchange takes place; an example is shown in Figure 10.2. The efficiency with which an oxygenator

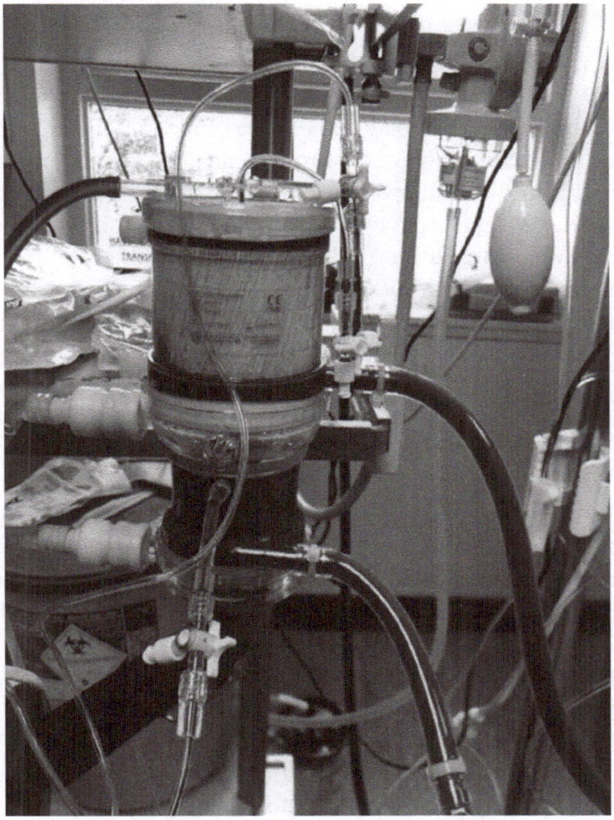

FIGURE 10.2 An example of a filter used in an ECMO machine to support gas exchange. Image provided by Dr Matthew Charlton, consultant anaesthetist, UK.

transfers oxygen to the blood is dependent on the surface area of the membrane and the time that the blood is in contact with the exchange membrane (similar in principle to the native lung), along with the fraction of oxygen in the sweep gas. A standard term 'rated flow' allows comparison between oxygenators. It is defined as the blood flow rate at which venous blood with saturation of 75% and haemoglobin of 120 g/l will exit the gas exchange device with a saturation of 95% (Brogan et al. 2017). Sweep gas flow rate determines carbon dioxide clearance by generating a continuous, favourable concentration gradient for the gas transfer to take place.

A heat exchanger surrounds the oxygenator allowing patient temperature regulation, and most typically working in its warming mode due to the exposure of blood to ambient temperatures during its transition through the extracorporeal circuit. However, cooling is also possible, and this is occasionally employed for reducing metabolic demand, during pyrexia, or for neuroprotection. Heat exchangers typically involve the circulation of water from a water bath maintained at a predetermined temperature.

10.3 THE KIDNEY

The kidney is a complex organ that is involved with filtration and excretion of waste substances in the body. They are critical in the overall maintenance of fluid balance and also contribute to endocrinological function of the body with a role in erythrocyte production, bone homeostasis, and the regulation of blood pressure. The role of filtration and excretion is undertaken by a series of ion pumps that can transport, actively or passively, ions and metabolites from blood flow into a waste system that creates urine (Palmer and Clegg 2019, 682–695). Alteration of the normal function of the kidney can lead to renal failure and this may be acute or chronic in nature. In end-stage renal disease, treatment options for renal replacement therapy include haemodialysis, peritoneal dialysis (either continuous ambulatory peritoneal dialysis or continuous automated peritoneal dialysis), or transplantation. Worldwide, the prevalence of end-stage renal disease exceeds 2 million individuals (Thomas 2019, 1–7).

Haemodialysis relies on the principle of solute diffusion across a semipermeable membrane. The movement of metabolic waste products occurs down a concentration gradient from the circulation to a dialysate. The rate of diffusion is affected by the concentration gradient, membrane surface area, pump speed, and the mass transfer coefficient of the membrane. The dialysate can be artificially manipulated depending upon the current state of the patients' blood and what needs to be filtered. This allows for finer control. Blood is extracted from a filter and passed through a dialysis machine before returning to the patient. Different dialysis membranes have different pore sizes and they can be further altered to remove different uremic toxins based on their molecular sizes (Cozzolino et al. 2019). Haemodialysis is undertaken several times a week depending upon the requirements of the patient. This is often performed at hospital in-centre haemodialysis units, an example of a dialysis machine is demonstrated in Figure 10.3, though it may be undertaken at a satellite unit; both mean time away from friends and family. Occasionally it may be performed at home. Peritoneal dialysis differs in that dextrose-containing, or amino acid-based solution is infused into the peritoneal cavity for a period of time before being removed. Dialysis occurs across a concentration gradient by diffusion and relies upon the balance between the movement of solute and water into the peritoneal cavity and absorption from the peritoneal cavity. As equilibrium is reached, the rate of diffusion diminishes (Kuo et al 2019, 86–95).

Transplantation of the kidney is undertaken for cases of advanced chronic renal failure. The aim is to transplant a functioning kidney such that dialysis is no longer required. Lifelong immunosuppression is used to prevent rejection. There are problems with all forms of renal replacement therapy and during the early days of end-stage renal failure, peritoneal dialysis may be more acceptable to the patient due to quality of life. Haemodialysis hinders mobility and limits activities of daily life. Peritoneal dialysis does the same but tends to affect the quality of life more than mobility. Both carry a risk of infection and failure of dialysis. Transplantation requires a carefully matched kidney and life-long immunosuppression. Thus, the

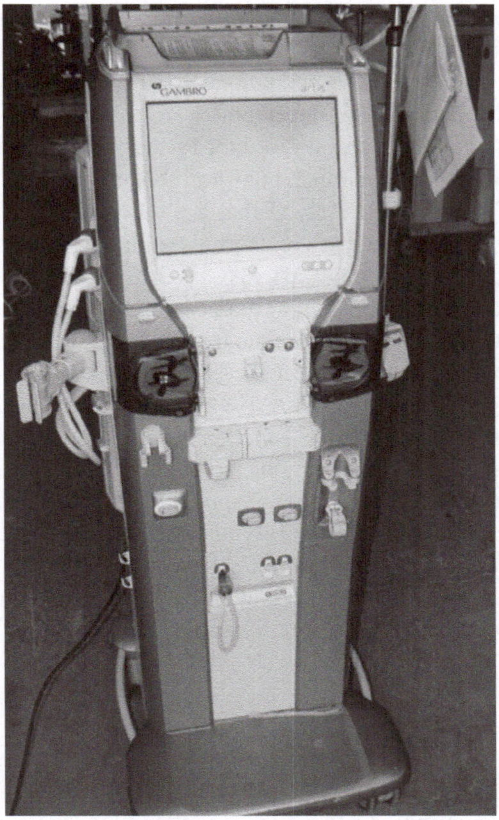

FIGURE 10.3 An example of a haemodialysis machine used in renal replacement therapy for patients with end-stage renal disease. Image provided by Dr Hussain Allawati, Consultant in General and Renal Medicine, New Zealand.

ability to design an artificial functioning kidney would have great promise (Kooman, Joles, and Gerritsen 2015, 373–376).

10.3.1 The Artificial Kidney and Associated Role of Textiles

An artificial kidney would be one that functions continuously, is able to remove toxic waste products indiscriminately, is portable, wearable, and light weight, and of low cost (Cheah et al. 2017, 1232–1240).

The single most important part of a wearable artificial kidney is the closed-system self-regenerative dialysate. To be able to achieve such design, the removal of diffused toxins from the dialysate would require nanoporous adsorbents with high adsorption capacity (Ronco, Davenport, and Gura 2008, S40–S47) and traditionally filtration has been undertaken by activated carbon. More recently, zeolites and polyethylene glycol-coated nanoporous silica have shown promising results against uraemic toxins. As the blood runs over the artificial filtration membrane, it is vitally important that the filter does not cause activation of the clotting cascade which would be a disaster for the patient. The development of hollow fibres to allow filtration (Saghafi et al. 2014, 962–970), has allowed for further development within this area. The textile needs to be biocompatible, non-thrombogenic and economic to use, and it is polyester (PET) and viscose rayon that are the two main fibre types used in mechanical kidneys. The ability to create fibres with nanopores to allow diffusion (e.g., by electrospinning webs and scaffolds) has enabled advancement in this area, particularly in tissue scaffold creation (Attanasio et al. 2016, 330–340). With progress in artificial intelligence, the role of smart textiles that can continually adapt to the internal physiological environment increases the likelihood of a personalised haemodialysis design (Hueso et al. 2018, 1–9). The ability of the textile to sense and respond to key stimuli is central to its function. There are some interesting developments for somewhat different applications on thermal stimuli effects for drug delivery in self-care garments (Wai Cheung, Yang and Li 2019, 2553–2568) that utilise non-woven fabrics made from crimped, synthetic polymer, staple hollow fibres (for their drug-holding ability) and incorporating silver-coated fibres into the non-woven fabric (for thermal stimulation). These may provide some ideas, in terms of finding an appropriate stimulus and a fibre/fibre formable to respond, for further progression of this avenue.

10.4 THE PANCREAS

The pancreas is an exocrine and endocrine organ that is involved in releasing digestive enzymes and secreting hormones that regulate blood glucose. Damage to the pancreas, such as in pancreatitis, can damage the cells that constitute the pancreas and impair its function. If the pancreas is globally affected, then pancreatic insufficiency occurs and both exocrine and endocrine functions are impaired. Diabetes mellitus, due to an inability to secrete insulin and/or regulate blood glucose occurs. In addition, malabsorption due to an inability to digest food occurs and the enzymes need to be replaced (Augustine et al. 2020, 1340–1343).

Diabetes mellitus refers to a group of common metabolic disorders that share the phenotype of hyperglycaemia. There are different types of diabetes mellitus based upon the causative factor. The two broad categories are type I and type II, though there are other types increasingly recognised. Type I diabetes mellitus develops as a result of autoimmunity against the insulin-producing beta cells of the pancreas. It results in near or total insulin deficiency. Type II diabetes mellitus is a group of disorders characterised by variable degrees of insulin resistance, impaired insulin secretion, and increased hepatic glucose production (NICE 2020). Those with type I diabetes mellitus are managed with exogenous insulin administration. Type II diabetes mellitus may be managed with lifestyle modification, medications, or insulin. Long-term complications include macrovascular and microvascular complications such as an increased risk of myocardial infarction, cerebrovascular accident, diabetic nephropathy, diabetic retinopathy and diabetic neuropathy (Mauricio, Alonso, and Gratacos 2020, 287–295). Tight blood glucose control reduces the risk of long-term diabetes-related complications although is limited by hypoglycaemia (Livingstone, Boyle, and Petrie 2020, 513–521).

10.4.1 The Artificial Pancreas and Associated Role of Textiles

The artificial pancreas addresses the unmet clinical need for improved glucose control. It is a closed-loop system that senses glucose blood levels and uses control algorithms to direct insulin delivery. It aims to improve glucose control whilst reducing the burden of hypoglycaemia and diabetes self-care (Thabit and Hovorka 2016, 1795–1805). One of the advantages it offers over the conventional injection regime is that it can respond to day-to-day and within-day glucose variability (Haidar et al. 2015, 17–26).

Regeneration of insulin-producing beta cells is a major goal for regenerative medicine. Scaffolds and tissue constructs may serve as adjuncts to allow cell growth and culture prior to transplantation. Interestingly, however, islet cells have the ability to engraft and function within the liver which thus means that they can be injected into the portal vein to lodge in the liver (Orlando et al. 2011, 223–232). One method to reduce rejection, and the need for immune suppressants, has been encapsulating the islet cells such that diffusion of nutrients, insulin, and waste can occur but infiltration by immune cells and antibodies is prevented. Alginate is commonly used for this purpose in a hydrogel sphere. Growth factors and medications may be added to engineer the properties favourably (Bochenek et al. 2018, 810–821; Kopan et al. 2018, 1354; Kumar, Joisher and Ganguly 2017, 334).

10.5 OTHER DEVICES FOR THE SUPPORT OF HOMEOSTASIS

Regenerative medicine has been directed at other tissues, such as heart muscle, liver, trachea, and skin, and scaffolds have been used to grow cells. This is a growing area of medicine with considerable scope for application clinically and the discovery of new materials with improved mechanical and biological function. Clay–polymer nanocomposites offer new opportunities for design; clay nanoparticles are biocompatible at doses significantly higher than most other nanoparticles and have non-toxic and absorbable degradation products. Studies have also demonstrated direct, beneficial, and concentration-dependent effects of clay nanoparticles on cellular adhesion, proliferation, and differentiation. This does, however, remain a field at the forefront of science and, as was the case ten years ago, there are still challenges that need to be overcome (Orlando et al. 2011, 223–232). A whole range of filters is available that use textile materials and are used within medical devices. For example, anaesthetic machines contain a range of filters (which may be ULPA or HEPA types, see Chapter 10, depending on the treatment being delivered) to ensure appropriate ventilation and a mixture of NaOH and CaO (soda lime) is used to remove carbon dioxide from the ventilatory system (Record and Beecroft 2019, 67–71).

10.6 TESTING OF EXTRACORPOREAL DEVICES

These potential embodiments fall under a number of regulations. In the USA one is required to refer to CFR21 – Food and Drugs: Sections 800–1050 (US Food and Drug Administration 2018). In the EU the devices fall into the new Medical Devices Regulations EU 2017/745 (European Commission 2021). In both cases, classification would depend on the specific application and on the intended use. However, a quick search on the FDA classification database will give an indication for the USA (US Food and Drug Administration 2021). In the EU one needs to utilise the classification rules given in Annex VIII of the EU 2017/745. In some cases, further regulations will need to be consulted and applied, especially where a device is powered and/or has computer-based components (such as – for example – electromagnetic compatibility testing). It is also worth noting that anything touching human tissue will need to have its biocompatibility evaluated to the latest version of ISO 10993. In these specific cases, there will be additional testing associated with function, performance, and intrinsic side effects. As their main function is to replace an organ, testing needs to be conducted to ensure that the said function is replaced within specified limits. In some cases, these limits will be specified within a specific standard; in others, the limits may be set by current knowledge. In either case, it is your responsibility to determine said performance specifications.

Regarding side effects, it must be remembered that these devices manipulate, move, and change the properties of fluids (be they liquid or vapour). It is important, therefore, that any materials selected behave as they should when in contact with the fluid and that any particulates from the device itself do not pass into the body – or any bacteria, viruses, or other sources of infection are not recirculated by default. All of these require functional tests to demonstrate that they are: as good as the organ it is replacing, as good as similar devices in the marketplace, or as good as it is feasible to achieve, the best of which would satisfy functional performance evaluation.

REFERENCES

Attanasio, Chiara, Marcela T. Latancia, Leo E. Otterbein, and Paolo A. Netti. "Update on renal replacement therapy: Implantable artificial devices and bioengineered organs." *Tissue Engineering Part B: Reviews* 22, no. 4 (2016): 330–340.

Augustine, P., R. Gent, J. Louise, M. Taranto, M. Penno, R. Linke, J. J. Couper et al. "Pancreas size and exocrine function is decreased in young children with recent-onset type 1 diabetes." *Diabetic Medicine* 37, no. 8 (2020): 1340–1343.

Bochenek, Matthew A., Omid Veiseh, Arturo J. Vegas, James J. McGarrigle, Meirigeng Qi, Enza Marchese, Mustafa Omami et al. "Alginate encapsulation as long-term immune protection of allogeneic pancreatic islet cells transplanted into the omental bursa of macaques." *Nature Biomedical Engineering* 2, no. 11 (2018): 810–821.

Bonacchi, Massimo. "Extracorporeal life support in polytraumatized patients." *International Journal of Surgery* 33 (2016): 213–217.

Brogan, Thomas V., Laurance Lequier, Robert Lorusso, Graeme MacLaren, and Giles Peek. *The ELSO Red Book*, 5th edition. Extracorporeal Life Support, 2017.

Cheah, Wee-Keat, Kunio Ishikawa, Radzali Othman, and Fei-Yee Yeoh. "Nanoporous biomaterials for uremic toxin adsorption in artificial kidney systems: A review." *Journal of Biomedical Materials Research Part B: Applied Biomaterials* 105, no. 5 (2017): 1232–1240.

Cozzolino, Mario, Lorenza Magagnoli, Paola Ciceri, Ferruccio Conte, and Andrea Galassi. "Effects of a medium cut-off (Theranova®) dialyser on haemodialysis patients: A prospective, cross-over study." *Clinical Kidney Journal* (2019).

European Commission. "Medical devices – Sector." 2021. Accessed March 8, 2021. https://ec.europa.eu/health/md_sector/overview:en.

Haidar, Ahmad, Laurent Legault, Virginie Messier, Tina Maria Mitre, Catherine Leroux, and Rémi Rabasa-Lhoret. "Comparison of dual-hormone artificial pancreas, single-hormone artificial pancreas, and conventional insulin pump therapy for glycaemic control in patients with type 1 diabetes: An open-label randomised controlled crossover trial." *The Lancet Diabetes & Endocrinology* 3, no. 1 (2015): 17–26.

Hueso, Miguel, Alfredo Vellido, Nuria Montero, Carlo Barbieri, Rosa Ramos, Manuel Angoso, Josep Maria Cruzado, and Anders Jonsson. "Artificial intelligence for the artificial kidney: Pointers to the future of a personalized hemodialysis therapy." *Kidney Diseases* 4, no. 1 (2018): 1–9.

Kooman, Jeroen P., Jaap A. Joles, and Karin GF Gerritsen. "Creating a wearable artificial kidney: Where are we now?." *Expert Review of Medical Devices* 12, no. 4 (2015): 373–376.

Kopan, Christopher, Tori Tucker, Michael Alexander, M. Rezaa Mohammadi, Egest J. Pone, and Jonathan Robert Todd Lakey. "Approaches in immunotherapy, regenerative medicine, and bioengineering for type 1 diabetes." *Frontiers in Immunology* 9 (2018): 1354.

Kumar, Nupur, Heer Joisher, and Anasuya Ganguly. "Polymeric scaffolds for pancreatic tissue engineering: A review." *The Review of Diabetic Studies: RDS* 14, no. 4 (2017): 334.

Kuo, Yi Ting, Chia Chun Lee, and Junne Ming Sung. "Dialysis therapy: Concept evolution and update." *Journal of Internal Medicine of Taiwan* 30, no. 2 (2019): 86–95.

Livingstone, R., J. G. Boyle, and J. R. Petrie. "How tightly controlled do fluctuations in blood glucose levels need to be to reduce the risk of developing complications in people with type 1 diabetes?" *Diabetic Medicine* 37, no. 4 (2020): 513–521.

Mauricio, Dídac, Núria Alonso, and Mònica Gratacòs. "Chronic diabetes complications: The need to move beyond classical concepts." *Trends in Endocrinology & Metabolism* 31, no. 4 (2020): 287–295.

NICE. "Type 1 diabetes in adults: Diagnosis and management (NG17)." 2020. Accessed February 6, 2020. https://www.nice.org.uk/guidance/ng17.

NICE. "Type 2 diabetes in adults: Management (NG28)." 2020. Accessed February 6th, 2020. https://www.nice.org.uk/guidance/ng28.

Orlando, Giuseppe, Pedro Baptista, Martin Birchall, Paolo De Coppi, Alan Farney, Nadia K. Guimaraes-Souza, Emmanuel Opara et al. "Regenerative medicine as applied to solid organ transplantation: Current status and future challenges." *Transplant International* 24, no. 3 (2011): 223–232.

Palmer, Biff F., and Deborah J. Clegg. "Physiology and pathophysiology of potassium homeostasis: Core curriculum 2019." *American Journal of Kidney Diseases* 74, no. 5 (2019): 682–695.

Record, Nicholas, and Christina Beecroft. "The anaesthetic machine." *Anaesthesia & Intensive Care Medicine* 20, no. 2 (2019): 67–71.

Ronco, Claudio, Andrew Davenport, and Victor Gura. "Toward the wearable artificial kidney." *Hemodialysis International* 12 Supplement 1 (2008): S40–S47.

Saghafi, R., M. Zarrebini, D. Semnani, and M. R. Mahmoudi. "Novel method for treatment of hollow fiber membranes using hypochlorite." *The Journal of The Textile Institute* 105, no. 9 (2014): 962–970.

Thabit, Hood, and Roman Hovorka. "Coming of age: The artificial pancreas for type 1 diabetes." *Diabetologia* 59, no. 9 (2016): 1795–1805.

Thomas, Bernadette. "The global burden of diabetic kidney disease: Time trends and gender gaps." *Current Diabetes Reports* 19, no. 4 (2019): 1–7.

US Food and Drug Administration. “Code of federal regulations – Title 21 – Food and drugs.” 2018. Accessed March 8, 2021. https://www.fda.gov/medical-devices/medical-device-databases/code-federal-regulations-title-21-food-and-drugs.

US Food and Drug Administration. “Product classification.” 2021. Accessed March 8th, 2021. https://www.accessdata.fda.gov/scripts/cdrh/cfdocs/cfPCD/PCDSimpleSearch.cfm.

Wai Cheung, Tin, Chenxiao Yang, and Li Li. “An integrated design of self-care textile wearables: Exploration of thermal-stimuli effects and drug delivery function.” *Textile Research Journal* 89, no. 13 (2019): 2553–2568.

11 Intelligent (SMART) Medical and Healthcare Textiles

Simon King and Holly Morris

11.1 INTRODUCTION

In a world of rapidly developing digitisation, automation, and smart control, even items as conventional and traditional as textiles are not immune. Smart textiles are quickly securing their position as essential items in many areas, revolutionising daily life from charging our portable electronic devices to delivering advanced medical care. Smart garments, powered by various means, are designed and engineered to deliver additional functionality on top of their conventional use, responding to input or environmental stimuli to serve or provide additional purpose. Some of the greatest impact of smart textiles is likely to be felt in the healthcare sector, with garments developed with the aim of allowing physicians to deliver all-year-round monitoring and improved care across a wide range of ailments, and the eventual target of providing treatments for the full spectrum of healthcare, be it preventative, curative, or palliative, and also in after-care. However, before these medical garments can be widely accepted, smart textiles face a number of challenges which must be overcome, not just with the conventional ones facing all medial textiles such as decontamination, disinfection, and sterilisation, but also with an emerging series of challenges, such as data security and accuracy.

11.2 SMART TEXTILES

Smart textiles/garments are textiles that can perform all, or one, of several functions; sensing the local surrounding environment and responding to environmental stimuli using integrated functions from the textile structure. The energy required to 'drive' the textile function may be derived from a mechanical, thermal, magnetic, chemical, kinetic, radiofrequency, or electrical stimulus (Dadhiwale 2015, 142–148).

The minimum requirement for a smart textile is the ability to sense environmental conditions or an external stimulus. Further functions the textile can perform help to classify the textile within the smart textile domain:

i) Passive smart textiles are those that can only sense the environmental conditions and stimuli

DOI: 10.1201/9781003170570-11

ii) Active smart textiles are those that sense and react to conditions and stimuli
iii) Very smart textiles sense, react, and adapt themselves accordingly
iv) Intelligent textiles are capable of responding or being activated to perform a function in a pre-programmed manner (Wu and Li 2019; Stoppa and Chiolerio 2014, 11957–11992)

Smart textiles and e-textiles (textiles with specified electronic properties included in the textile fibres/yarn) differ from other smart wearables already in wide use such as the Fitbit™ (Fitbit Inc., San Francisco USA), in that emphasis in the smart textile is on the integration of sensors and electronics in the textile/finished product itself, rather than that being carried as a separate electronic device. A smart textile system has five functional components: sensors, actuators, data processing, energy source, and communication (Tyler et al. 2019, 299–384). Currently, power-generating devices, sensors, and transmitters are being woven or knitted into the fabric, stitched onto the garment, embroidered, or printed directly onto fabrics, with varying degrees of success. The accent is not only on their physical flexibility, but on their correct positioning, effectiveness, consistency in the sensing, recording, and transmitting of physiologically important data, and their durability. Conductivity of, or between the active textile components in smart textiles is key in transferring the electrical energy needed to drive the device or for carrying the signal generated by the sensor to the transmitter or recording device. Given that electroconductive textiles have applications not only as medical textiles, but also in energy harvesting, electromagnetic shielding, in heating pads, and in a range of sensors, technology has rapidly developed to enable conductive textile yarns to be manufactured in various ways (Maiti, Das, and Sen 2017, 1–52) such as:

i) Inherently conductive metallic filament materials such as stainless steel or silver used alone or embedded in a non-conductive substrate for its protection (Cheng, Ueng, and Dixon 2001, 732–738)
ii) Non-conductive fibres such as polyethylene or polypropylene incorporating conductive fillers, such as metal powders, nanowires or graphene during melt spinning or solvent spinning, with solvent spinning providing the best outcomes (King et al. 2018, 207–214; Maiti, Das, and Sen 2017, 1–52)
iii) Carbon fibres (Hasan et al. 2011, 1603–1616)
iv) Intrinsically conductive polymers such as polythiophene or its more easily processable derivative, poly(3,4-ethylene dioxythiophene)-poly(styrene sulfonate) or (PEDOT:PSS) (Akerfeldt 2015), polypyrrole (PPy) (Maity and Chatterjee 2015, 6) or polyaniline (PANI) (Muthukumar, Thilagavathi, and Kannaian 2016, 283–290) are used as coatings on non-conductive fibres because in filament form they are very stiff.
v) Non-conductive or weakly conductive fibres given a conductive coating with a dispersion such as carbon black, a metal coating or treatment with carbon nanotubes (CNTs; tubes of graphene) or cotton fibres with a graphene coating, is in continuing development (Chatterjee, Nivas Kumar, and Maity 2017, 1910–1916)

Each of these approaches has its advantages and disadvantages in both final material quality, performances, and commercial scalability (Stoppa and Chiolerio 2014, 11957–11992).

Depending on the desired application for the smart textile, material characteristics are often key. Research at the University of Otago has already highlighted the importance of fibre type, yarn, and the fabric structure used in socks and the resulting underlying skin health. The key determinant for fabric behaviour on cyclic loading was whether the fabric was dry or damp; where damp fabrics absorbed less energy, retained less thickness during compression, and recovered less than compared to dry fabrics. Whilst the structure of the fabric was deemed less important in comparison but still posed a small influence in this example (Van Amber et al. 2015, 26–35). Fabric structure has been shown to be of importance in other applications; for example, the ability to 3D knit and braid fabrics containing integrated chemical and electrochemical sensors allows for the creation of garments that can replace bulky analytical devices (Farajikhah et al. 2020, 1–9).

In addition to manufacturing fabrics with electroconductive yarns, the development of stimuli-responsive materials with shape-changing behaviours is also highly desirable as it allows for products to be designed wherein substantial sections of it can respond to stimuli (Tyler et al. 2019, 299–384). Shape-memory materials that have the ability to change shape when exposed to an external stimulus (e.g., moisture, stress, temperature, pH) then return to the original shape when that stimulus is removed, have been incorporated into medical devices (Gök, Bilir, and Gürcüm 2015, 2160–2169; British Plastics Federation 2020). Research from the University of Minnesota has seen the development of a prototype garment that allows for dynamic compression of varying location and intensity for managing sensory processing disorders (Duvall et al. 2019).

Chromic materials may sense and change colour in response to a stimulus, as illustrated in Figure 11.1 (Ramlow, Andrade, and Immich 2020, 1–20). Thermochromic fabrics potentially may highlight patients or locations within patients that have a raised or lowered temperature, a feature possibly useful in the management of sepsis. Chemochromic (chemically sensitive) materials may have applications in the detection of pH changes or changes to constituents of bodily fluids, for example, in dialysis where it is critical to ensure the correct balance of constituents in returning blood. More recent applications of chemochromic materials include facemasks which change colour with the detection of pathogens or after a period of exposure to CO_2, prompting the wearer to replace the mask with a clean one for continued protection (Yenisafak 2021).

Phase change materials which may change from one state to another in an exothermic or endothermic reaction are already used in specialist industries. For example, NASA exploited phase change material to ensure thermal regulation in extremes of temperature (NASA 2016) and it is a matter of time until this effectively crosses into the healthcare domain. Designing with bio-fabricated textiles, materials grown from live microorganisms such as bacteria, yeast, algae or fungi, potentially offer a sustainable and compostable solution to single-use medical devices (Tyler et al. 2019, 299–384).

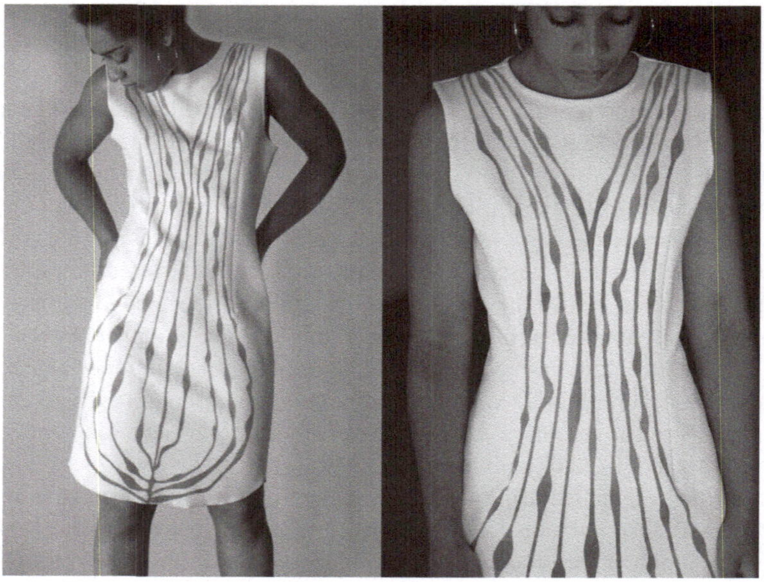

FIGURE 11.1 A fashion dress garment containing thermochromic compounds that changes colour in response to heat. Reproduced with permission granted by FabTextiles Team 2017: Anastasia Pistofidou, Clara Davis, and Rose Ekwe.

The first smart shirt was developed in the 1990s for use by medical staff in combat situations; optical fibres woven through the fabric were connected to sensors that monitored vital signs to detect and assess inflicted wounds (O'Connor 2010, 50–67). Since the release and successful use of that smart shirt, much research has been directed towards smart textiles and potential benefits that sensors embedded in garments may have in healthcare. For example, the EU project BIOTEX, developed a range of e-textile sensors that can measure sweat rate, electrolyte concentration, and the pH of the sweat from the wearer, allowing for potential monitoring of both the fluid and electrolyte status of patients (Cherenack, and Van Pieterson 2012, 0901301; Coyle 2010, 364–370). The BIOTEX textiles consist of a multi-layered flexible braided structure of 120 μm-enamelled copper wire as the conductor and 19 tex air-jet spun single viscose rayon yarns as the hygroscopic dielectric. It was developed as a moisture sensor which would work because of capacitance changes within the braid caused by changes in relative humidity in the adjacent environment. Enamelled copper wires (6 in total) were braided to function as the central core, which was then overbraided with 12 of the viscose rayon yarns and that assembly openly overbraided by six of the enamelled copper wires to form an outer conductor. This construction was porous enough to allow moisture to penetrate through to the viscose rayon dielectric, whilst not so densely packed as to reduce the overall electrical capacitance too significantly. Unlike thin film devices, the properties of the braided structure were such as to enable it to be compatible with and directly incorporated into other textiles, such as bandages or clothing, and it was found to be highly sensitive for relative humidities between 22% and 94% (Wendler et al. 2020, 469–477).

Another type of smart textile intended for use within healthcare involves the use of organic electrochemical transistors (OECTs). These devices consist of one electrically conductive polymer as the 'channel' and another acting as a 'gate,' with the two separated by an electrolyte solution. In this configuration, the electrical current passing through the channel can be modulated by the gate via an applied voltage, which influences the channel by varying the electrostatic field generated by the applied voltage. This electrostatic field controls the electrical current passing through the channel by inducing electrochemical reactions within the polymer, which causes changes to the charge-carrier concentration in the transistor channel material thereby altering the conductivity of the channel. An OECT was developed which consisted wholly of the flexible conductive polymer PEDOT: PSS (Akerfeldt 2015) and this was screen printed onto/embedded into a flexible fabric made of woven cotton/Lycra®, this enabled non-invasive monitoring of biomarkers in external body fluids (Gualandi et al. 2016, 1–10; Castano and Flatau 2016, 121–146).

Applications of smart textiles in healthcare range from surgical uses of a single fibre, to complex wearable constructions and auxiliary systems for personalised care (Mečņika et al. 2014, 150–161). The ability to identify declining health within a patient and subsequently alert healthcare providers creates the potential for smart textiles to be used in preventive medicine and in managing pre-existing disease, whether as an inpatient or within the wider community. To achieve the required performance, sensors may be embedded directly into the fabric or embedded into a coating applied to the fabric surface (Ciocchetti et al. 2015, 602–615) which allows production of devices that can capture a myriad of data, including physiological variables; the measurement of cardiorespiratory parameters, electromyography, and electroencephalography can be achieved with garments and fabrics already available (Coosemans, Hermans, and Puers 2006, 48–53; Coyle 2002, 297–300). The devices typically consist of a sensor to monitor physiological parameters, conductive yarns, and an interface that can interpret and collect incoming data prior to transmission to a remote location, for example, *via* Bluetooth® (Bluetooth Special Interests Group, Kirkland, Washington, USA) (Zheng, Ha, and Zhang 2017, 283–294). An American company produced one of the earliest examples of these garments which allowed for physiological measuring, marketed as LifeShirt® (VivoMetrics, Vivosense, San Diego, USA). This garment included attachments that monitored blood pressure, electroencephalogram, temperature, and pulse oximetry. Whilst no longer available for sale, production of this garment did highlight the possibilities for future design and the breadth of clinical application for which design and manufacture may be suitable (Heilman and Porges 2007, 300–305). Since then, more recent garments have been produced for a range of applications, including home monitoring for episodes of sleep apnoea (Azouz et al. 2018, 104–107; Guo et al. 2013, 499–509), transcutaneous electrical nerve stimulation (TENS) (Li et al. 2010, 279–286), posture monitoring for spinal repair (Wang et al. 2015, 5736–5739), flexible joint monitoring garments for joint therapy (Abro et al. 2019, 262–274) and diabetic foot ulcer monitoring (Raviglione et al. 2017, 894–898). Other approaches have included incorporation of sensors in the form of fibre optics, this has further allowed for the development of socks which can be used to monitor pressure changes and temperature to provide some measure of pre-ulcerative inflammation and possibly predict the likelihood of diabetic foot ulceration (Najafi et al. 2014).

Outside of healthcare, the sporting industry also has a keen interest in smart textiles, not just for athlete healing after some unfortunate incident but also for position tracking, performance and engagement monitoring, providing real-time data on strength, agility, and fatigue. In these cases, garments which respond to material stresses caused by compression, such as in the sole of a footballer's boot, are typically employed (Mao et al. 2019, 3310). Such compression garments have also attracted experts in the field of vascular pathology (MacRae, Cotter, and Laing 2011, 815–843). Compression garments are typically comprised of a piezoelectric active material such as polyvinylidene fluoride (PVDF) which create a voltage signal when subject to compression or kinetic movements. Such garments can be engineered to be extremely sensitive, detecting movements as small as those from an unborn foetus, to detecting larger more aggressive movements in contact sports, as illustrated in Figure 11.2 (Forouharshad et al. 2019, 1900364). For orthopaedics and sports medicine, in a similar fashion to the compression garments, a knee sleeve with inbuilt

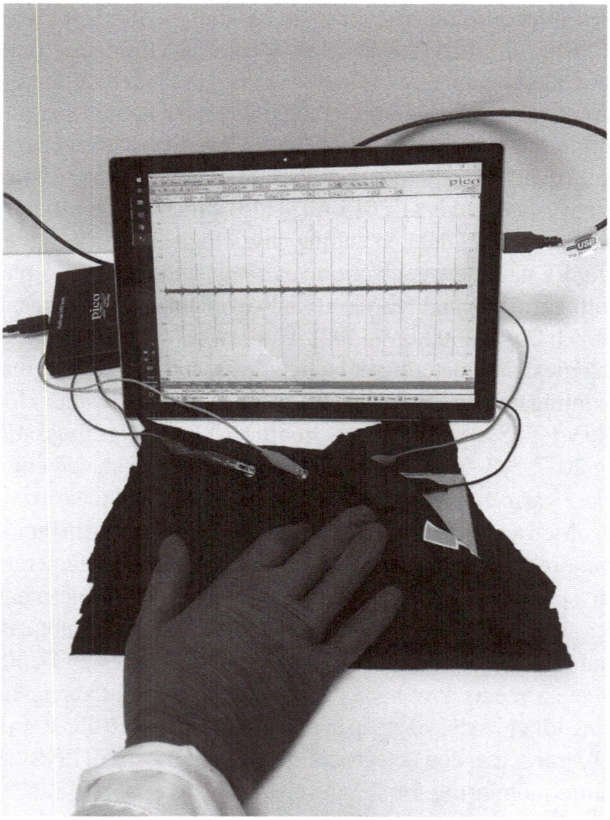

FIGURE 11.2 A piezoelectric smart textile being developed for foetal monitoring garments. Small levels of kinetic stimulus from the solenoid onto the garment give rise to electrical pulses read on the computer. Reproduced with permission granted by Radical Fibres Ltd, UK, 2020.

goniometers was trialled. The textile goniometer coupled two knitted piezoresistive layers on either side of an electrically insulating layer, an arrangement which would appear to have many potential applications for post-operative physiotherapy in orthopaedics and sports medicine, allowing for direct collection of movement data for either continual monitoring or remote healthcare (Grassi et al. 2017, 5927–5936; Tognetti et al. 2015, 28435–28455; Wong et al. 2015, 2747–2760). Historical methods for measuring joint movement included using optical fibre Bragg-Grating sensing (Lakho et al. 2019, 3433–3446) and still proves to be a useful technique for monitoring posture and pressure (Abro et al. 2020, 386–394).

Often, medical garments for monitoring and sensing movement have the potential to be applied to yield end-of-care improvements to quality of life. As a result, attention has been directed at how smart textiles may improve prosthetics for amputees. For example, electronic skin has sensory capabilities whilst textile-based sensors can be easily worn over prosthetics whilst retaining the appearance of being a regular garment, as in Figure 11.3. Flexible, stretchable piezoresistive fabrics are available for a range of pressure-sensing applications that can be incorporated into robotic limbs for direct feedback to the wearer (Leong et al. 2016, 335–346). Such textiles can also incorporate infection control management systems aimed at preventing the onset of any infection by continuing wounds or use of the prosthetic, as well as posing key benefits to a wider range of general medical garments, such as bandages, bedding, and dressings (Rajendran and Anand 2016).

Being able to monitor physiological variables and continually communicate the relevant information by electronic means has the potential to revolutionise healthcare by enabling remote monitoring of patients, thus reducing overall admissions to hospital, the duration of stay, and perhaps identifying early onset of disease. For example, within the UK alone, in 2018, 1 in every 250 pregnancies end in stillbirth, roughly equating to 3,000 babies/year (Tommys 2020). Between 30% and 55% of women whose pregnancies end in stillbirth experience reduced foetal movements in the preceding week (Norman et al. 2018, 1629–1638). Smart garments incorporating foetal movement monitoring sensors could allow for continual foetal movement monitoring by an automated system, alerting remote healthcare experts in real time to any perceived movement issues, ideally without alerting the expectant mother

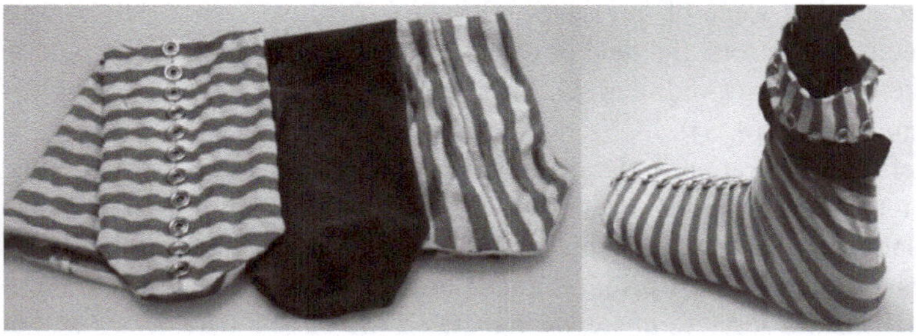

FIGURE 11.3 Prototype of a textile-based sensing sock. Reproduced with permission granted by Media Interaction Lab, University of Applied Sciences, Upper Austria.

and avoiding unnecessary stresses caused by false alarms experienced with current alternatives. Smart textile technologies such as these may not only save lives but also reduce the strain on the healthcare sector through automated and remote care. In a fiscally tight public healthcare sector, benefits may accrue to businesses engaging in the development of textile products for remote healthcare monitoring. In 2019, the global smart textile industry was estimated to reach US$5.55 billion US dollars by 2025 with a projected compound annual growth rate of 30.4% (Grand View Research 2019), owing to a combination of the rising geriatric population, ongoing technological advancements, and stringent legislative framework mandating the use of medical textiles. However, before smart textiles can be widely accepted and utilised to a far broader scope, there are several challenges which need to be overcome:

i) Acceptance by both patient and health professional needs to be achieved
ii) Sterility, stability, and the efficacy of the sensing function in the presence of any form of moisture such as bodily fluids, need to be considered
iii) Efficacy following cleaning requires investigation when the product is designed for re-use (Rotzler et al. 2020, 1–12)
iv) The security of the data being collected and (possibly) transmitted must be assured
v) Backup procedures must be in place if the smart textile malfunctions
vi) What happens at the end of the textile's useable life and the environmental impact of any residues need to be optimised

All of the above factors are critical to the success of smart textiles in healthcare. There are also important ethical considerations surrounding the information/data collected and forwarded through the use of garments which include connectivity as one of their functions. For example, who will own the data, how it will be stored and for how long, and who will have access to it are critical issues to settle prior to implementation. If data from patients in the community are sent to a central point, there needs to be sufficient adequately trained staff to collect and interpret the data, and it needs to be established who will be responsible for making decisions on identification and management of abnormal parameters. Whilst there has already been work directed at some of the issues relevant to medical textile sensors and wearable electronic sensors, the field of research is wide and ever evolving and requires continuous attention (Andreoni, Barbieri, and Piccini 2011, 269–285; Hughes-Riley, Dias, and Cork 2018, 34).

Careful consideration in data handling must also include future-proofing of the data set itself, ensuring that the designed systems remain entirely functional as software platforms evolve. Whilst this may sound trivial, data management on this level remains a key concern. A prime example of the potential impacts of these issues is in the UK health services misreporting COVID-19 patient data, as a result of using an outdated version of Microsoft Excel to perform analysis (BBC News 2020). From a clinicians' point of view, bedside skills and the importance of a thorough history and examination ought never to be negated just because of the existence of readily accessible and measurable data.

REFERENCES

Abro, Zamir Ahmed, Chengyu Hong, Nanliang Chen, Yifan Zhang, Rafique Ahmed Lakho, and Sohail Yasin. "A fiber Bragg grating-based smart wearable belt for monitoring knee joint postures." *Textile Research Journal* 90, no. 3–4 (2020): 386–394.

Åkerfeldt, Maria. "Electrically conductive textile coatings with PEDOT: PSS." PhD diss., Högskolan i Borås, 2015.

Andreoni, Giuseppe, Massimo Barbieri, and Luca Piccini. "A review of the intellectual property right in the field of wearable sensors and system." *International Journal of Educational Computing Research* 18, no. 3/4 (2011): 269–285.

Azouz, Aymen Ben, Ahmed Issa, Peter Knief, Thomas Kane, Shirley Coyle, Richard Costello, Kevin G. McGuigan, and Dermot Diamond. "Evaluation of use of wearable sensor garment in home screening for sleep apnea events." In *2018 International Conference on Promising Electronic Technologies (ICPET)*. IEEE, 2018, pp. 104–107.

BBC News. "Excel: Why using Microsoft's tool caused covid-19 results to be lost." 2020. Accessed January 6, 2021. https://www.bbc.co.uk/news/technology-54423988.

British Plastics Federation. "Shape memory polymers – A complete guide." 2020. Accessed December 31, 2020. https://www.bpf.co.uk/plastipedia/applications/shape-memory-polymer.aspx.

Castano, Lina M., and Alison B. Flatau. "Smart textile transducers: Design, techniques, and applications." In *Industrial Applications for Intelligent Polymers and Coatings*, 121–146. Cham: Springer, 2016.

Chatterjee, Arobindo, M. Nivas Kumar, and Subhankar Maity. "Influence of graphene oxide concentration and dipping cycles on electrical conductivity of coated cotton textiles." *The Journal of The Textile Institute* 108, no. 11 (2017): 1910–1916.

Cheng, K. B., T. H. Ueng, and G. Dixon. "Electrostatic discharge properties of stainless steel/polyester woven fabrics." *Textile Research Journal* 71, no. 8 (2001): 732–738.

Cherenack, Kunigunde, and Liesbeth van Pieterson. "Smart textiles: Challenges and opportunities." *Journal of Applied Physics* 112, no. 9 (2012): 091301.

Ciocchetti, Marco, Carlo Massaroni, Paola Saccomandi, Michele A. Caponero, Andrea Polimadei, Domenico Formica, and Emiliano Schena. "Smart textile based on fiber bragg grating sensors for respiratory monitoring: Design and preliminary trials." *Biosensors* 5, no. 3 (2015): 602–615.

Coosemans, Johan, Bart Hermans, and Robert Puers. "Integrating wireless ECG monitoring in textiles." *Sensors and Actuators A: Physical* 130 (2006): 48–53.

Coyle M. Ambulatory cardiopulmonary data capture. In *2nd Annual International IEEE-EMBS Special Topic Conference on Microtechnologies in Medicine and Biology*, 297–300. Proceedings (Cat. No. 02EX578) 2002 May 2. IEEE, 2002.

Coyle, Shirley, King-Tong Lau, Niall Moyna, Donal O'Gorman, Dermot Diamond, Fabio Di Francesco, Daniele Costanzo et al. "BIOTEX—Biosensing textiles for personalised healthcare management." *IEEE Transactions on Information Technology in Biomedicine* 14, no. 2 (2010): 364–370.

Dadhiwale, A. "Smart textiles--Part I." *Man-Made Textiles in India* 43, no. 4 (2015).

Duvall, Julia C., Nicholas Schleif, Lucy E. Dunne, and Brad Holschuh. "Dynamic compression garments for sensory processing disorder treatment using integrated active materials." *Journal of Medical Devices* 13, no. 2 (2019).

Farajikhah, Syamak, Jaecheol Choi, Dorna Esrafilzadeh, Jenny Underwood, Peter C. Innis, Brett Paull, and Gordon G. Wallace. "3D textile structures with integrated electroactive electrodes for wearable electrochemical sensors." *The Journal of The Textile Institute* (2020): 1–9.

Forouharshad, Mahdi, Simon G. King, Wesley Buxton, Philip Kunovski, and Vlad Stolojan. "Textile-compatible, electroactive polyvinylidene fluoride electrospun mats for energy harvesting." *Macromolecular Chemistry and Physics* 220, no. 24 (2019): 1900364.

Gök, Mustafa O., Mehmet Z. Bilir, and Banu H. Gürcüm. "Shape-memory applications in textile design." *Procedia-Social and Behavioral Sciences* 195 (2015): 2160–2169.

Grand View Research. "Smart textile market size worth $5.55 billion by 2025." 2019. Access December 31, 2020. *https://www.grandviewresearch.com/press-release/global-smart-textiles-industry.*

Grassi, Angela, Francesca Cecchi, Martina Maselli, Marloes Röling, Cecilia Laschi, and Matteo Cianchetti. "Warp-knitted textile as a strain sensor: Characterization procedure and application in a comfortable wearable goniometer." *IEEE Sensors Journal* 17, no. 18 (2017): 5927–5936.

Gualandi, I., M. Marzocchi, A. Achilli, D. Cavedale, A. Bonfiglio, and B. Fraboni. "Textile organic electrochemical transistors as a platform for wearable biosensors." *Scientific Reports* 6, no. 1 (2016): 1–10.

Guo, Li, Lena Berglin, Urban Wiklund, and Heikki Mattila. "Design of a garment-based sensing system for breathing monitoring." *Textile Research Journal* 83, no. 5 (2013): 499–509.

Hasan, Mir Mohammad Badrul, Olaf Diestel, and Chokri Cherif. "Electro-mechanical properties of friction spun conductive hybrid yarns made of carbon filaments for composites." *Textile Research Journal* 81, no. 15 (2011): 1603–1616.

Heilman, Keri J., and Stephen W. Porges. "Accuracy of the LifeShirt®(Vivometrics) in the detection of cardiac rhythms." *Biological Psychology* 75, no. 3 (2007): 300–305.

Hughes-Riley, Theodore, Tilak Dias, and Colin Cork. "A historical review of the development of electronic textiles." *Fibers* 6, no. 2 (2018): 34.

King, Simon G., Nicholas J. Terrill, Andrew J. Goodwin, Robert Stevens, Vlad Stolojan, and S. Ravi P. Silva. "Probing of polymer to carbon nanotube surface interactions within highly aligned electrospun nanofibers for advanced composites." *Carbon* 138 (2018): 207–214.

Lakho, Rafique Ahmed, Zhang Yi-Fan, Jiang Jin-Hua, Hong Cheng-Yu, and Zamir Ahmed Abro. "A smart insole for monitoring plantar pressure based on the fiber Bragg grating sensing technique." *Textile Research Journal* 89, no. 17 (2019): 3433–3446.

Leong, Joanne, Patrick Parzer, Florian Perteneder, Teo Babic, Christian Rendl, Anita Vogl, Hubert Egger, Alex Olwal, and Michael Haller. "proCover: Sensory augmentation of prosthetic limbs using smart textile covers." In *Proceedings of the 29th Annual Symposium on User Interface Software and Technology*, 335–346, 2016.

Li, Li, Wai Man Au, Yi Li, Kam Man Wan, Sai Ho Wan, and Kwok Shing Wong. "Design of intelligent garment with transcutaneous electrical nerve stimulation function based on the intarsia knitting technique." *Textile Research Journal* 80, no. 3 (2010): 279–286.

MacRae, Braid A., James D. Cotter, and Raechel M. Laing. "Compression garments and exercise." Sports Medicine 41, no. 10 (2011): 815–843.

Maiti, Syamal, Dipayan Das, and Kushal Sen. "Flexible non-metallic electro-conductive textiles." *Textile Progress* 49, no. 1 (2017): 1–52.

Maity, Subhankar, and Arobindo Chatterjee. "Textile/polypyrrole composites for sensory applications." *Journal of Composites* 2015 (2015).

Mao, Yupeng, Mailun Shen, Bing Liu, Lili Xing, Song Chen, and Xinyu Xue. "Self-powered piezoelectric-biosensing textiles for the physiological monitoring and time-motion analysis of individual sports." *Sensors* 19, no. 15 (2019): 3310.

Mečņika, Viktorija, Melanie Hoerr, Ivars Krieviņš, and Anne Schwarz. "Smart textiles for healthcare: Applications and technologies." *Rural Environment, Education, Personality* 7 (2014): 150–161.

Muthukumar, N., G. Thilagavathi, and T. Kannaian. "Polyaniline-coated foam electrodes for electroencephalography (EEG) measurement." *The Journal of The Textile Institute* 107, no. 3 (2016): 283–290.

Najafi, Bijan, Gurtej Singh Grewal, Saman Parvaneh, Jacqueline Lee-eng, Robert A. Menzies, Talal K. Talal, and David G. Armstrong. "Validation of an optical fiber based smart textile: A clinical tool for predicting diabetic foot ulceration." In *Qatar Foundation Annual Research Conference Proceedings*, Volume 2014 Issue 1, vol. 2014, no. 1, p. HBPP0345. Hamad bin Khalifa University Press (HBKU Press), 2014.

NASA. "Phase Change Material Heat Exchanger (PCM HX)." 2016. Accessed December 31, 2020. https://www.nasa.gov/directorates/spacetech/image-feature/phase_change-material_heat_exchanger.

Norman, Jane E., Alexander E. P. Heazell, Aryelly Rodriguez, Christopher J. Weir, Sarah J. E. Stock, Catherine J. Calderwood, Sarah Cunningham Burley et al. "Awareness of fetal movements and care package to reduce fetal mortality (AFFIRM): A stepped wedge, cluster-randomised trial." *The Lancet* 392, no. 10158 (2018): 1629–1638.

O'Connor, Kaori. "How smart is smart? T-shirts, wellness, and the way people feel about "medical" textiles." *Textile* 8, no. 1 (2010): 50–66.

Rajendran, Subbiyan, and Subhash C. Anand. "Smart textiles for infection control management." In *Advances in Smart Medical Textiles*, 93–117. Woodhead Publishing, 2016.

Ramlow, Heloisa, Karina Luzia Andrade, and Ana Paula Serafini Immich. "Smart textiles: An overview of recent progress on chromic textiles." *The Journal of The Textile Institute* (2020): 1–20.

Raviglione, Andrea, Roberto Reif, Maurizio Macagno, Davide Vigano, Justin Schram, and David Armstrong. "Real-time smart textile-based system to monitor pressure offloading of diabetic foot ulcers." *Journal of Diabetes Science and Technology* 11, no. 5 (2017): 894–898.

Rotzler, Sigrid, Christine Kallmayer, Christian Dils, Malte von Krshiwoblozki, Ulrich Bauer, and Martin Schneider-Ramelow. "Improving the washability of smart textiles: Influence of different washing conditions on textile integrated conductor tracks." *The Journal of The Textile Institute* (2020): 1–12.

Stoppa, Matteo, and Alessandro Chiolerio. "Wearable electronics and smart textiles: A critical review." *Sensors* 14, no. 7 (2014): 11957–11992.

Tognetti, Alessandro, Federico Lorussi, Nicola Carbonaro, and Danilo De Rossi. "Wearable goniometer and accelerometer sensory fusion for knee joint angle measurement in daily life." *Sensors* 15, no. 11 (2015): 28435–28455.

Tommy's. "Stillbirth statistics." 2020. Accessed December 31, 2020. https://www.tommys.org/baby-loss-support/stillbirth-information-and-support/stillbirth-statistics.

Tyler, David, Jane Wood, Tasneem Sabir, Chloe McDonnell, Abu Sadat Muhammad Sayem, and Nick Whittaker. "Wearable electronic textiles." *Textile Progress* 51, no. 4 (2019): 299–384.

Van Amber, Rebecca R., Bronwyn J. Lowe, Brian E. Niven, Raechel M. Laing, and Cheryl A. Wilson. "Sock fabrics: Relevance of fiber type, yarn, fabric structure and moisture on cyclic compression." *Textile Research Journal* 85, no. 1 (2015): 26–35.

Wang, Qi, Wei Chen, Annick AA Timmermans, Christoforos Karachristos, Jean-Bernard Martens, and Panos Markopoulos. "Smart rehabilitation garment for posture monitoring." In *2015 37th Annual International Conference of the IEEE Engineering in Medicine and Biology Society (EMBC)*, 5736–5739. IEEE, 2015.

Wendler, Johannes, Daniel Maraite, Andreas Nocke, and Chokri Cherif. "Novel textile moisture sensors based on multi-layered braiding constructions." *Textile Research Journal* 90, no. 3–4 (2020): 469–477.

Wong, Charence, Zhi-Qiang Zhang, Benny Lo, and Guang-Zhong Yang. "Wearable sensing for solid biomechanics: A review." *IEEE Sensors Journal* 15, no. 5 (2015): 2747–2760.

Wu, Jennifer Xiaopei, and Li Li. "An introduction to wearable technology and smart textiles and apparel: terminology, statistics, evolution, and challenges." In *Smart and Functional Soft Materials*. IntechOpen, 2019.

Yenisafak. "Turkish firm produces smart masks using artificial intelligence." 2021. Accessed January 6, 2021. https://www.yenisafak.com/en/technology/turkish-firm-produces-smart-masks-using-artificial-intelligence-3519386,

Zheng, J., C. Ha, and Z. Zhang. "Design and evaluation of a ubiquitous chest-worn cardiopulmonary monitoring system for healthcare application: A pilot study." *Medical & Biological Engineering & Computing* 55, no. 2 (2017): 283–294.

12 Case Studies

12.1 CASE STUDY ONE: PPE AND PLANNING FOR EMERGENCIES

The aim of this case study is to bring together details about epidemics and associated events to help government officials, healthcare managers and administrators, and healthcare practitioners to become better prepared for emergency situations such as those which arose as a consequence of the COVID-19 pandemic. Its three components, '2020 Vision,' '2020 Hindsight,' and 'Beyond 2020' work together to set the context and to provide a guide to the type of information needed to begin the development of an Emergency Management Plan. The idea is that shortages of PPE during future crises will not be experienced again to the extent that they were during the COVID-19 pandemic.

12.1.1 2020 Vision: Epidemics and Shortages of PPE

12.1.1.1 Early Warnings

a) ***Outbreaks: Previous Epidemics***

In any pandemic-type emergency, each country will have to put its own peoples' needs first. What this means is that for PPE, there needs to be sufficient PPE-dedicated manufacturing capacity within each country or region itself, not just to satisfy its ongoing needs but its likely emergency levels of requirement as well. Several significant epidemics have occurred in recent years: Ebola, SARS, H1N1, MERS, and most recently, the COVID-19 pandemic. With widespread and growing levels of air travel together with recognition at the time of the SARS epidemic in 2003 that cross-infection occurred during flights (Olsen *et al.* 2003, 2416–2422), a suitable preventative ventilation method having been found to help limit transmission within the passenger cabin (You *et al.* 2019, 840–853) and an air purification system with the capability to reduce the levels of bacteria, viruses, and fungi in the air (97%–99%) and at the highest level (99%) on surfaces (Airius 2021; Fink & Ellis 2011) but neither widely enough installed as yet, it continues to be essential that healthcare officials and government bodies remain on high alert for warnings about possible spread when a substantial epidemic occurs anywhere in the world. It is also important for them to be engaged and honest about their preparedness for emergencies, and not to act in a covert fashion to conceal incompetence. For David Tkachuk, deputy chair of a Senate Committee looking into the mismanagement of Canada's

DOI: 10.1201/9781003170570-12

emergency response system in Canada in 2008, that kind of behaviour provoked him into preparing a colourful report: "Emergency preparedness in Canada: how the fine arts of bafflegab and procrastination hobble the people who will be trying to save you when things get really bad." expressing the frustration caused by inability to admit failure by those responsible (CBC 2020a).

b) ***Vulnerability of supply***

12.1.1.2 Single Use vs Reusable

The guidance on how to make the choice in a justifiable way has been available for some years (Zins 2006, 73–80). Essentially, the advice is to reserve the use of disposable devices for types of items not used in volume (Walton 1986, 213–217). PPE is a volume product so, to avoid the potential for shortages to rise during a crisis, the selected items should be reusable, and if reusable items are not available, research efforts need to be devoted to developing a reusable form of that device. Regarding filter face pieces, preparatory work was reported on such a respirator device in the USA 8 years ago, namely the 'B95: A new respirator for health care personnel' (Gosch. *et al.* 2013, 1224-1230) but for whatever reason, the B95 had not appeared in time to mitigate the respirator shortage crisis caused by COVID-19 combined with the N95 being single use only. Is the development of a reusable respirator which performs as well as the single-use disposable N95 too difficult a task to achieve? Apparently not. The production of a reusable N95 mask to counteract shortages experienced during the COVID-19 epidemic is being undertaken by Precision ADM, a manufacturing company in Winnipeg that won a bid to make 1 million reusable N95 masks for the Manitoba government. The masks, designed by two Manitoba doctors, can be used up to 30 times with disinfecting after each use (CBC 2020b), and a team from Shinshu Uinversity in Japan and Pohang University of Science and Technology in Korea have shown that replacing the web-blown layer in a respirator with a nanofibre filter layer enabled its repeated decontamination and re-use (Ullah et al. 2020, 7231–7241).

12.1.1.3 Quantity Issues

A full ten years ahead of the COVID-19 pandemic and just prior to the H1N1 outbreak, researchers from NIOSH in the United States together with members of staff from a highly respected US Federal Government contractor, USAAF researchers and an academic from the University of Nebraska repeated the warning given in 2006 by the US Institute of Medicine, Committee on the Development of Reusable Facemasks for Use During an Influenza Pandemic (Institute of Medicine 2006) in their own papers, that supplies of PPE would run short in an epidemic (90 million N95 surgical respirators would be needed), and laid down a set of demonstration methods to form the basis for the development of N95 respirator decontamination and reuse. Reuse would help because despite the creation of a stockpile, the total quantities required would still be difficult to provide (Bergman *et al.* 2010, 33-41 and Viscusi *et al.* 2009a, 815-827). The

FDA commissioned Battelle to work on the respirator topic and they reported on the development of a decontamination and reuse treatment in 2016, so the FDA was prepared ahead of the COVID-19 crisis (Battelle, 2016). However, despite recognising the COVID-19 emergency on February 4th 2020, the Secretary of the Department of Health and Human Services was slow in authorising emergency use of medical devices, that is not until 27th March 2020 (U.S. Department of Health and Human Services 2020a and 2020b) and that delay prevented the FDA up until that point, releasing their 'Emergency Use Authorisation' (FDA 2020). Without Emergency Use Authorisation' hospitals in the USA would be left open to litigation had they unilaterally decided to implement respirator decontamination and reuse until that had happened.

12.1.1.4 Quality Issues

With rapid globalisation in supply not being accompanied by similar worldwide rapidity in the development of and insistence by governments on appropriate levels of corporate responsibility for business and industry, it is not sensible to rely on manufacturers and suppliers to assure quality, as illustrated by the check run by the Health & Safety Executive in the UK in 2017, which showed that for FFP3 masks (respirators) 50% of the items tested were defective (HSE 2016). The European Safety Federation and 3-M, a widely respected manufacturer of N95 and other respirators, have also both uncovered dishonesty and serious quality breaches (European Safety Federation 2020 and Manufacturing.net 2020).

12.1.1.5 Supply Issues

The USA, Canada, and the UK do have national stockpiles, but to function properly, they require proper management; stock rotation, and withdrawal for use of product from the stockpile before the expiry date, rather than wasteful disposal. There need be no rush to accomplish those steps. For example, considerable leeway is available to accomplish the required rotation and replacement in the case of respirators, where it has been shown that one essential component, the electret, is capable of maintaining the charge essential for its operation for at least ten years (Viscusi *et al.* 2009b, 815-827). A particularly messy situation was uncovered in Canada when the contents of a stockpile in Ottawa, part of the National Emergency Stockpile System consisting mostly of N95 respirators purchased in 2009 and disposable gloves, were thrown away in mid-2019 as out of date, following failure to continually draw on its contents for normal use and to replenish and rotate its stock.

12.1.1.6 Supply-Chain Management Issues

Overreliance on overseas manufacturers led to serious shortages of all kinds of PPE in Western countries. Even if the supply-chain management were as sophisticated, and both quality and quantity in supply were as highly supervised as in the operations carried out by fashion-retail companies, which it was not, it is still highly unlikely that adequate levels of supply could have been maintained, but warnings and notice of the need for action would definitely have emerged earlier.

12.1.1.7 Decontamination and Reuse Issues

If a country or region finds itself in the unfortunate position of approving only single-use devices, hospitals are vulnerable to litigation if they begin to decontaminate and reuse without the appropriate signal coming from the approval organisation to go ahead with specified decontamination methods. Given the emergence of an epidemic, such approval needs to be swift enough to ensure continued adequate supply of PPE items. For N95 respirators it was about four and a half months (March 24, 2020) before any such approval was allowed to emerge through the FDA. In the UK it was March 27, 2020, when guidance on what to do in the case of shortages of FFP3 respirators emerged, which was not to carry out decontamination and reuse, but just to use FFP2 respirators instead (UK Health and Safety Executive 2020). There had however, been strong and detailed guidance on decontamination and reuse of N95 respirators published ten years earlier (Bergman *et al.* 2010, 33-41 and Viscusi *et al.* 2009b, 815-827) so although that information was open to all to read and respond perhaps it was not read by those responsible for maintaining adequate supplies of PPE. Whether the attention paid to those published works was adequate or not can be determined from whether there were any plans to cope with severe PPE shortages in each country as the pandemic progressed. Regarding the UK and USA and parts of Europe, especially Italy, there were shortages, so if any attention was paid in those places, it was clearly inadequate.

For the USA, decontamination and reuse of respirators was never an open-ended matter, and given that it was thought that there was no longer any shortage in supply, on April 30, 2021, the FDA revoked the emergency use authorisation (EUA) of the Battelle CCDS™, its Critical Care Decontamination System (Battelle 2016), which was authorised for use in decontaminating compatible N95 respirators for multiple user reuse by healthcare personnel. The Battelle CCDS™ service had been provided at no charge to healthcare providers through 60 sites in the eastern United States, on the basis of funding by government agencies. The FDA revoked the EUA in response to Battelle's request for voluntary withdrawal of the authorisation. In response to changing customer needs, as of March 31, 2021, Battelle has ceased all Battelle CCDS decontamination site operations and marketing activities. What many might consider a far better response with longer term significance, this time based in Canada, has been to undertake design and development of a reusable N95 mask to counteract shortages such as those experienced in Manitoba. Precision ADM, a manufacturing company in Winnipeg, won a bid to make 1 million reusable N95 masks for the Manitoba government. The masks, designed by two Manitoba doctors, can be used up to 30 times with disinfecting after each use, according to a news release from the province (CBC 2020a).

12.1.2 2020 Hindsight: Prepare for the Next Healthcare Crisis

a) ***Learn from the Most Recent Healthcare Crisis***

- It is worth having an emergency response arrangement to compensate for the inability of normal arrangements to cope with a crisis (FDA 2020).

- It could be worthwhile establishing a better way of ensuring that the equipment being provided by suppliers is up to standard and not overpriced, rather than relying solely on self-monitoring by suppliers themselves (PULSE 2020 and UK Department for Business, Energy & Industrial Strategy 2020) such as that developed by Project N95.org (Project N95 2020).
- It could be worthwhile publishing a blacklist of disreputable, profiteering suppliers who could not be trusted during the crisis to provide N95, FFP 2, or FFP3 devices that were up to standard. It is in everyone's interest that the list is made public as was the case with the EU, otherwise lives may again be put at risk by the suppliers on the blacklist if potential users are kept in ignorance of their incompetence. (European Safety Federation 2020, HSE 2016 and Manufacturing.net 2020).

b) ***Learn from Best Practice in Other Regions/Countries***

- USA:

  NIOSH-sponsored research into decontamination and reuse of N95 respirators (Bergman *et al.* 2010, 33-41 and Viscusi *et al.* 2009a, 815-827 and Viscusi *et al.* 2009b, 381-386)

  The establishment of N95.org to guide consumers in the selection of respirators with better reliability than 'Trusted Sources' lists (N95.org 2020)

  The 'BREATHE' Project aimed at developing a better, standard compliant and reusable N95-type respirator, the B95 (Gosch. *et al.* 2013, 1224-1230)

  FDA Emergency response preparedness (FDA 2020)
- Canada:

  Development of Reusable N95 respirators (CBC 2020b)
- UK:

  HSE early warnings about defective FFP3 masks (but failure to name the suppliers of the defective masks) (HSE 2016)

  Excellence in systematic provision of coronavirus vaccination reducing level of demand on PPE (Reuters 2021)
- EU:

  Blacklisting and openness in making public the list of the unreliable FFP2 suppliers providing defective and below-standard FFP2 masks
- Switzerland:

  Sustainable decontamination and reuse of FFP2-type respirators at one-tenth of the cost of a new device (Widmer & Richner 2020, 1-4)
- China:

  Expertise in effective lockdown (BBC 2021)
- Korea

  Reliable and effective KF94 respirators at half the price of an N95

  Effective at the process of lockdown (Baskar 2021)
- Japan and Korea

  Wearing of masks (The Japan Times 2020).

Development of reusable respirators by replacement of web-blown layer with nanofibre web; able to be decontaminated with 75% ethanol wash (Ullah et al. 2020, 7231–7241)

- Australia

  Emergency management planning guidance and templates (Australian Government 2021)

12.1.3 Beyond 2020: Planning

It is essential to urgently prepare an Emergency Management Plan to try to stay well ahead of the next emergency, because such a plan becomes much more effective with practice than simply struggling to cope with events as they arise and progress, especially if regular communication and training about the plan and its requirements and implementation are undertaken to prepare staff at all levels. Whatever the size of the healthcare unit you are responsible for or work in, there should be an emergency management plan for it and if not, there should be an overarching plan for the organisation which includes sufficient detail to guide what should happen within your unit as well as the organisation as a whole. If the overarching plan does not include such detail, it is your responsibility to make sure that is enhanced so that for the future, it does. Perhaps the simplest way to accomplish such an adjustment is to develop a full plan for the unit then to use this to check whether the overarching plan needs editing. An excellent template to use for the task is available from the Australian Government's website about how to prepare an emergency management plan (Australian Government 2021). It is focused on business, but it is a small step to adjust it to meet the requirements of a healthcare organisation which is part of a national or regional health service rather than one which is a private/profit-making healthcare business operation.

It should prove much easier for you, rather than some distant official or administrator, to include in the plan those matters which are most important to enable you to continue with your day-to-day operations. However, having drafted out your plan, it is of paramount importance that communication takes place with senior management and that you persuade them to include your sub-plan in their overarching organisational plan. Regarding PPE, assuring supply is key and there are plenty of indicators about what to include from both the 'Vision' and 'Hindsight' sections above, but stipulating the required rate of response to each element of supply and establishing the ability for this to be achieved in times of crises is key to its success.

a) ***Preparation of the Emergency Management Plan***

There are three parts to an emergency management plan:

- **The continuity plan** – helps you prepare your healthcare unit or organisation for an emergency by identifying risks to critical areas and how to best protect them.

- **The emergency action plan** – helps you and your staff know what to do during an emergency situation.
- **The recovery plan** – guides your healthcare unit or organisation's recovery after an emergency.

The website provides detailed guidance about how to complete the three plans using the template provided and draws attention to the need to keep the Emergency Management Plan up to date.

b) ***Training in Implementation of the Plan***

Frequent rehearsal of the elements within the Emergency Action Plan is essential so that they can become a part of regular practice. An even better way of ensuring that the actions needed to minimise some effects of a crisis are followed is to make them part of everyday practice; this may take somewhat longer to achieve and may need to be addressed first in the unit or organisation's strategic planning, see below.

c) ***Using the Emergency Management Plan to enhance Strategic Planning***

The Emergency Management Plan is likely to make it easier to highlight those aspects of the day-to-day operation of the unit and its resource needs which would benefit from enhancement and make the response to an emergency more effective and more reliable. Such enhancements may take some time to put in place hence the need for them to become part of the longer term planning by setting them down with a workable timescale for their introduction attached and including that in the unit or organisation's strategic plan. One such example would be to move away from the use of disposables for high-volume items of PPE (Walton 1986) whilst a second might be to undertake laundering of the reusables in house using one of the emerging low-cost low-temperature disinfection and laundering systems (JLA 2021) and a third would be to press for the acceptance and approval of decontamination and reuse of respirators (for organisations outside the USA at least), and particularly for the FFP and FFP3 devices so that organisations based in the UK and Europe can reap the benefit (Widmer & Richner 2020, 1-4). The steps requested can be justified on several counts, namely:

i) Increased safety and reliability
ii) Reduced cost
iii) Reduced environmental impact

REFERENCES

Airius. "NPBI™ Technology Neutralises SARS-CoV-2". 2021. Accessed June 9th, 2021. https://www.airius.co.uk/all-resources/npbi-technology-neutralises-sars-cov-2/.

Australian Government. "How to Prepare An Emergency Management Plan." 2021. Accessed May 16, 2021. https://business.gov.au/risk-management/emergency-management/how-to-prepare-an-emergency-management-plan.

Baskar, P. "Coronavirus FAQ: Why Am I Suddenly Hearing So Much About KF94 Masks?". 2021. Accessed May 16, 2021. https://www.npr.org/sections/goatsandsoda/2021/01/22/959683338/coronavirus-faq-why-am-i-suddenly-hearing-so-much-about-kf94-masks?t=1621281361381.

Battelle. "N95 FFR Decontamination for Reuse Final Report July 22, 2016 "REPORT for Bioquell HPV Decontamination for Reuse of N95 Respirator". 2016. Accessed May 16, 2021. https://www.fda.gov/media/136386/download.

BBC. "Wuhan Lockdown: A Year of China's Fight Against the Covid Pandemic." 2021. Accessed January 22nd, 2021. https://www.bbc.co.uk/news/world-asia-china-55628488.

Bergman, Michael S., Dennis J. Viscusi, Brian K. Heimbuch, Joseph D. Wander, Anthony R. Sambol, and Ronald E. Shaffer. "Evaluation of multiple (3-cycle) decontamination processing for filtering facepiece respirators." *Journal of Engineered Fibers and Fabrics* 5, no. 4 (2010): 155892501000500405.

CBC. "Health Minister Reviewing Management of Canada's Emergency Stockpile: "Experts Criticize Ottawa for Mismanaging and Destroying Millions of N95 Masks." 2020a. Accessed May 16th, 2021. https://www.cbc.ca/news/canada/saskatchewan/heath-minister-emergency-stockpile-1.5530081.

CBC. "Shift to Reusable PPE 'an Immediate Need' for Public Health — But Transition Won't be Simple, Experts Say". 2020b. Accessed May 16th, 2021. https://www.cbc.ca/news/canada/manitoba/reusable-ppe-covid-19-manitoba-1.5628089.

European Safety Federation. "COVID19 Suspicious Certificates for PPE - Updated 09/07/2020". Accessed May 16th, 2021. 2020. https://www.eu-esf.org/covid-19/4513-covid-19-suspicious-certificates-for-ppe.

FDA. "Emergency Use Authorisation". 2020. Accessed May 16th, 2021. https://www.fda.gov/medical-devices/coronavirus-disease-2019-covid-19-emergency-use-authorizations-medical-devices/decontamination-systems-personal-protective-equipment-euas.

Fink R.G. & Ellis, W. B. 2011 "Device, system and method for an advanced oxidation process using photohydroionization" US Patent No. US7988923B2, August 2nd 2011 assigned to RGF Environmental Group, Inc., Riviera, Beach, FL. USA

Gosch, Megan E., Ronald E. Shaffer, Aaron E. Eagan, Raymond J. Roberge, Victoria J. Davey, and Lewis J. Radonovich Jr. "B95: A new respirator for health care personnel." *American Journal of Infection Control* 41, no. 12 (2013): 1224–1230.

HSE. "RR1087 - Market Surveillance of FFP3 Disposable Respirators (first published 2016)." 2016. Accessed May 16th, 2021. https://www.hse.gov.uk/research/rrhtm/rr1087.htm.

Institute of Medicine. "Committee on the development of reusable facemasks for use during an influenza pandemic." In *Reusability of Facemasks During an Influenza Pandemic: Facing the Flu*. Washington, DC: The National Academies Press, 2006.

JLA. "OTEX Laundry Disinfection System". 2021. Accessed May 16th, 2021. https://jla.com/otex/laundry.

Manufacturing.net. "3M Has Probed Over 4,000 Cases of N95 Fraud, Filed 18 Lawsuits."(17 July 2020). 2020. Accessed May 16th, 2021. https://www.manufacturing.net/laws-regulations/news/21140427/3m-has-investigated-over-4000-cases-of-n95-mask-fraud.

Olsen, Sonja J., Hsiao-Ling Chang, Terence Yung-Yan Cheung, Antony Fai-Yu Tang, Tamara L. Fisk, Steven Peng-Lim Ooi, Hung-Wei Kuo et al. "Transmission of the severe acute respiratory syndrome on aircraft." *New England Journal of Medicine* 349, no. 25 (2003): 2416–2422.

Project N95. 2020. Accessed July 20th, 2020. https://www.projectn95.org/supply.

PULSE. "PPE: Suppliers approved by the British Safety Industry Federation – April; Directory of PPE suppliers approved by the British Safety Industry Federation for meeting safety standards, 9 April 2020". 2020. Accessed May 16th, 2021. http://www.pulsetoday.co.uk/clinical/clinical-specialties/respiratory-/ppe-suppliers-approved-by-the-british-safety-industry-federation-april/20040597.article.

Reuters. "UK Sets New Daily COVID Vaccination Record in 'Mammoth Team Effort. 2021. March 21st, 2021." Accessed May 16th, 2021. https://www.reuters.com/article/uk-health-coronavirus-britain-vaccinatio-idUSKBN2BD0JQ.

The Japan Times. "The History Behind Japan's Love of Face Masks". 2020. Accessed May 16th, 2021. https://www.japantimes.co.jp/news/2020/07/04/national/science-health/japans-history-wearing-masks-coronavirus/.

UK Department for Business, Energy & Industrial Strategy. "Guidance: CE Marking: 'How a Product Complies with EU Safety, Health and Environmental Requirements, and How to Place a CE Marking on Your Product'." 2020. Accessed May 17th, 2021. https://www.gov.uk/guidance/ce-marking.

UK Health and Safety Executive. "HSE Rapid Evidence Review Publication Version 27 March 2020". 2020. Accessed May 17th, 2021. https://www.hse.gov.uk/news/assets/docs/face-mask-equivalence-aprons-gown-eye-protection.pdf.

Ullah, S., A. Ullah, J. Lee, Y. Jeong, M. Hashmi, C. Zhu, K. Il Joo, H. J. Cha, and I.S. Kim. "Reusability Comparison of Melt-Blown vs Nanofiber Face Mask Filters for Use in the Coronavirus Pandemic." *ACS Applied Nano Materials* 3 no.7 (2020): 7231–7241. https://doi.org/10.1021/acsanm.0c01562.

U.S. Department of Health and Human Services. "Determination of a Public Health Emergency and Declaration that Circumstances Exist Justifying Authorizations Pursuant to Section 564(b) of the Federal Food, Drug, and Cosmetic Act, 21 U.S.C. § 360bbb-3. 85 FR 7316". 2020a. Accessed June 9th, 2021. https://www.federalregister.gov/documents/2020/02/07/2020-02496/determination-of-public-health-emergency.

U.S. Department of Health and Human Services. "Declaration that Circumstances Exist Justifying Authorizations Pursuant to Section 564(b) of the Federal Food, Drug, and Cosmetic Act, 21 U.S.C. § 360bbb-3, 85 FR 17335". 2020b. Accessed June 9th, 2021. https://www.fda.gov/media/135787/download.

Viscusi, Dennis J., Michael S. Bergman, Benjamin C. Eimer, and Ronald E. Shaffer. "Evaluation of five decontamination methods for filtering facepiece respirators." *Annals of Occupational Hygiene* 53, no. 8 (2009a): 815–827.

Viscusi, Dennis J., Mike Bergman, Edward Sinkule, and Ronald E. Shaffer. "Evaluation of the filtration performance of 21 N95 filtering face piece respirators after prolonged storage." *American Journal of Infection Control* 37, no. 5 (2009): 381–386.

Walton, J. R. "A new controversy in respiratory equipment management: Reusables versus disposed disposables versus reused disposables." *Respiratory Care* 31, no. 3 (1986): 213–217.

Widmer, Andreas F., and Gilles Richner. "Proposal for a EN 149 acceptable reprocessing method for FFP2 respirators in times of severe shortage." *Antimicrobial Resistance & Infection Control* 9, no. 1 (2020): 1–4.

You, Ruoyu, Chao-Hsin Lin, Daniel Wei, and Qingyan Chen. "Evaluating the commercial airliner cabin environment with different air distribution systems." *Indoor Air* 29, no. 5 (2019): 840–853.

Zins, Howard M. "Environmental, cost and product issues related to reusable healthcare textiles." *Research Journal of Textile and Apparel* 10, no. 4 (2006): 73–80

12.2 CASE STUDY TWO: AORTODUODENAL FISTULA AFTER ENDOVASCULAR ANEURYSM REPAIR

Aortoenteric fistula (AEF) is an abnormal communication between the aorta and gut, most commonly between the aorta and duodenum (ADF) (O'Mara et al. 1977, 556–566). Although uncommon, they carry a high mortality due to their bleeding potential. An aortoenteric fistula may be caused by compression, from an aneurysm that eventually leads to a connection forming between the two structures, or infection. Less commonly, they may be caused by a prosthetic graft eroding into the gut (secondary). Although absent in up to a third of cases, gastrointestinal (GI) bleeding should raise suspicion (Reilly et al. 1984, 36–44). A presentation would normally involve gastrointestinal signs on a background of cardiovascular or aneurysmal disease. This case focuses on ADF in a patient with a previous aneurysm repair.

A 79-year-old male presented acutely with a fresh rectal bleed on a background of ruptured infrarenal abdominal aortic aneurysm (AAA) which was repaired endovascularly 8 years prior. Unfortunately, aortic graft infection followed requiring lifelong antibiotic therapy. During this admission he also developed melaena (digested blood in the stool). Gastroscopy identified altered blood in the stomach and duodenum, but no obvious source of bleeding. CT angiogram also did not identify an obvious bleeding point but did show the duodenum closely adherent to the graft (Figures 12.1 and 12.2). He became haemodynamically unstable and was taken to theatre for acute surgical exploration for the suspected bleeding origin.

Intraoperatively, it was evident that the aortic stent had eroded through the aortic wall at the proximal end, adhering to the third part of the duodenum with ADF identified. The graft was excised (Figure 12.3) and an antibiotic impregnated. Dacron graft was handsewn. The duodenum was then mobilised, directly closed, and reinforced with an omental patch.

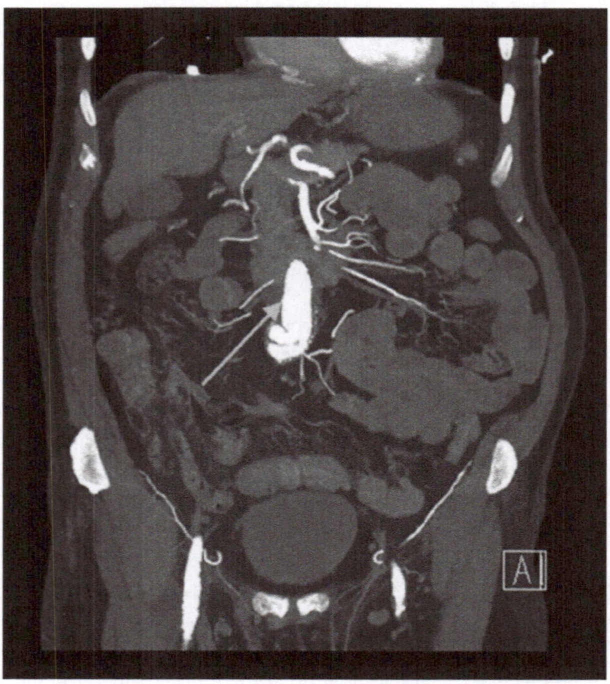

FIGURE 12.1 CT imaging showing aortic graft in contact with duodenum (D3) in coronal view.

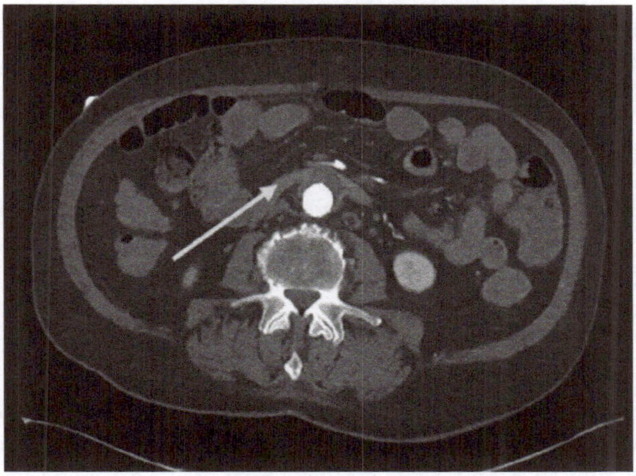

FIGURE 12.2 CT imaging as Figure 12.1 in cross-section. D3 is in close proximity to the anterior surface of the aortic graft.

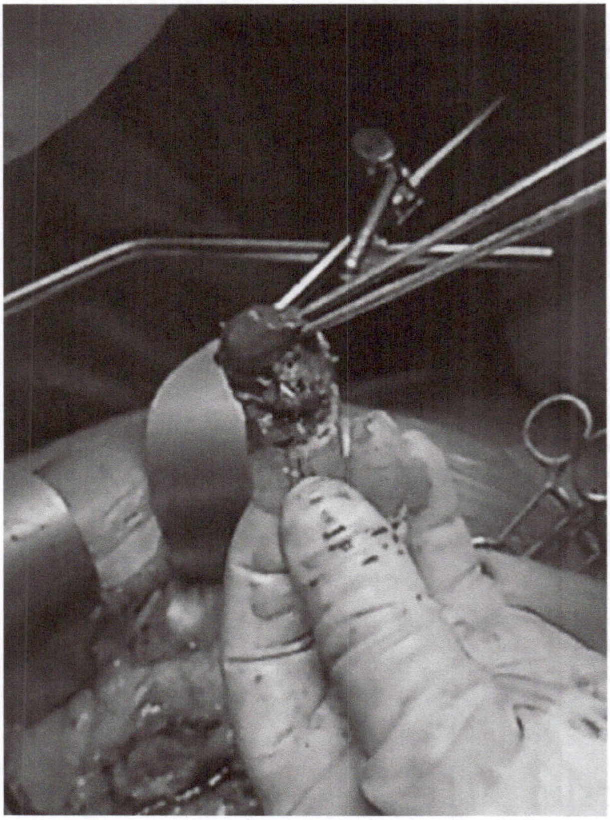

FIGURE 12.3 Proximal aortic graft excised intra-operatively.

Post-operatively he was weaned from ICU to high dependency setting but became unwell with overwhelming sepsis. Unfortunately, he developed multi-organ failure and passed away.

12.2.1 Discussion

This case highlights one of the complications possible from aortic grafting and the high mortality associated with graft infections. Diagnosis of an aortoenteric fistula is. Particularly challenging with CT angiogram being recommended as first-line imaging for confirmation of the diagnosis. It does not exclude the diagnosis (Hughes et al. 2007, 398–402). This accounts for the diagnostic difficulty experienced even with a history of aneurysms.

Either open or endovascular (via the vessel) repair can be performed. Endovascular repair by stent-graft could be carried out; however if due to an infective cause, there would undoubtedly be a high incidence of reinfection post-operatively (Antoniou et al. 2009, 782–789). It is important to note that repair of the AEF may be achieved by either of these two approaches. If secondary to an infective process, it has been suggested that more definitive surgical repair can be undertaken once the patient's condition has improved (Thomson et al. 2009, 267–269).

This case demonstrates the risks associated with graft repair. Foreign material, such as a woven implant, can erode through adjacent tissue structures and create false passages and connections between structures. The importance of preventing infection should not be underestimated – biofilms can develop upon implants and require removal of implant or lifelong antibiotics. With new and advancing technology, the ability to manufacture grafts that mimic the biology of the surrounding vessel wall or an implant with antimicrobial properties may help to mitigate the complications described above.

REFERENCES

Antoniou, G. A., S. Koutsias, S.A. Antoniou, A. Georgiakakis, M.K. Lazarides, and A.D. Giannoukas "Outcome after endovascular stent graft repair of aortoenteric fistula: A systematic review". *Journal of Vascular Surgery* 49, no. 3 (2009): 782–789.

Hughes, F.M., D. Kavanagh, M. Barry, A. Owens, D.P. MacErlaine, and D.E. Malone "Aortoenteric fistula: A diagnostic dilemma". *Abdominal Imaging* 32, no. 3 (2007): 398–402.

O'Mara, C., and A.L. Imbembo. "Paraprosthetic-enteric fistula". *Surgery* 81, no. 5 (1977): 556–566.

Reilly, L.M., H. Altman, R.J. Lusby, R.A. Kersh, W.K. Ehrenfeld, and R.J. Stoney. "Late results following surgical management of vascular graft infection". *Journal of Vascular Surgery* 1, no. 1 (1984): 36–44.

Thomson, V.S., K.G. Gopinath, E. Joseph, and G. Joseph. "Primary aorto-enteric fistula: A rare complication of abdominal aortic aneurysm". *Journal of Postgraduate Medicine* 55, no. 4 (2009): 267–269.

12.3 CASE STUDY THREE: NASAL HAEMOSTASIS

Nasal packing may be used in a variety of causes of nasal haemorrhage. Absorbable textiles allow blood to be absorbed and for expansion of the textile to fit the cavity it is filling and to provide pressure over the bleeding point, with the aim of blood cessation. They must still be able to be removed without triggering further bleeding or trauma to the nasal mucosa unless an absorbable is utilised. Following are two clinical examples for which they may be used.

A 36-year-old woman with asthma and allergic nasal polyps is scheduled for endoscopic sinus surgery to improve her breathing. She has a very aggressive disease and there is a lot of inflammation noted during surgery to remove her polyps, resulting in bleeding from the nasal lining. During the SARS-CoV-2 pandemic, the operating surgeon has tried to minimise patient movements and aerosol generation to reduce the risk of potential exposure to the virus. An absorbable haemostatic dressing was therefore used over and above traditional removable nasal packing materials to provide tamponade, facilitate clot formation, and avoid the need for uncomfortable pack removal and associated coughing and sneezing which could generate aerosol.

An 85-year-old man with high blood pressure who also takes Aspirin for a previous stroke presents to the emergency department with epistaxis (a nose bleed). The doctors have attempted chemical cautery with silver nitrate but the combination of Aspirin and high blood pressure prevents it from being successful initially. A choice of nasal tampons is available. Given the difficulty stopping the bleeding, the doctor chooses an inflatable nasal tampon with a carboxymethylcellulose lining over a hydroxylated PVA tampon. This allows extra pressure to be applied to the bleeding site, but the carboxymethylcellulose lining prevents the tampon from adhering to the nasal wall and dislodging a precarious blood clot upon removal 24 hours later. The site of bleeding is successfully cauterised the following day (Figure 12.4).

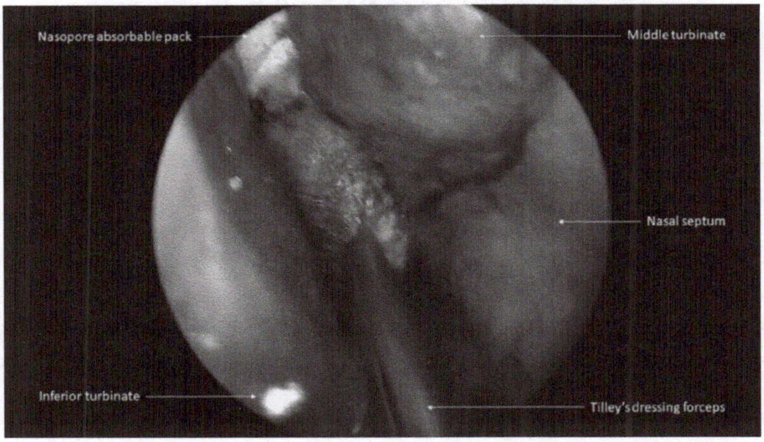

FIGURE 12.4 Using textile to assist haemorrhage control in the nasal cavity.

12.4 CASE STUDY FOUR: CATARACT

Opacification of the normal lens is called a cataract and is the commonest cause of blindness in the world. Cataracts are mainly caused by aging, but may also be due

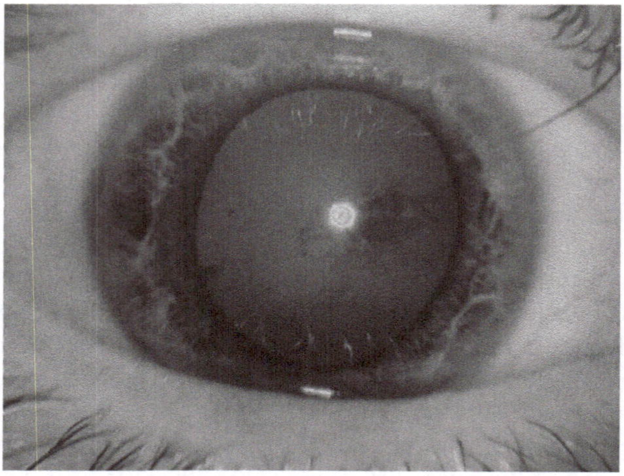

FIGURE 12.5 Cataract.

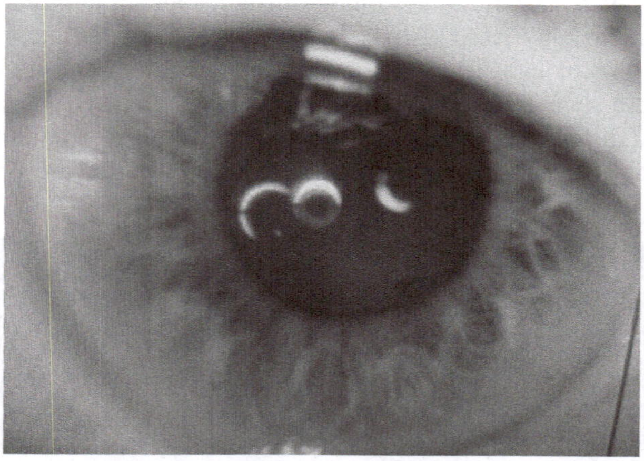

FIGURE 12.6 Intraocular lens used for correction.

to various other causes, for example, trauma, diabetes, sun exposure, medications. Cataracts develop gradually and cause clouding of the vision, as demonstrated in Figure 12.5.

The treatment of cataract is the removal of the cataractous lens and replacing it with an intraocular implant, as demonstrated in Figure 12.6. The most commonly used technique is phacoemulsification, which is a suture-less procedure where the nucleus of the lens is broken into smaller fragments and aspirated. In some rare cases when there is a wound leak or needing to extend the wound to implant an unfoldable intraocular lens, the wound is closed using 8–0 polyglactin 910 or 10–s0 nylon suture. Similarly, in conditions such as a dense, matured cataract where phacoemulsification is unsuitable, the lens is removed using wider corneal excision and the wound is closed using 10–0 nylon monofilament suture. These sutures are chosen as they glide through the tissue easily and can be removed at a later date (Figure 12.6).

12.5 CASE STUDY FIVE: RISK ANALYSIS TABLE

A small company conducts a risk analysis of the delivery procedure. A hazard identified is that their device may not have been identified as delivered; this has the effect that they may receive a complaint that would require investigation.

First notice that another column has been added to the table 'company' – this has been done for clarity. As stated earlier, you can simply use the 'bystander' column to represent the company as the 'effect' clearly states the hazard is related to the company (not being paid is an issue for the company). Also, note that your values of L and S will have different interpretations. You just need to associate S with the table as given before – so Death, for example, could be closure of the company, or loss of clearance to market.

This case study illustrates that risk is relative. When dealing with humans, it is associated with injury and death. When dealing with companies, it is more associated with critical outcomes. It is possible for a potential hazard to have an effect that is both liable to cause physical injury to a patient, an end-user, or bystander as well as harming the company's reputation, bank balance, and registration status.

RISK ANALYSIS

Characteristic	Hazard 2.1.2					Lifecycle Phase				Design, Manufacture, and Supply				Comment	FDA request letter ref x.y.z
Failure/Hazard	Delivery not recorded as delivered														
Effect	Company may receive a complaint														
Root Cause(s)	Hazard Relevance √ = relevant					Estimation of Risk: Likelihood x Severity at start of lifecycle phase L x S = RPN			Risk reduction activities (Grey Black Zones) (if practical): Comment if required (White Only)	Estimation of **residual risk** at the end of this lifecycle phase			Can the risk be reduced further? (Grey)	Action proposed to protect from residual risk; implementation and verification of efficacy?	Additional hazards introduced by risk control measures? If so, what action taken?
	Patient	End-User	Bystander	Company	Environment	L	S	RPN		L	S	RPN			
Item not delivered at all				✓		**3**	**4**	**12**	Delivered by hand by company personnel or by reputable delivery company	**1**	**4**	**4**	**AFAP: clinical benefit outweighs the residual risk**	**None**	**No additional hazard.**
Item delivery not recorded				✓		3	4	12	Delivery note has signature and date	**1**	**4**	**4**	**AFAP: clinical benefit outweighs the residual risk**	**None**	**No additional hazard.**
Item delivery not recorded				✓		3	4	12	Delivery by Delivery Company can be tracked	**1**	**4**	**4**	**AFAP: clinical benefit outweighs the residual risk**	**None**	**No additional hazard.**

13 Medical Textiles
The State of the Art

Historically, as has been the case in medicine generally, commendable advances have been made in the field of medical textiles, but typically, innovation has been beset by tradition so the adoption of new approaches, devices, and materials has been stilted. The field of surgery has been particularly innovative in the application of textiles because their structures and flexibility offer solutions to several of the problems which arise during the demanding and often urgent work being undertaken. The medical field, typically that which is pharmaceutical based, is also benefitting, for example from pharmaceuticals encapsulated in fibre or filament implants and also from the high-performance fibre filters for bodily fluids, crucial components in artificial organ support. However, there is still significant room for improvements such as fibres that do not trigger coagulation cascade and are biocompatible as these will allow for inbuilt organs rather than the patient having to be attached to a large extra-corporeal device such as a dialysis machine.

Of what were perhaps the two most significant ideas of the 19th century about how to improve patient recovery following surgical treatment, namely antisepsis and asepsis, it is reasonable to say that on the whole, antisepsis has been able to demonstrate greater patient benefit whilst for asepsis, the wearing of gloves has shown significant beneficial effect since its inception in the early 20th century. A feature associated with the adoption of the aseptic concept which should not be ignored, is the psychological reassurance provided to patients by a well-cared for, clean and hygienic environment in the healthcare setting, not least because it confers the impression of a responsible, professional approach to their work by healthcare staff members.

Antiseptic agents were successfully introduced by Lister not only into the operating environment but also into sutures to reduce the incidence of surgical site infection which continued to beset surgery in the 19th century. Much improved (less toxic) types of agents were introduced for the same purpose over time and with the more recent introduction of nanotechnology, nanoparticulate antimicrobial agents such as silver are often incorporated because of their enhanced ability to release the active agent (silver ions) in a controlled manner over time compared with larger particles, wires, or coatings. Although antimicrobial agents which give positive results in standard test methods for antibacterial action for medical textiles are effective in this particular setting, and, together with other finishes in wound dressings, the same does not apply when the agents are used as treatments intended to confer antimicrobial action against contaminants on garments worn for personal protection by

DOI: 10.1201/9781003170570-13

healthcare workers, or for treated items of uniform clothing. Test methods for the detection of pathogens, those used to establish the effectiveness of implanted devices treated with antibacterial agents and those used to determine the effectiveness of barrier materials against the penetration of pathogens including viruses appear to work well enough, but the largely dry conditions appropriate to personal protective equipment during use and uniform clothing during wear are very different from those applied in most standard test procedures and the agent is less likely to be effective (OECD 2019, 35). Properly designed trials undertaken in realistic situations are few and far between but the trials which have been carried out show that existing antimicrobial treatments are ineffective in the practical setting. However, there will always be a need for fabrics able not only to act as barriers but also to deactivate pathogens and therefore to keep staff and patients safe despite contamination during their treatment, so good researchers should recognise that for fabrics and garments to be able to demonstrate the antimicrobial action necessary to prevent cross-contamination, testing must be done under conditions which adequately represent those experienced by surgeons and healthcare professionals during their work. A new start needs to be made, but reassuringly, the groundwork was prepared some years ago and set down in the 'Three-Tier' protocol published by the OECD in 2008 in their *Guidance Document on the Evaluation of the Efficacy of Antimicrobial Treated Articles with Claims for External Effects* (OECD 2008) where Tier 1 concerns 'Proof of Principle,' Tier 2 'Simulated Use,' and Tier 3 'In-Use Evaluation.' It is high time that the protocol was put into proper use and it is at Tier 2 where current test methods fall seriously short. Realistic, reliable, laboratory-based Tier 2 test methods now need to be developed for medical textiles and validated for their alignment with practice (e.g., through their capacity to reliably predict outcomes from earlier clinical trials) before they could be considered for acceptance as standards. The OECD does give guidance on the development of appropriate Tier 2 test methods in their 2019 document *Guidance Document on Use and Development of Tier-2 Laboratory Based Tests Used to Substantiate Claims for Efficacy of Biocide Treated Articles* (OECD 2019) as detailed in Chapter 5, and this is what more researchers now need to build on to develop effective antimicrobial PPE.

Asepsis comes into its own when airborne pathogens are a particular issue, but fully-effective patient and practitioner arrangements are difficult to achieve unless complete and separate methods of enclosure of both parties are adopted, for example by sealed full-body suits coupled with independent air supply. There is a conflict, currently, between the demands for items of clothing which provide an effective barrier and the comfort of the wearer, and these continue to apply even when the three-layer laminates with a microporous PTFE central layer are used, so there is considerable room for improvement of the barrier fabrics to enhance their comfort. With respirators (filtering face pieces), the more efficient filters provide a greater barrier to the passage of air and make breathing difficult, so work needs to be done to maintain their high efficiency whilst enabling easy breathing. The incorporation of nanofibre webs within the mask layers allows for thickness reduction and that appears promising in this regard. Even so, there continues to be a need for improved, reusable, and more versatile respirators and protective clothing against airborne pathogens for healthcare workers, patients, and members of the general public, as has been amply demonstrated most recently during the COVID-19 pandemic. However, that was a need which had already been highlighted much earlier (following the SARS epidemic in 2003 and prior to the H1N1 influenza epidemic in 2009). Suffice it to say that whatever steps were taken to ensure adequacy of supply, they were insufficient, which goes to illustrate that when such warnings are issued, and methods for the avoidance of a crisis are identified, it is of paramount importance that not just other researchers, but also government officials, healthcare managers, and administrators pay more attention to research outcomes and take the necessary action to minimise all possible damage before crises occur. The 'BREATHE' project for the development of a reusable respirator (Gosch et al. 2013) needs to be properly addressed in the USA and other countries need to follow a similar path to Manitoba in Canada (CBC 2020), where a reusable respirator has been developed which will be produced locally. Although research is a key component in moving things forward, on its own, it is insufficient in enabling healthcare to benefit from innovation. Moreover, it has to be realised that those who were lazy and incompetent in preparing for the pandemic eventuality are unlikely to come forward to take any criticism or accept any responsibility for inaction, and the unacceptability of claims that the third serious epidemic in 20 years was a 'learning experience' should be made clear. The need for an appropriately well-developed and regularly rehearsed emergency management plan to deal with emerging crises cannot be overstressed, and there is no excuse for procrastination in this regard because detailed guidance on its development is available from the Australian Government website. Such a plan needs to take account of the need to be able to provide adequate supplies of PPE of all kinds, and where reusable items are unavailable, steps need to be taken (including the provision of funding support) to ensure their early development. The widespread use of disposable items has continued to be promoted and a throwaway culture has been nurtured and grown in the healthcare sector, with little concern for cost or indeed for the environment. Any healthcare unit whether it is situated in a developing or developed country should at the very least pay attention to cost. The application of low-temperature disinfecting laundry systems such as those which make use of ozone generated within the device itself can make a further cost-saving contribution (JLA 2021; OPL 2021). Lack of such attention is a quality-management issue that needs to be swiftly corrected. Many items can be recycled or remanufactured for reuse at a saving of between 40% and 60% and this can be done by outsourcing to companies specialising in those types of activity, so it is difficult to argue not to do it. All healthcare facilities need therefore to develop and implement a policy of reuse. For items currently designed to be for single use, concerted efforts need to be made to ensure their replacement through the design and implementation of reusable versions of those items. It is an unhealthy contradiction that if healthcare across the world were considered as a country in its own right, it would be the world's 5th largest polluter. Much of the filth it discharges into the atmosphere from burning single-use items in its incinerators or by dumping them into landfills has the potential to damage the very health the sector is supposed to be supporting. Such environmentally-unfriendly activity by the healthcare sector needs to be brought to a halt, urgently.

Recent modelling of air circulation and the associated distribution of pathogens in the USA and the UK both in a problematic environment (aircraft passenger cabin) and a healthcare setting (hospital ward) illustrate the need for action to prevent (or at least limit) transmission. Whatever PPE is being deployed in the healthcare environment, a wider environmental adjustment to support the achievement of a more hygienic healthcare environment through air filtration, purification, exposure to microbiocidal agents and coupling with UVC or far-UV to ensure that pathogens are not being circulated continues to deserve concerted effort. The microbiocidal textile finishing agent able to demonstrate effectiveness in the filter of an air filtration device, an N-halamine (Ren et al. 2018), deserves further investigation, perhaps not only in air filtration but also for items of PPE, as other candidate antimicrobial agents such as silver nanoparticles and covalently bound quaternary ammonium compounds coupled with silane treatments, the kind of multifunctional finishes sought by practitioners, do not appear to perform in the practical setting.

Nanofibre production by electrospinning is becoming a better established part of medical textiles especially with the improved control exerted over the filaments as they emerge into the electrostatic field and travel to the collector. This control enables the formation of yarns with fibres neatly arranged side by side. The advantage is that such yarns have greater integrity than those made from mats/webs and a micro-sized circular loom has been used for making miniature woven nanofibre stents which have subsequently been successfully implanted. A micro-sized braiding machine has also been developed and used for braiding multiple conducting nano-width metal wires for use in a device for precision stimulation of nerves. Nanofibre yarns continue to possess the capacity for greater impact in medical devices, particularly in implants, where they offer the opportunity to provide a much better match to the dimensions, consistencies, and textures of the wide variety of tissue types being treated/repaired, especially in relation to structures such as scaffolds for tissue engineering, but with their large surface areas, they also have significant drug-holding capacity. Particular attention needs to be paid in this regard to ways of suppressing any initial surges in drug release and nano-engineering and molecular imprinting of the nanofibre surfaces offers the opportunity to exert fine control over the rate of release.

Of the range of traditional and high-performance fibre types used in medical textiles, synthetic absorbable polymers continue to have significant impact particularly in sutures and mesh, because suitable selection means that an implanted device can provide its temporary support whilst healing takes place, before being absorbed so that no further surgery is required for its removal. Where continuous support is required over long periods of time, non-absorbable polymers such as PET have been used, but problems with non-absorbable meshes have emerged over the longer term and these now need to be addressed. Electroactive fibre types are expected to enjoy greater use when smart textiles and garments become better developed. Super absorbable polymers in fibre form deserve mention because of their value not only in improving patient comfort by de-bulking hygiene items such as diapers and bed mats but also in making it possible for such items to be repeatedly laundered and reused.

Standards, specifications, and clinical trials of medical devices must always remain at the forefront of the medical textile device designer's mind and appropriate test regimes and record-keeping need to be applied from the earliest stages to improve the possibility of approval. Some new entrants into the smart textiles market, including those keen to make use of artificial intelligence within the items, appear to be unable to justify or prove the credibility of their design so there should be an accreditation process that follows accepted definitions of what that device is supposed to be and do. Regarding garments, a lot of work has been undertaken concerned with the modelling to determine the effectiveness of tests and the successful operation of pressure garments but there is still room for improvement here in particular for the treatment of burns patients and there needs to be a collaboration between disciplines to make better progress. Orthotics will always be needed, and the focus of attention needs to be on new materials that can offer improved fit and aesthetics. Data protection and security for smart garments which transfer information about the wearer to central units should always be a matter of concern, but there is such great value in being able to remotely monitor patients that appropriate arrangements need to be identified and supported. These are rapidly-moving topic areas, so designers should play a role in ensuring that appropriate ISO tests are up to date and relevant and bring attention to the bodies responsible for the development of standards whenever the need arises to overhaul obsolete standards.

REFERENCES

CBC. "Shift to reusable PPE 'An Immediate Need' for public health — But transition won't be simple, experts say." 2020. Accessed June 28, 2020. https://www.cbc.ca/news/canada/manitoba/reusable-ppe-covid-19-manitoba-1.5628089.

Gosch, M. E., Ronald E. Shaffer, Aaron E. Eagan, Raymond J. Roberge, Victoria J. Davey, and Lewis J. Radonovich Jr. 2013 "B95: A new respirator for health care personnel." *American Journal of Infection Control* 41, no. 12: 1224–1230.

JLA. "Ozone laundry disinfection." 2021. Accessed May 7, 2021. https://jla.com/otex/laundry.

OECD. "Guidance document on Use and development of tier-2 laboratory based tests used to substantiate claims for efficacy of biocide treated articles"; Environment, Health and Safety Publications Series on Testing and Assessment No. 287 Series on Biocides No. 13; p. 35 Section 77; Inter-Organisation Programme for the Sound Management of Chemicals, Environment Directorate, 2019. OECD, March 1, 2019. https://www.oecd.org/officialdocuments/publicdisplaydocumentpdf/?cote=env/jm/mono(2018)20&doclanguage=en.

OECD. "Guidance document on the evaluation of the efficacy of antimicrobial treated articles with claims for external effect." 2008. ENV/JM/MONO(2008)27, November 18, 2008. https://www.oecd.org/env/ehs/pesticides-biocides/41692131.pdf.

OPL. "Ozone laundry systems." 2021. Accessed June 22, 2021. https://opl-ltd.co.uk/ozone-laundry-systems/.

Ren, Tian, Teresa V. Dormitorio, Mingyu Qiao, Tung-Shi Huang, and Jean Weese. "N-halamine incorporated antimicrobial nonwoven fabrics for use against avian influenza virus." *Veterinary Microbiology* 218 (2018): 78–83.

Index